Endocrine Disorders During Pregnancy

Guest Editors

RACHEL PESSAH-POLLACK, MD
LOIS JOVANOVIČ, MD

ENDOCRINOLOGY AND METABOLISM CLINICS OF NORTH AMERICA

www.endo.theclinics.com

Consulting Editor
DEREK LEROITH, MD, PhD

December 2011 • Volume 40 • Number 4

SAUNDERS an imprint of ELSEVIER, Inc.

W.B. SAUNDERS COMPANY
A Division of Elsevier Inc.

1600 John F. Kennedy Boulevard • Suite 1800 • Philadelphia, Pennsylvania 19103-2899

http://www.theclinics.com

ENDOCRINOLOGY AND METABOLISM CLINICS OF NORTH AMERICA Volume 40, Number 4
December 2011 ISSN 0889-8529, ISBN-13: 978-1-4557-7982-6

Editor: Rachel Glover
Developmental Editor: Donald Mumford

Endocrinology and Metabolism Clinics of North America (ISSN 0889-8529) is published quarterly by Elsevier Inc., 360 Park Avenue South, New York, NY 10010-1710. Months of issue are March, June, September, and December. Periodicals postage paid at New York, NY and additional mailing offices. Subscription prices are USD 313.00 per year for US individuals, USD 536.00 per year for US institutions, USD 158.00 per year for US students and residents, USD 393.00 per year for Canadian individuals, USD 656.00 per year for Canadian institutions, USD 456.00 per year for international individuals, USD 656.00 per year for international institutions, and USD 233.00 per year for international and Canadian and foreign students/residents. To receive student/resident rate, orders must be accompanied by name of affiliated institution, date of term, and the signature of program/ residency coordinator on institution letterhead. Orders will be billed at individual rate until proof of status is received. Foreign air speed delivery is included in all *Clinics* subscription prices. All prices are subject to change without notice. **POSTMASTER:** Send address changes to *Endocrinology and Metabolism Clinics of North America*, Elsevier Health Sciences Division, Subscription Customer Service, 3251 Riverport Lane, Maryland Heights, MO 63043. **Customer Service: Telephone: 1-800-654-2452** (U.S. and Canada); **1-314-447-8871** (outside U.S. and Canada). **Fax: 1-314-447-8029. E-mail: journalscustomerservice-usa@elsevier.com** (for print support); **journalsonlinesupport-usa@elsevier.com** (for online support).

Reprints. For copies of 100 or more, of articles in this publication, please contact the Commercial Rights Department, Elsevier Inc., 360 Park Avenue South, New York, NY 10010-1710; phone: (+1) 212-633-3813; fax: (+1) 212-462-1935; e-mail: reprints@elsevier.com.

Endocrinology and Metabolism Clinics of North America is covered in *MEDLINE/PubMed (Index Medicus)*, *EMBASE/Excerpta Medica*, *Current Contents/Clinical Medicine*, *Current Contents/Life Sciences*, *Science Citation Index*, *ISI/BIOMED*, *BIOSIS*, and *Chemical Abstracts*.

Printed and bound by CPI Group (UK) Ltd, Croydon, CR0 4YY

Transferred to Digital Print 2011

Contributors

CONSULTING EDITOR

DEREK LEROITH, MD, PhD
Chief, Division of Endocrinology, Metabolism, and Bone Diseases, Department of Medicine, Mount Sinai School of Medicine, New York, New York

GUEST EDITORS

RACHEL PESSAH-POLLACK, MD
Division of Endocrinology, Mount Sinai School of Medicine, New York, New York

LOIS JOVANOVIČ, MD
CEO and Chief Scientific Officer, Sansum Diabetes Research Institute, Santa Barbara, California

AUTHORS

DIMA ABDELMANNAN, MD, FRCP
Assistant Professor, Division of Clinical and Molecular Endocrinology, Department of Medicine, Louis Stokes Cleveland Department of Veterans Affairs Medical Center, Case Western Reserve University School of Medicine, Cleveland, Ohio

TAKAKO ARAKI, MD
Division of Endocrinology and Metabolism, Beth Israel Medical Center and Albert Einstein College of Medicine, New York, New York

DAVID C. ARON, MD, MS
Professor of Medicine, Division of Clinical and Molecular Endocrinology, Department of Medicine, Louis Stokes Cleveland Department of Veterans Affairs Medical Center, Case Western Reserve University School of Medicine, Cleveland, Ohio

LEWIS E. BRAVERMAN, MD
Section of Endocrinology, Diabetes, and Nutrition, Boston University School of Medicine, Boston, Massachusetts

KENNETH D. BURMAN, MD
Chief, Section of Endocrinology, Department of Medicine, Washington Hospital Center; Professor, Department of Medicine, Georgetown University Hospital, Washington, DC

PETER DAMM, MD, DMSc
Professor, Department of Obstetrics, Center for Pregnant Women with Diabetes, Rigshospitalet, University of Copenhagen, Copenhagen Ø, Denmark

JODIE DODD, MBBS, PhD, FRANZCOG, CMFM
Professor, Maternal Fetal Medicine Specialist; NHMRC Practitioner Fellow, The Robinson Institute, Australian Research Centre for Health of Women and Babies, School of Paediatrics and Reproductive Health, University of Adelaide, North Adelaide, South Australia, Australia

RONY ELIAS, MD
The Ronald O. Perelman and Claudia Cohen Center for Reproductive Medicine, Weill Cornell Medical College, New York, New York

YAKOV GOLOGORSKY, MD
Resident, Department of Neurosurgery, Mount Sinai Hospital, New York, New York

MARIBETH INTURRISI, RN, MS, CNS, CDE
Coordinator and Nurse Consultant, Region 1&3, California Diabetes and Pregnancy Program; Assistant Clinical Professor, Family Health Care Nursing, University of California; Diabetes Nurse Educator, Department of Maternal-Fetal Medicine, Sutter Pacific Medical Foundation at California Pacific Medical Center, San Francisco, California

JANE KOSTANDINOV, NP, RN
Nurse Practitioner, Department of Neurosurgery, Mount Sinai Hospital, New York, New York

CHRISTOPHER S. KOVACS, MD, FRCPC, FACP, FACE
Professor of Medicine, Obstetrics & Gynecology, and BioMedical Sciences, Faculty of Medicine–Endocrinology, Health Sciences Centre, Memorial University of Newfoundland, St John's, Newfoundland, Canada

DOROTA A. KRAJEWSKI, MD
Section of Endocrinology, Department of Medicine, Washington Hospital Center and Georgetown University Hospital, Washington, DC

ANGELA M. LEUNG, MD, MSc
Section of Endocrinology, Diabetes, and Nutrition, Boston University School of Medicine, Boston, Massachusetts

NANCY C. LINTNER, RN, MS, ACNS, RNC-OB
Clinical Nurse Specialist, Diabetes and Pregnancy Program, Division of Maternal-Fetal Medicine, Department of Obstetrics and Gynecology, University of Cincinnati College of Medicine, Cincinnati, Ohio

ELISABETH R. MATHIESEN, MD, DMSc
Professor, Department of Endocrinology, Center for Pregnant Women with Diabetes, Rigshospitalet, University of Copenhagen, Copenhagen Ø, Denmark

LISA J. MORAN, BSc, BND (Hons), PhD
NHMRC Research Fellow, The Robinson Institute, Research Centre for Reproductive Health, School of Paediatrics and Reproductive Health, University of Adelaide, North Adelaide, South Australia, Australia

SORIAYA MOTIVALA, MD
Resident, Department of Neurosurgery, Mount Sinai Hospital, New York, New York

VICTORIA NISENBLAT, MD
PhD Candidate, The Robinson Institute, School of Paediatrics and Reproductive Health, University of Adelaide, North Adelaide, South Australia, Australia

ROBERT J. NORMAN, BSc (Hons), MBChB (Hons), MD, FRANZCOG, FRCPA, FRCPath, FRCOG, CREI
Director, The Robinson Institute; Professor of Reproductive and Periconceptual Medicine, Research Centre for Reproductive Health, School of Paediatrics and Reproductive Health, University of Adelaide, North Adelaide, South Australia, Australia

ELIZABETH N. PEARCE, MD, MSc
Section of Endocrinology, Diabetes, and Nutrition, Boston University School of Medicine, Boston, Massachusetts

LEONID PORETSKY, MD
Division of Endocrinology and Metabolism, Beth Israel Medical Center and Albert Einstein College of Medicine, New York, New York

KALMON D. POST, MD
Chair Emeritus, Professor, Department of Neurosurgery, Mount Sinai Hospital, New York, New York

LENE RINGHOLM, MD, PhD
Department of Endocrinology, Center for Pregnant Women with Diabetes, Rigshospitalet, University of Copenhagen, Copenhagen Ø, Denmark

ZEV ROSENWAKS, MD
The Ronald O. Perelman and Claudia Cohen Center for Reproductive Medicine, Weill Cornell Medical College, New York, New York

JANET SCHLECHTE, MD
Professor of Medicine, Division of Endocrinology and Metabolism, Department of Internal Medicine, University of Iowa, Iowa City, Iowa

ELLEN W. SEELY, MD
Department of Medicine, Brigham and Women's Hospital, Boston, Massachusetts

AMAL SHIBLI-RAHHAL, MD
Assistant Professor of Clinical Medicine, Division of Endocrinology and Metabolism, Department of Internal Medicine, University of Iowa, Iowa City, Iowa

CAREN G. SOLOMON, MD, MPH
Department of Medicine, Brigham and Women's Hospital, Boston, Massachusetts

KIMBERLEE A. SOREM, MD
Medical Director, Region 1&3, California Diabetes and Pregnancy Program; Maternal Fetal Medicine Specialist, Medical Director, Sweet Success Program, Sutter Pacific Medical Foundation at California Pacific Medical Center, San Francisco, California

Contents

methods to assess iodine sufficiency, the importance of adequate iodine nutrition, studies of iodine supplementation during pregnancy and lactation, the consequences of hypothyroidism during pregnancy, the current status of iodine nutrition in the United States, the global efforts toward achieving universal iodine sufficiency, and substances that may interfere with iodine use.

Adrenal disorders may manifest during pregnancy de novo, or before pregnancy undiagnosed or diagnosed and treated. Adrenal disorders may present as hormonal hypofunction or hyperfunction, or with mass effects or other nonendocrine effects. Pregnancy presents special problems in the evaluation of the hypothalamic-pituitary-adrenal axis in addition to the usual considerations. The renin-angiotensin-aldosterone axis undergoes major changes during pregnancy. Nevertheless, the common adrenal disorders are associated with morbidity during pregnancy and their management is more complicated. A high index of suspicion must be maintained for these disorders lest they go unrecognized and untreated.

Pregnancy and lactation cause a substantial increase in demand for calcium that is met by different maternal adaptations within each period. Intestinal calcium absorption more than doubles during pregnancy, whereas the maternal skeleton resorbs to provide most of the calcium content of breast milk during lactation. These maternal adaptations also affect the presentation, diagnosis, and management of disorders of calcium and bone metabolism. Although some women may experience fragility fractures as a consequence of pregnancy or lactation, for most women, parity and lactation do not affect the long-term risks of low bone density, osteoporosis, or fracture.

The pituitary gland undergoes much anatomic and physiologic variation during pregnancy. Pituitary disease may have a significant impact on a patient prior to conception as well as throughout her pregnancy. It is imperative to provide care to patients affected by pituitary disease with a multidisciplinary approach involving endocrinologists, obstetricians and, when appropriate, neurosurgical care, as this group of disorders can represent a substantial level of morbidity and mortality for both mother and fetus.

Prolactin-secreting pituitary tumors are a common cause of amenorrhea and infertility in premenopausal women. The goals of therapy are to normalize prolactin, restore gonadal function and fertility, and reduce tumor size, and dopamine agonists are the preferred therapy. Clinically significant tumor enlargement during pregnancy is uncommon and dependent on tumor size and prepregnancy treatment.

Hypertension is a common complication of pregnancy. Preeclampsia, in particular, is associated with substantial risk to both the mother and the fetus. Several risk factors have been recognized to predict risk for preeclampsia. However, at present no biomarkers have sufficient discriminatory ability to be useful in clinical practice, and no effective preventive strategies have yet been identified. Commonly used medications for the treatment of hypertension in pregnancy include methyldopa and labetalol. Blood pressure thresholds for initiating antihypertensive therapy are higher than outside of pregnancy. Women with prior preeclampsia are at increased risk of hypertension, cardiovascular disease, and renal disease.

Polycystic ovary syndrome (PCOS) is a disease of complex and still poorly understood cause and of variable phenotypes. It is characterized by anovulation, hyperandrogenism, and polycystic ovaries. Infertility is commonly present. A variety of methods has been used successfully to achieve pregnancy in women with PCOS. Maintenance of pregnancy is complicated by a higher rate of premature spontaneous abortions and high risk of gestational diabetes, hypertension, and preeclampsia. However, with careful monitoring and treatment, the outcome of pregnancy in most women with PCOS is excellent.

Overweight and obesity are significant and increasing health problems associated with increased risks of morbidity, quality of life, and metabolic and reproductive health consequences. In women, being overweight or obese is associated with impaired fertility and decreased chance of conception both in natural and assisted reproductive technology births. During pregnancy, overweight and obesity are associated with increased risk of adverse maternal and infant health outcomes. Attention to weight loss before conception may improve fertility and maternal and infant health outcomes during pregnancy.

VISIT US ONLINE!
Access your subscription at:
www.theclinics.com

Foreword

Management of Endocrine Disorders During Pregnancy

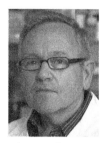

Derek LeRoith, MD, PhD
Consulting Editor

Pregnancy is associated with numerous alterations of normal physiological processes and many disorders predate the pregnancy, whereas others are affected by the pregnancy. This issue is devoted to those common endocrine disorders that endocrinologists encounter in their practice and those involved in clinical research on these topics.

Drs Inturrisi, Lintner, and Sorem, in their article, discuss the diagnosis and treatment of hyperglycemia in pregnancy. Conceptually, pregnant women with hyperglycemia, whether beginning prior to the pregnancy with a diagnosis of diabetes, or discovered during pregnancy, called gestational diabetes, should be treated in a similar manner. The occurrence is very high and should be suspected and tested for in all women. Complications to the mother and fetus are generally the result of poor control of the metabolic state.

It is clear that uncontrolled hyperglycemia during pregnancy has deleterious effects on the mother and infant and it behooves us to attempt to maintain a normal blood glucose both during the preconceptual period as well as during the pregnancy. Hypoglycemia should similarly be avoided. In general, diet, exercise, and insulin are the mainstay of therapy, while oral agents such as metformin and sulfonylureas have been tested, although not yet recommended, as their effects on the fetus, if any, are uncertain. Drs Mathiesen, Ringholm, and Damm also point out that management of blood pressure and screening for retinopathy and nephropathy is no less critical.

As discussed in their article, Drs Krajewski and Burman make a strong case for maintaining normal thyroid function in pregnancy to ensure the delivery of a normal infant. Perturbations of thyroid function, whether hypothyroid or hyperthyroidism, are deleterious to the fetus and newborn. Hyperthyroidism is treated with thionamides, whereas radioiodine is contraindicated to avoid fetal hypothyroidism. Since thyroid function tests vary during pregnancy, when treating hypothyroidism, constant monitoring is essential for appropriate thyroid hormone replacement.

Endocrinol Metab Clin N Am 40 (2011) xi–xiii
doi:10.1016/j.ecl.2011.09.004
0889-8529/11/$ – see front matter © 2011 Elsevier Inc. All rights reserved.

In their article, Drs Leung, Pearce, and Braverman describe the critical role of an adequate iodine supply required for normal thyroid function during both pregnancy and lactation to ensure normal fetal and postnatal development, especially development of the nervous system. They describe a number of substances that can interfere with normal iodine metabolism as well as present evidence that pregnancy may be associated with an inadequate intake even in the United States; guidelines suggest supplementation with multivitamins containing 150 ug iodine daily during pregnancy.

Because of the hormonal changes that occur during pregnancy, diagnosing hypo- or hyperadrenalism presents a challenge to the clinician. Thus, as discussed by Drs Abdelmannan and Aron, evaluating the hypothalamic-pituitary-adrenal axis as well as the changes in total and free cortisol and alterations in the renin-aldosterone system requires special expertise. Hypoadrenalism may present prior to pregnancy and thus maintenance of normal cortisol levels becomes critical. Alternatively, it may occur during pregnancy following adrenal hemorrhage. Their article gives the clinician a clearer understanding of these issues.

During pregnancy, there are some significant shifts in calcium metabolism. As Dr Kovacs describes in his article, intestinal calcium absorption increases to accommodate the demand made by the placenta and fetus, whereas, during lactation, the increased demand is dealt with by resorption from the skeletal calcium pool. While these changes may affect women during pregnancy, reestablishment of the skeleton occurs rapidly once lactation is complete. Thus, in most cases, the changes in pregnancy are temporary and seldom leave long-lasting effects in calcium homeostasis or bone loss.

Many organs and physiological processes change dramatically during pregnancy and the pituitary is no exception. Enlargement of the pituitary is generally due to hypertrophy and hyperplasia of the prolactin-producing lactotrophs. As discussed in the article by Drs Motivala, Gologorsky, Kostandinov, and Post, the enlargement generally recedes postpartum. They also discuss rare but important issues such as lymphocytic hypophysitis that may occur peripartum, Sheehans syndrome that may occur as a result of postpartum pituitary necrosis secondary to severe hemorrhage, and pituitary apoplexy, with all their sequelae.

Drs Shibli-Rahhal and Schlechte discuss the effect of prolactin on fertility. Hyperprolactinemia, often caused by pituitary adenomas, is commonly associated with abnormal gonadal function clearly affecting both menstruation, with amenorrhea being the symptom, as well as infertility, a serious consequence for young women. Reductions in prolactin levels, either by effective medication or by surgery, often relieves the amenorrhea and infertility. Since the pituitary often enlarges during pregnancy, special attention should be paid to women with prolactinomas who become pregnant as a result of effective medical therapy. The main downside of dopamine agonist therapy is that, while very effective, cessation of therapy often results in remission of the hyperprolactinemia and tumor regrowth.

There are numerous causes of hypertension in pregnancy. Some are associated with preexisting conditions, such as obesity, the metabolic syndrome, and diabetes, in addition to renal causes. On the other hand, preeclampsia, a serious condition, is also common, although, as discussed by Drs Solomon and Seely, the cause is not yet defined. In their article, they discuss screening and management of hypertension and particularly address which antihypertensive medications are appropriate and which can affect the fetus.

Drs Araki, Elias, Rosenwaks, and Poretsky describe the prevalence and clinical diagnosis of polycystic ovarian syndrome. Almost 7%–8% of women suffer from the syndrome that is the commonest cause of infertility in women. Polycystic ovarian syndrome is, of course, a state of hyperandrogenism, but also includes insulin resistance and a measurable elevation in luteinizing hormone. Insulin resistance can be overcome in 50% of women by weight loss and exercise but others need treatment, such as clomiphene, GnRH, or, better still, metformin, that lowers insulin resistance; similarly, so do the thiazolidinediones and GLP-1 agonists. Finally, aromatase inhibition may also be successful. Overall, metformin, sometimes in combination with other medications, gives the best results for ovulation and pregnancy.

Obesity represents a significant factor in reproductive health in women, in addition to the health consequences associated with cardiovascular complications, for example. Obese women are less fertile and attention to weight may help in conception, both with natural methods and with assisted technology. As discussed by Drs Moran, Dodd, Nisenblat, and Norman, even during pregnancy obese women and their offspring are at increased risk for adverse events. Weight loss, of course, is still the best way to prevent these complications.

The readers of this issue will undoubtedly appreciate the value of the articles in this issue as much as I did. They have been written by experts in the field, whose time and efforts are greatly appreciated by the issue editors, Drs Pessah-Pollack and Jovanovič, and me. In particular, the authors have presented basic concepts as well as practical clinical advice.

Derek LeRoith, MD, PhD
Division of Endocrinology, Metabolism, and Bone Diseases
Department of Medicine
Mount Sinai School of Medicine
One Gustave L. Levy Place
Box 1055, Altran 4-36
New York, NY 10029, USA

E-mail address:
derek.leroith@mssm.edu

Preface

Endocrine Disorders During Pregnancy

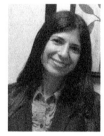 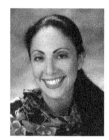

Rachel Pessah-Pollack, MD   Lois Jovanovič, MD
Guest Editors

Although it has been only 5 years since the last publication of the *Endocrinology and Metabolism Clinics of North America* issue devoted to Endocrine Disorders During Pregnancy, our knowledge and management of endocrine disorders during pregnancy have evolved and changed. We view pregnancy as a continuum, starting with preconception planning, continuing with gestation of the fetus, and culminating in the postpartum period. We have chosen to represent these phases and selected topics that cover a wide range of the subspecialties primarily within adult endocrinology, but also diseases faced by adolescents, and importantly, the effect these diseases can have on the health of the baby.

Given the challenge women often face with conception, we have dedicated articles to address reproductive dysfunction during pregnancy. With the rise of obesity in the United States and around the world, the prevalence of reproductive dysfunction secondary to obesity is rising; thus, we included an article investigating this powerful relationship. Another section focuses on the hormonal milieu in polycystic ovarian syndrome and the challenge of achieving a successful pregnancy. Optimistically, the article highlights treatment regimens that are proven to be more efficacious and that increase the likelihood of a successful pregnancy. We have included an article on the pathophysiology and evaluation of hyperprolactinemia and infertility, because of its prevalence, particularly with the use of medications today with a side effect of hyperprolactinemia.

With the surge in cases of newly diagnosed type 2 diabetes mellitus, we include a section specifically addressing pregestational diabetes and highlighting the challenges of treatment both before and during pregnancy. Hyperglycemia in pregnancy is given a specific article and focuses on the diagnosis and management of diabetes during pregnancy as well as the need for postpartum care. The management of pituitary tumors during pregnancy and how treatment differs compared with the nonpregnant state are included. The article on iodine deficiency during pregnancy is timely and

Endocrinol Metab Clin N Am 40 (2011) xv–xvi
doi:10.1016/j.ecl.2011.09.003
0889-8529/11/$ – see front matter © 2011 Elsevier Inc. All rights reserved.

relevant, particularly given the NHANES data highlighting the increased risk for iodine deficiency in reproductive age women. Finally, thyroid disorders during pregnancy are a "hot" topic as well as an important one. We devote a special section to the evaluation of both hyper- and hypothyroidism during pregnancy and evaluate the controversy over screening for thyroid dysfunction during pregnancy.

The challenge of diagnosing endocrine disorders during pregnancy is often camouflaged by the normal symptoms and disorders seen during pregnancy. The article on adrenal disorders during pregnancy provides diagnostic clues to how to make the diagnosis during pregnancy of Cushing's syndrome as well as other adrenal disorders. Maternal adaptations during pregnancy and lactation also affect the diagnosis and management of disorders of calcium and bone metabolism, as well as vitamin D deficiency, which is presented in the section of bone and mineral disorders. The differential diagnosis of hypertension during pregnancy is complex; therefore, we devoted an article to the evaluation of hypertensive disorders during pregnancy.

It has been an immense pleasure and honor to work with and learn from renowned experts who specialize in the management of the pregnant woman. Largely because of our colleagues' dedication and enthusiasm for this issue, it has been a privilege to serve as guest editors. We trust you will find these articles both informative and enlightening and this issue will provide valuable insight into the complex management of the pregnant woman.

Rachel Pessah-Pollack, MD
Mount Sinai School of Medicine
Division of Endocrinology
One Gustave L. Levy Place, Box 1055
New York, NY 10029, USA

Lois Jovanovič, MD
Sansum Diabetes Research Institute
2219 Bath Street
Santa Barbara, CA 93105, USA

E-mail addresses:
Rpessahpollack@gmail.com (R. Pessah-Pollack)
ljovanovic@sansum.org (L. Jovanovič)

Diagnosis and Treatment of Hyperglycemia in Pregnancy

Maribeth Inturrisi, RN, MS, CNS, CDE[a,b,c,]*,
Nancy C. Lintner, RN, MS, ACNS, RNC-OB[d], Kimberlee A. Sorem, MD[a,e]

KEYWORDS

- Gestational diabetes mellitus • Type 2 diabetes
- Large for gestational age • Blood glucose
- Oral glucose tolerance test • Self-monitoring of blood glucose
- American Association of the College of Endocrinologists
- Certified diabetes educators

Gestational diabetes mellitus (GDM) has been defined as any degree of glucose intolerance with onset or first recognition during pregnancy.[1] This definition is a misnomer in that it includes unrecognized overt diabetes that may have existed before pregnancy and hyperglycemia that is diagnosed concurrently with pregnancy. Those with suspected type 2 diabetes mellitus (T2DM) have been referred to as "hyperglycemia in pregnancy," despite evidence of severe hyperglycemia consistent with preexisting T2DM. Because the term "gestational diabetes mellitus" is confusing, the authors recommend use of the term "hyperglycemia in pregnancy," as defined by the Endocrine Society.[2]

SIGNIFICANCE

The prevalence of hyperglycemia in pregnancy varies in direct proportion to the prevalence of type 2 diabetes in a given population or ethnic group. Whereas in 1964 the prevalence of hyperglycemia in pregnancy was 1% to 4%,[3] the current estimate is 7%

The authors have nothing to disclose.

[a] Region 1 & 3, California Diabetes and Pregnancy Program, San Francisco, CA, USA
[b] Family Health Care Nursing, University of California, San Francisco, CA, USA
[c] Department of Maternal-Fetal Medicine, Sutter Pacific Medical Foundation at California Pacific Medical Center, San Francisco, CA, USA
[d] Diabetes and Pregnancy Program, Division of Maternal-Fetal Medicine, Department of Obstetrics and Gynecology, University of Cincinnati College of Medicine, 231 Albert Sabin Way, 5553, PO Box 670526, Cincinnati, OH 45267–0526, USA
[e] Sweet Success Program, Sutter Pacific Medical Foundation at California Pacific Medical Center, 3700 California Street, G321, San Francisco, CA, USA
* Corresponding author. 2 Koret Way, PO Box 0606, San Francisco, CA 94143–0606.
E-mail address: maribeth.inturrisi@nursing.ucsf.edu

to 14%.[3] In 1964, the number of adults estimated to have type 2 diabetes in the United States was 2.3 million and in 2011 estimates were as high as 25.6 million, indicating that type 2 diabetes in America is increasing in an epidemic pattern. Likewise, hyperglycemia in pregnancy is a silent epidemic. If current trends continue, by 2050 one in three Americans will have diabetes.[3]

Hyperglycemia in pregnancy shares the pathophysiology of type 2 diabetes (increased insulin resistance and hyperinsulinemia) and confers an increased lifetime risk for future type 2 diabetes for both the mother and her newborn. Hyperglycemia in pregnancy is not just a pregnancy problem. Soon after giving birth, 90% to 95% of women with hyperglycemia in pregnancy are diabetes-free by a standard 2-hour 75-g oral glucose tolerance test (OGTT). By 6 to 12 weeks, 4% to 9% are diagnosed with T2DM. More than 20% have impaired glucose tolerance or impaired fasting glucose or both (prediabetes). By 36 months, 30% have metabolic syndrome (dysglycemia, abnormal lipid profile, hypertension, and central adiposity). By 5 years, 50% have T2DM. The cumulative risk over 10 years is 2.6% to 70%.[4] Fetal, neonatal, and adult consequences of uncontrolled maternal hyperglycemia include a variety of serious short- and long-term consequences (**Table 1**).

Detection and diagnosis of hyperglycemia in pregnancy provides an opportunity to assist women to establish healthy lifestyle habits and give them tools to reduce maternal and fetal risks (see **Table 1**) by facilitating normoglycemia. Providers who manage diabetes care during pregnancy are in the unique position to educate women about a healthy lifestyle and prevention of T2DM. The primary goals of hyperglycemia in pregnancy diagnosis are to reduce the short- and long-term risks associated with mild to moderate hyperglycemia during pregnancy through healthy lifestyle education.[5,6]

SCREENING

For decades, the American Diabetes Association (ADA) published a two-step glucose screening and diagnosis of hyperglycemia in pregnancy that was solely based on the woman's risk for developing T2DM in the future.[7] The recommendations included the avoidance of screening in women considered low risk: less than 25 years of age, normal body weight, no family history of diabetes, and not a member of an ethnic or racial group at high risk for diabetes. The Fifth International Workshop on Gestational Diabetes in November 2005 recommended that hyperglycemia in pregnancy risk assessment should be ascertained at the first prenatal visit. The American College of Obstetricians and Gynecologists (ACOG) recommends that all pregnant patients

Table 1
Fetal, neonatal, and adult consequences of uncontrolled maternal hyperglycemia during pregnancy

Short Term (Fetal and Neonatal)	Long Term (Adult)
LGA	Obesity
Organomegaly	Visceral adiposity
Neonatal hypoglycemia	Hyperinsulinemia
Transient tachypnea, respiratory distress	Insulin resistance
Birth trauma (Erb palsy, asphysia, fractured bones)	T2DM
Feeding abnormalities	Cardiovascular disease
	Metabolic syndrome

be screened for hyperglycemia in pregnancy, whether by patient history, clinical risk factors, or a laboratory test to determine blood glucose (BG) levels early in pregnancy.[8] In 1996, the US Preventive Services Task Force concluded that evidence was insufficient to recommend for or against routine screening for hyperglycemia in pregnancy, and this recommendation remained unchanged in 2003.[9] Two subsequently published studies show benefit (particularly a reduction in macrosomia) when women are treated for hyperglycemia in pregnancy versus no treatment.[5,6]

Most American providers have used a two-step method involving a nonfasting 1-hour 50-g oral glucose screen (glucose loading test) with a subsequent diagnostic 3-hour 100-g OGTT for those who failed the initial screen. Screening reduces the number of women who would have to be subjected to a fasting plus 3-hour 100-g OGTT. Using a plasma glucose threshold greater than or equal to 140 mg/dL for screening has a sensitivity of 80% and specificity of 90% for a positive OGTT. Lowering the threshold to greater than or equal to 130 mg/dL increases the sensitivity to 90% but also increases the number of women requiring diagnostic testing by 60%. ACOG and ADA endorse either cut point.[5,6]

DIAGNOSIS

Women who fail the 1-hour glucose loading test screen take a 3-hour 100-g glucola OGTT and are considered to have hyperglycemia in pregnancy if two of the four values equal or exceed the cut points of fasting BG 95 mg/dL, 1-hour after 100-g glucola of 180 mg/dL, 2-hour of 155 mg/dL, and 3-hour of 140 mg/dL.[10] If hyperglycemia in pregnancy is not diagnosed, the OGTT should be repeated at 24 to 28 weeks gestation or any time a patient presents with signs or symptoms suggestive of hyperglycemia.[11] Women with an abnormal 3-hour OGTT who are less than 24 weeks gestation may have undiagnosed T1DM, T2DM, or prediabetes but the diagnosis of preexisting diabetes or prediabetes can only be made definitively after delivery regardless of the severity of hyperglycemia.[11]

This method remained the gold standard in the United States with changes in the glucose cutoffs as glucose assays changed and the use of plasma replaced whole blood. Internationally, more than 10 different ways of diagnosing hyperglycemia in pregnancy included one- or two-step procedures primarily using a 2-hour 75-g OGTT but with a variety of different cut points and numbers of abnormal values required to diagnose hyperglycemia in pregnancy. Until now, no worldwide standard existed for the diagnosis of hyperglycemia in pregnancy.

THE HYPERGLYCEMIA AND ADVERSE PREGNANCY OUTCOME STUDY

For the last 50 years, the diagnosis of hyperglycemia in pregnancy has been based on the 100-g, 3-hour OGTT that predicts the risk of the mother developing diabetes in the future.[12] Physicians have not had useful guidelines to link the diagnosis of hyperglycemia in pregnancy to neonatal outcomes. The Hyperglycemia and Adverse Pregnancy Outcome (HAPO) Study is a basic epidemiologic investigation designed to clarify unanswered questions about the association between various levels of glucose during the third trimester of pregnancy that indicate that the mother, fetus, and newborn are at increased risk for adverse outcomes. This 7-year international study was conducted in 15 centers in nine countries with 23,325 women participating in the study.

The women were given a 2-hour 75-g OGTT at 24 to 28 weeks of gestation. Providers and patients were blinded to the results unless they exceeded predefined cutoff values requiring treatment. The cutoffs were as follows: fasting BG greater than 105 mg/dL or 2-hour greater than 200 mg/dL or random BG at 34 weeks greater than 160 mg/dL. The women who exceeded the cutoffs were removed from the study and treated for diabetes. The remainder received routine prenatal care, a random BG at 34 weeks, and fetal kick counts. Primary outcomes included those listed in **Boxes 1** and **2**.[10]

Results indicated that there is a continuous, positive, independent relationship between maternal BG and percent newborn body fat, and between cord C-peptide concentrations and percent newborn body fat.[11] This suggests that the relationship between maternal glycemia and fetal fat deposition is mediated by fetal insulin production. The association between hyperglycemia and poor outcomes was continuous, making it difficult to identify threshold criteria below which no risk is present. The task of translating these associations into diagnostic criteria was assigned to a committee of experts formed by the International Association of Diabetes in Pregnancy Study Groups (IADPSG). In March 2010, the group published recommendations for a global method of diagnosing hyperglycemia in pregnancy using glucose cutoffs based on an odds ratio of 1.75 for having one of the primary adverse outcomes listed in **Box 1**.[11] **Table 2** provides a comparison of the old and new methods for diagnosing hyperglycemia in pregnancy. The 2011 ADA Standards of Medical Care published the IADPSG recommended method as the standard method of diagnosing hyperglycemia in pregnancy discontinuing all other methods.[12] This was in concert with many countries.

PREGNANCY: A DIABETOGENIC STATE

Normal pregnancy can be viewed as a progressive condition of insulin resistance, hyperinsulinemia, and mild postprandial hyperglycemia mediated by increasing placental secretion of antiinsulin hormones including, progesterone, human placental lactogen, cortisol, growth hormone, and tumor necrosis factor (TNF)-α. This prepares the mother for the increased demands of the fetus for amino acids and glucose in the latter half of pregnancy. Mild postprandial hyperglycemia serves to increase the amount of time that maternal glucose levels are elevated above the basal after a meal, thereby increasing the flux of ingested nutrients from mother to the fetus and enhancing fetal growth.[13]

The fetal demand for glucose in the third trimester is met during maternal fasting by hepatic glucose production, which increases 15% to 30% by late third trimester. The liver begins to supply glucose within 5 to 6 hours of the last meal when absorption of nutrients from the intestinal tract ceases. Depletion of glycogen stores results from this accelerated hepatic glucose production. Lower fasting values (55–65 mg/dL) offset the postprandial elevations resulting in 24-hour mean glucose values similar to nongravid women.[14]

Fetal growth accelerates in the last trimester of pregnancy. During the last trimester, the fetus is constantly feeding while the mother alternates between fasting and

---

Box 1
HAPO study primary neonatal outcomes

- Birth weight above the 90th percentile for gestational age
- Primary cesarean delivery
- Clinically diagnosed neonatal hypoglycemia
- Cord-blood serum C-peptide level above the 90th percentile

Data from The HAPO Study Cooperative Research Group. Hyperglycemia and adverse pregnancy outcomes. N Engl J Med 2008;358:1991–2002.

Box 2
Objectives of medical nutrition therapy in diabetes and pregnancy

- Determine energy needs

- Set appropriate weight goals

- Develop an individualized, nutritionally balanced meal plan

- Provide education concerning nutrition-related lifestyle issue

- Counsel on the importance of normoglycemia before, during, and after pregnancy

- Evaluate adherence to the meal plan

Adapted with permission from the California Department of Public Health, California Diabetes and Pregnancy Program Sweet Success Guidelines for Care 2006. Funding for the development of the original materials was provided by the Federal Title V block grant from the California Maternal, Child and Adolescent Health Division.

---

feeding. Glucose is transported across the placenta from the mother to the fetus by facilitated diffusion. The concentration of glucose within the fetus is approximately 15% to 20% lower than maternal glucose.[13] Insulin does not cross the placenta. The fetus synthesizes its own insulin starting at 9 to 12 weeks gestation. From gestational weeks 9 to 15, maternal insulin requirements decrease. Reasons for this decrease are not well understood.

Fetal β cells respond to an increase in glucose and amino acids. Amino acids are transported against a concentration gradient from the maternal to fetal circulation. The fetal concentration of amino acids is three to four times that of the maternal concentration.

Late pregnancy has also been characterized as a catabolic phase or a period of accelerated starvation, which consists of an earlier switch from carbohydrate to fat metabolism (lipolysis) with fasting.[14] This metabolic response to fasting develops in 14 to 18 hours in pregnant women (accelerated starvation) and in 2 to 3 days in the nonpregnant state.[13] Ketones also cross the placenta in the direction of the concentration gradient. Ketones may be used as an alternate fuel for the fetus when glucose is not available. The hyperglycemia in pregnancy diet is designed to provide frequent

Table 2
Diagnosing hyperglycemia in pregnancy

	Old Method[10]	New Method[11]
24–28 wk gestation	Screen high-risk or all women	Universal testing of all pregnant women
Screen	1-h 50-g glucose load, nonfasting, glucose loading test; if ≥130 or 140, proceed to diagnostic test	None
Diagnostic test	After 8- to 12-h fast, obtain fasting; provide 100-g glucose load; then obtain 1-, 2-, and 3-h venous BG	After 8- to 12-h fast, obtain fasting, provide 75-g glucose load, then obtain 1- and 2-h venous BG
Diagnosis of GDM	If two of the following values meet or exceed: fasting 95 mg/dL, 1-h 180 mg/dL, 2-h 155 mg/dL, 3-h 140 mg/dL	If any 1 value meets or exceeds fasting 92 mg/dL, 1-h 180 mg/dL, 2-h 153 mg/dL

Data from American Diabetes Association. Standards of medical care in diabetes–2011. Diabetes Care 2011;34(Suppl 1):S11–61.

sources of small amounts of carbohydrate by encouraging small frequent meals and a bedtime snack.

HEALTHY EATING

The cornerstone for diabetes management is healthy eating and appropriate physical activity. The diagnosis of hyperglycemia in pregnancy gives women the opportunity to focus on healthy eating and staying active to improve their lifestyle for better health. The goal of the hyperglycemia in pregnancy meal plan is to attain and maintain euglycemia and adequate nutrition for the growth and development of the fetus. The achievement of these goals is based on the individualized medical nutrition therapy (MNT) plan developed by the woman and the registered dietitian. Registered dieticians should be central to the management team and should be included in the initial assessment and on an ongoing basis.

Creating a Meal Plan

Calories for pregnancy should be comprised of 40% to 50% carbohydrates, including high-fiber fruits and starches and milk as tolerated; 20% protein; and 35% fat, preferably unsaturated and monosatuarated types.[15] Although caloric needs are determined, they no longer dominate the meal plan. The American Dietetic Association has abandoned the 1800- to 2200-calorie ADA diet. Instead, a carbohydrate-controlled meal plan that is culturally appropriate and individualized to take into account the individual's body habitus and physical activity is recommended to achieve treatment goals. The Institute of Medicine (IOM) has set dietary reference intakes as the minimum nutrient requirements for pregnancy.[16] The hyperglycemia in pregnancy meal plan should be built around these requirements. Women should be taught to read labels and recognize total carbohydrates and serving sizes. Ideally, they should keep food and BG records that allow providers to suggest strategies that lead to optimal nutrition and glycemic control. Nutritional interventions should emphasize overall healthy food choices, portion control, and cooking practices that can be continued throughout life. The carbohydrates should be distributed in three meals and several snacks to decrease postprandial hyperglycemia and the risk of between-meal hypoglycemia. Aspartame has been determined to be safe as a nonnutritive sweetener in pregnancy except in women with phenylketonuria. Saccharin does cross into placental circulation but there is no evidence of harmful fetal effects.[17]

Because healthy eating is central to adopting a healthy lifestyle, emphasis on nutrition education is fundamental. Assessment and reevaluation of the meal plan by a registered dietician should occur at the first hyperglycemia in pregnancy visit and then on an ongoing basis thereafter, and finally in the postpartum period. Dietary adjustments are needed as a woman learns how certain foods influence her BG. "Principles of Healthy Eating during Pregnancy" modified from the California Diabetes and Pregnancy Program Sweet Success Guidelines for Care 2002, provides a general guide in Box 3.

WEIGHT MANAGEMENT

In normal pregnancy, expected weight gain varies according to the prepregnancy weight. The IOM recommendations for nonpregnant women are listed in Table 3.[18]

After the release of the 2009 IOM guidelines, some investigators and experts expressed concern that higher weight gains among a population of normal and overweight women would not reduce adverse infant outcomes and would put women at risk for delivering macrosomic infants and for postpartum weight retention.[19] Since

---

Box 3
Principles of healthy eating during pregnancy

Distribute carbohydrates intake among three meals and three snacks spaced at 2.5- to 3-hour intervals. Skipping meals or snacks can result in hypoglycemia, ketone production, or overeating later in the day. Bedtime snack should provide 15–30 g of carbohydrates and approximately 7–15 g of protein

Sample distribution of carbohydrates (individualize)

Dietary reference intakes = 175 g carbohydrates per day in pregnancy

Breakfast   Lunch   Dinner
15------------30-------------- 45-------------15----------------45----------30 = 180 g carb

Macronutrient distribution:

- Carbohydrates: ~40%–50%; ideally, carbohydrates should be combined with protein.

- Fat: <30%; use nuts, peanut butter, canola oil, or olive oil as primary sources of fat

- Protein: ~30%; look for lean meats, fish (check safety)

Avoid high glycemic foods at breakfast:

- Processed, ready to eat cold cereals (instant cereals)

- Milk

- Fruit

- Fruit juice

- A breakfast that consists of whole grain starch plus protein is suggested

Limit fruit

- Two to three fruit servings per day

Encourage nonstarchy vegetables

- Greens, tomatoes, carrots, and so forth, at least five servings per day

Protein

- 71 g/day: meat, poultry, fish, eggs, cheese, tofu, and so forth

Fats

- Minimum three servings per day: nuts, oils, and so forth; watch for excess calories with fats

Adapted with permission from the California Department of Public Health, California Diabetes and Pregnancy Program Sweet Success Guidelines for Care 2006 Updates by the California Diabetes and Pregnancy Program. Funding for the development of the original materials was provided by the Federal Title V block grant from the California Maternal, Child and Adolescent Health Division.

---

then, several studies have observed that the infants of women with pregnancy weight gains within the IOM recommendations are relatively less likely to be at the extremes of birth weight for a given gestational age.[19] In one study, women who gained more than recommended by the IOM were three times more likely to have an infant with large for gestational age (LGA) and nearly 1.5 times more likely to have an infant with hypoglycemia or hyperbilirubinemia, compared with women whose weight gain

Table 3	
IOM Guidelines for total gestational weight gain[a]	
Body Mass Index Category	**Weight Gain Ranges**
Underweight <18.5	28–40 lb
Normal 18.5–24.9	25–35 lb
Overweight 25–29.9	15–25 lb
Obese ≥30	11–20 lb

[a] Certain Asian populations may need lower body mass index cut points for each body mass index category and this might impact weight gain goals for pregnancy.[76]

Data from Institute of Medicine Report Brief. Weight gain during pregnancy reexamining the guidelines 2009. Available from: http://www.iom.edu/w/media/Files/Report%20Files/2009/Weight-Gain-During-Pregnancy-Reexamining-the-Guidelines/Report%20Brief%20-%20Weight%20Gain%20During%20Pregnancy.pdf. Accessed September 3, 2011.

was in the recommended range.[20] In another study, weight gain ranges based on adverse obstetric and neonatal outcome data were lower than the IOM recommendations, and the differences were most pronounced for overweight or obese women.[21] Excess gestational weight gain can be associated not only with fetal LGA but also with unhealthy maternal postpartum weight retention.[22]

Weight gain or loss should be monitored closely and the meal plan should be adjusted accordingly. Plotting weekly body weights on a weight gain grid specific to body mass index classification is encouraged to facilitate recognition of inadequate or excess weight gain. Sample weight gain grids for pregnancy are available online based on the 2009 IOM recommendations at http://www.cdph.ca.gov/pubsforms/forms/Pages/MaternalandChildHealth.aspx.

Obesity

No discussion of weight during pregnancy can be adequate without a discussion of obesity. Obesity has reached epidemic proportions globally, with more than 1 billion adults overweight, at least 300 million of them clinically obese. The epidemic of T2DM has paralleled the epidemic of obesity. The likelihood of developing T2DM and hypertension rises steeply with increasing body fat. Confined to older adults for most of the twentieth century, this disease now affects obese children even before puberty. Approximately 90% of people with diabetes have T2DM, and of these, 85% are obese or overweight.[23] The strong presence of obesity in a population makes it certain that a significant number of women with pregestational diabetes (type 1 and type 2 diabetes) and women who subsequently develop hyperglycemia in pregnancy will enter pregnancy obese. Obese women are at increased risk for morbidity and mortality during pregnancy.[24] Several studies have demonstrated that the risk of congenital malformations, especially neural tube defects, is double among obese women compared with fetus of normal-weight women, after correcting for diabetes as a potential confounding factor.[25,26] An increased incidence of miscarriage and intrauterine fetal demise has also been associated with obesity even in the absence of diabetes.[27–29]

Obesity confers a certain elevated level of insulin resistance and inflammation that may mediate these adverse outcomes. When combined with hyperglycemia, morbidities increase. Even lactation can be negatively impacted because overweight or obese women were found to have a lower prolactin response to suckling, and thus diminished milk production.[30] Limited or no weight gain in obese pregnant women has favorable pregnancy outcomes.[31] Obese women with hyperglycemia in pregnancy treated with diet therapy who achieved targeted levels of glycemic control nevertheless had a twofold to threefold higher risk for adverse pregnancy outcomes compared with overweight and normal-weight patients with well-controlled hypergly-cemia in pregnancy. In obese women with body mass index greater than 30 and hyperglycemia in pregnancy, achievement of targeted levels of glycemic control was associated with enhanced outcome only in women treated with insulin.[32] Several studies show a protective effect of reduced gestational weight gain and even weight loss on LGA births and cesarean delivery for obese women.[33] An upper limit on gesta-tional weight gain should be considered to prevent comorbidities among obese women but controversy remains as to whether the 2009 IOM recommendation of 20 lb should be that upper limit.[31] Weight loss during pregnancy has not been recommen-ded in the past, but women who are obese and adhere to the meal plan prescribed for managing diabetes during pregnancy are likely to lose weight while maintaining a healthy, nutrient-rich diet. The issue of starvation ketones emerges with weight loss. No correlation exists between ketonuria and ketonemia. Ketonemia is unlikely to exist when the meal plan includes at least 1800 calories and small frequent meals. However, obese women who want to become pregnant should be counseled about the increased risks, including gestational diabetes, associated with obesity and preg-nancy. Immediate referral to a dietitian to address safe weight loss before pregnancy should occur.

Some women may choose bariatric surgery as a method of weight loss. Several studies have indicated that previous bariatric surgery in patients with GDM is not asso-ciated with adverse perinatal outcomes.[34] Many individuals who had T2DM no longer require medication to maintain normoglycemia. When screening for gestational dia-betes, an alternate method for testing is necessary. Administration of a standard glucose solution would precipitate "dumping syndrome." Women with previous bari-atric surgery may need to test their blood sugars fasting and after meals for several days to determine if they are experiencing hyperglycemia. Some providers have used continuous glucose monitoring systems to help with diagnosis.[35]

Staying Active

Research over the past 22 years has focused on the safety of physical activity during pregnancy. The overwhelming results of most studies show primarily beneficial effects on the maternal–fetal unit and very few negative effects.[36] The role of physical activity for pregnant women with diabetes has also gained acceptance and has become an essential part of the treatment plan.

Exercise facilitates the glucose uptake that regulates glucose transport and intracel-lular metabolism and sustains insulin sensitivity and improves glucose clearance.[37,38] Furthermore, exercise regulates hepatic glucose output, evidenced in fasting BG levels and the counterregulatory hormones.[39] Additionally, weight-bearing exercise may moderate insulin resistance, improve caloric expenditure, favorably alter basal metabolic rate, and enhance weight loss. The effect of exercise on decreasing glucose and insulin concentrations is greatest with low-intensity, prolonged exercise that uses a large muscle mass shortly (<2 hours) after mixed caloric intake.[38] Regular exercise during pregnancy decreases TNF-α originating from the placenta, a substance that directly correlates with the level of insulin resistance throughout pregnancy.[38]

The ADA suggests that "women without medical or obstetric contraindications be encouraged to start or continue a program of moderate exercise as part of the treat-ment" of hyperglycemia in pregnancy.[40] The American College of Sports Medicine recommends that every adult accumulate at least 30 minutes of moderate-intensity aerobic activity on most, preferably all, days of the week.[36] Walking is the most popular form of aerobic exercise for adults, and walking at a normal-to-brisk pace constitutes moderate-intensity exercise. Walking is also an activity that many women can fit into their lifestyles, even when pregnant. To reduce postmeal glucose excursions, three 10-minute walks can meet this requirement. Many women with gestational diabetes find this regimen reduces or in some cases eliminates the need for insulin therapy. A 10-minute activity session timed at 30 minutes after each meal may help to control postmeal glucose excursions and reduce the need for insulin.

Monitoring BG

The consideration of glycemic goals in the pregnant diabetic woman must take into account the normal glucose ranges in nondiabetic pregnant women. Recently reexamined with the use of continuous glucose monitoring systems, mean fasting BG values have been shown to range from 61 to 75 mg/dL decreasing over the course of gestation.[41] In diabetic and nondiabetic pregnancies, maximal postprandial glucose excursions occur between 60 and 90 minutes after meal ingestion and correlate more closely with 1- than 2-hour postprandial measurements.[42] Understanding these nondiabetic pregnancy values, normal glucose ranges (**Table 4**) provide additional support to the previous observation that the LGA risk increases with increasing maximal postprandial hyperglycemia.[43]

During a healthy pregnancy, mean fasting blood sugar levels decline progressively to a remarkably low value of 75 ± 12 mg/dL. However, peak postprandial blood sugar values rarely exceed 126 mg/dL. Meticulous replication of the normal glycemic profile during pregnancy has been demonstrated to reduce the LGA rate. **Table 5** shows the commonly held BG targets for hyperglycemia in pregnancy.

Daily BG self-monitoring, compared with weekly office-based testing, is associated with a reduction in the incidence of LGA infants in women with hyperglycemia in pregnancy.[44] Women should be taught to check their BG using a home meter. The frequency of testing is determined by whether or not they need medication and how well their blood sugars are controlled. Suggested frequencies are listed in **Box 4** but can be modified depending on the individual circumstances.

Because of the high frequency of self-monitoring blood glucose testing required in pregnancy, the use of alternative-site self-monitoring blood glucose testing is appealing, but the dynamically changing BG concentrations after eating may be identified at finger sites before being detected at the forearm or thigh sites. Because there

Table 4	
Ambulatory glycemic profile and postprandial glucose levels in nondiabetic pregnancies	
Mean blood glucose (mg/dL)	83.7 ± 18
Fasting glucose (mg/dL)	75 ± 12
Preprandial glucose (mg/dL)	78 ± 11
Peak postprandial glucose value (mg/dL)	110 ± 16
Peak postprandial time (min)	70 ± 13
Mean blood glucose of 3-h postprandial measurements (mg/dL)	98 ± 12
1-h postprandial glucose value (mg/dL)	105 ± 13
2-h postprandial glucose value (mg/dL)	97 ± 11
3-h postprandial glucose value (mg/dL)	84 ± 14
Mean blood glucose at nighttime (mg/dL)	68 ± 10

Data from Yogev Y, Ben-Haroush A, Chen R, et al. Diurnal glycemic profile in obese and normal weight nondiabetic pregnant women. Am J Obstet Gynecol 2004;191:949–53.

Table 5		
Blood glucose targets for hyperglycemia in pregnancy		
Fasting and premeal	60–89 mg/dL[a]	95 mg/dL[b]
Peak postprandial	100–129 mg/dL[a]	140 mg/dL[b]

[a] Handelsman Y, Mechanick JI, Blonde L, et al. American Association of Clinical Endocrinologists Medical Guidelines for Clinical Practice for developing a diabetes mellitus comprehensive care plan. Endocr Pract 2011;17(Suppl 2):1–53.
[b] American College of Obstetricians and Gynecologists Committee on Practice Bulletins–Obstetrics. ACOG Practice Bulletin. Clinical management guidelines for obstetrician-gynecologists. Number 30, September 2001 (replaces Technical Bulletin Number 200, December 1994). Gestational diabetes. Obstet Gynecol 2001;98(3):525–38.

are no studies that have evaluated the use of BG values from alternative sites in pregnancy, alternative-site self-monitoring blood glucose testing must be discouraged.

TREATMENT OF HYPERGLYCEMIA IN PREGNANCY

Although some women can attain normoglycemia through MNT and exercise alone, insulin or oral agents may be required for women to control BG levels during pregnancy. The percentage of women with hyperglycemia in pregnancy requiring insulin varies based on the population served. In 2009, the California Diabetes and Pregnancy Program Data System reported that of approximately 11,400 women with hyperglycemia in pregnancy, treated in the Sweet Success Program, about 40% (~4500) required medication in addition to meal plan and exercise to achieve normalization of BG during pregnancy complicated by hyperglycemia in pregnancy.[45]

When considering medication therapy for hyperglycemia in pregnancy, a number of considerations are important as described in **Box 5**.

Insulin has been the gold standard for achieving tight control during pregnancy. Initiating insulin with mild-to-moderate hyperglycemia can be accomplished with a simple approach as described in **Table 6**. For more severe hyperglycemia, dose calculations are similar to overt T2DM based on weight and gestational age.

A certified diabetes educator should teach the woman the safe and effective way to administer insulin and should follow-up in a few days. Compliance and success with insulin therapy has been positively correlated with provider contact.

Hyperglycemia in Pregnancy and Oral Glucose-Lowering Agents

Although insulin has been the gold standard for treatment of hyperglycemia during pregnancy, there are disadvantages that make some women refuse or comply poorly with the treatment plan when the treatment includes insulin. Some women restrict carbohydrate intake severely to avoid requiring insulin. The effects of severe

Box 4
Self-monitoring blood glucose suggested frequencies
Fasting
1 hour postprandial
Bedtime
Preprandial, when indicated
3 AM, when indicated

Box 5
When to initiate medication therapy for hyperglycemia in pregnancy

When BGs are greater than 20% beyond target despite meal plan and exercise adherence:

- Three or more elevated fasting BGs and/or
- Six or more postmeal elevations in 1 week

Before starting the woman with hyperglycemia in pregnancy on insulin evaluate for:

- Persistent fasting plasma BG ≥90 mg/dL (three or more in 1 week)
- BG records that indicate a pattern (six or more in 1 week) of elevations despite adherence to the meal plan and exercise
- The degree of elevation above the target values: mild to moderate
  - Fasting plasma BG 90–120 mg/dL, postmeals 130–180 mg/dL
- Estimated LGA fetus >90th percentile or abdominal circumference >70th percentile on ultrasound (Buchanan et al, 2007)

---

restriction are not known, but women with an average BG of less than 87 mg/dL have an increased risk of a small-for-gestational-age infant.[46] There is some evidence that when carbohydrates have been severely restricted the pancreas is underdeveloped leading to T2DM in the offspring later in life.[47] Some women fear injections will be painful, hurt the fetus, or cause a reliance on injections for a lifetime. Although none of this is true, some women remain fearful and resist therapy. Insulin therapy is associated with risks of hypoglycemia and increase in appetite and weight.

As an alternative to insulin some providers are choosing to use oral medications, such as glyburide and metformin (glucophage), based on studies supporting relative safety and efficacy.[48,49] Langer and colleagues[48] have found that glyburide, a sulfonylurea drug, did not seem to pass through the placenta in the laboratory. The researchers speculated glyburide would be safe to use during pregnancy and designed a study to test the efficacy. Their randomized study of 404 women with gestational diabetes who received either insulin injections or glyburide pills confirmed this hypothesis. The outcomes in each group were similar. The percentage of newborns that were large for their gestational age was similar in both groups of women. In addition, there were no statistically significant differences in the infants' rates of birth defects, lung complications, or low blood sugar.

Table 6
Starting doses of insulin with mild hyperglycemia

Elevated fasting blood sugars	0.2 units/kg NPH at bedtime
Elevated postbreakfast	Insulin to carbohydrate ratio is ~2:15 at breakfast (2–4 units) rapid-acting analog
Elevated postlunch or postdinner	Insulin to carbohydrate ratio is ~1:15 at lunch (3–5 units) rapid-acting analog prelunch and predinner

Adapted with permission from the California Department of Public Health, California Diabetes and Pregnancy Program Sweet Success "Diabetes and Pregnancy Pocket Guide for Professionals" 2008 by the California Diabetes and Pregnancy Program. Funding for the development of the original materials was provided by the Federal Title V block grant from the California Maternal, Child and Adolescent Health Division.

The researchers also did not detect glyburide in the umbilical-cord blood of the 12 newborns that were tested. Only eight of the women taking glyburide needed to switch to insulin to control their gestational diabetes. The number studied was insufficient to show statistical difference in this subgroup. The incidence of fetal LGA in both groups was greater than 12%. Glycemic control was not optimal in either group. Although the protocol in the study allowed for up to 10-mg glyburide twice a day, other authors have cautioned against such a high dose because hypoglycemia can accompany glyburide use.[50,51] **Box 6** describes one approach to dosing glyburide during pregnancy.

Although glyburide works by stimulating insulin secretion, it is also associated with risks of maternal hypoglycemia and weight gain. Metformin, an oral biguanide, may be a possible alternative to insulin for women with hyperglycemia in pregnancy who are unable to cope with the increasing insulin resistance of pregnancy. In another study, Rowan and associates[49] showed similar perinatal mortality and morbidity for women treated with metformin compared with insulin. There are data from over 30 years ago reporting use of metformin in women with hyperglycemia in pregnancy or T2DM in pregnancy in South Africa with no reports of adverse outcomes.[52] However, metformin does cross the placenta and little is known concerning long-term effects resulting from fetal exposure. There are ongoing studies. It should be noted that a total of 30% of metformin-treated women with hyperglycemia in pregnancy ultimately required insulin for adequate glucose control. **Box 7** provides a sample protocol for metformin use in pregnancy.

As with insulin, optimum care involves provider follow-up at frequent short intervals (every 3 days) until an adequate dose is achieved. As pregnancy progresses insulin resistance increases and doses need to be adjusted.

Box 6
Glyburide protocol for hyperglycemia in pregnancy

Begin with 1.25 mg/day either in the AM or PM depending on individual needs

After 2–3 days without achieving target blood sugars, increase by 1.25 mg so total dose at one time is 2.5 mg/day AM or PM

Next (after 2–3 days without achieving targets) add 2.5 mg to the opposite time of day so the patient is taking 2.5 mg twice daily

Increase every 3 days by 1.25–2.5 mg total until targets are reached or maximum daily dose is 20 mg per day

Maintain meal plan and exercise therapy

Comply with recommended self-monitoring blood glucose schedule

Conduct fetal surveillance as recommended for patients using insulin therapy

Be aware that hypoglycemia can occur

Adhere to MNT meal and snack regimen to avoid hypoglycemia

Ensure that the woman can recognize and treat hypoglycemia

Monitor weight and assess for appropriate weight gain because weight gain has been associated with this agent

Adapted with permission from the California Department of Public Health, California Diabetes and Pregnancy Program Sweet Success "Diabetes and Pregnancy Pocket Guide for Professionals" 2008 by the California Diabetes and Pregnancy Program. Funding for the development of the original materials was provided by the Federal Title V block grant from the California Maternal, Child and Adolescent Health Division.

> **Box 7**
> **Metformin protocol for hyperglycemia in pregnancy**
>
> Start at a dose of 500 mg once or twice daily with food or at bedtime depending on the target pattern of hyperglycemia
>
> Increase by 500 mg every 3–5 days over a period of 1–2 weeks, to meet glycemic targets up to a maximum daily dose of 2500 mg
>
> Obtain serum creatinine at start of therapy if renal dysfunction is suspected; metformin is cleared in the kidneys
>
> Common side effects are nausea, vomiting, diarrhea, loss of appetite, stomach fullness, constipation, and heartburn
>
> Drug should be discontinued before major surgery, or radiologic studies involving contrast materials
>
> Metformin is associated with mild weight loss
>
> *Adapted with permission from* the California Department of Public Health, California Diabetes and Pregnancy Program Sweet Success "Diabetes and Pregnancy Pocket Guide for Professionals" 2008 by the California Diabetes and Pregnancy Program. Funding for the development of the original materials was provided by the Federal Title V block grant from the California Maternal, Child and Adolescent Health Division.

Hypoglycemia

Hypoglycemia is the result of insulin excess and compromised physiologic defenses against falling plasma glucose concentrations. Hypoglycemia has been classified as" asymptomatic" or "biochemical," which is particularly common, and "symptomatic" or "severe," which requires the assistance of another individual. The biochemical definition is a BG less than or equal to 70 mg/dL because in nondiabetic individuals, a BG of 65 to 70 mg/dL stimulates counterregulatory hormones epinephrine and glucagon but after repeated episodes of low BG, this response is blunted.[53] Episodes of hypoglycemia are infrequent but do occur when insulin or glyburide are used. When taking either of these agents, women must not further restrict their carbohydrates or skip meals and snacks to prevent hypoglycemia. The treatment of hypoglycemia as described in **Box 8** is limited to those women taking insulin or glyburide, and the recommendation is to eat a meal or snack containing a carbohydrate and a protein.

> **Box 8**
> **Hypoglycedmia and the Rule of 15's**
>
> Feeling low? Got symptoms? Check BG
>
> If BG >50 mg/dL <70 mg/dL, treat with 15-g fast-acting carbohydrates (4 glucose tablets with water or 8 oz nonfat milk or 4 oz juice)
>
> Check BG in 15 minutes
>
> BG should increase at least 15 points
>
> If not 15 points higher, repeat treatment
>
> Once BG is >70 mg/dL, have a 15 g carbohydrate snack with 7 g protein
>
> *Adapted with permission from* the California Department of Public Health, California Diabetes and Pregnancy Program Sweet Success "Diabetes and Pregnancy Pocket Guide for Professionals" 2008 by the California Diabetes and Pregnancy Program. Funding for the development of the original materials was provided by the Federal Title V block grant from the California Maternal, Child and Adolescent Health Division.

Hyperglycemia

The Pedersen hypothesis, based on a glucocentric view of the pathophysiology of diabetes during pregnancy, theorizes that hyperglycemia mediates hyperinsulinemia in the fetus. Because insulin does not cross the placenta, spikes in maternal BG cause spikes in fetal BG, which stimulate fetal insulin production.[52] This process works well to encourage normal fetal growth when BG levels are in a normal range; however, high glucose levels produce high fetal insulin levels, promoting visceral fat deposition, abnormal growth, delay in lung maturation, and an overresponsive fetal pancreas.

Hyperglycemia is also known to cause oxidative stress and proinflammatory responses. The effects of these processes on the fetus are not well known. In adults with diabetes, hyperglycemia impairs the immune response and causes vascular damage that eventually results in end-organ disease.

As pregnancy progresses particularly in the third trimester, hyperglycemia increases as insulin resistance becomes greater. Increasing levels of progesterone, human placental growth hormones, and cytokines, such as TNF-α, are among the placental substances responsible for insulin resistance. Normoglycemia is more difficult to achieve without meticulous attention to meal plan, exercise, and for some, medication. Healthcare providers need to recognize situations that increase the risk for hyperglycemia, anticipate them, and assist women to adjust the variables that control BG levels to maintain normoglycemia (**Box 9**).

For example, individuals often have certain foods that trigger spikes in BG, such as sourdough bread, white rice, or cereal and milk at breakfast. Recognizing these patterns and intervening to avoid hyperglycemia is an integral part of problem solving. Obtaining BG measurements at the appropriate time and frequency allows evaluation of the appropriate intervention.

Reducing Risks

The three main goals of antepartum fetal surveillance are avoidance of fetal deaths, early detection of fetal compromise, and prevention of unnecessary premature birth and cesarean section. Fetal death in the final weeks of pregnancy has been associated with poor glycemic control, hydramnios, and fetal macrosomia.[54] All women with hyperglycemia in pregnancy are encouraged to do kick counts beginning around 26 to 28 weeks gestation.

NONPLACENTAL INCREASED INSULIN NEEDS IN THE ANTEPARTUM PERIOD

Although specific detrimental outcomes of temporary hyperglycemia are not fully known, it is known that the fetal pancreas is stimulated to overproduce insulin in

---

Box 9
High-risk situations for hyperglycemia

Stress

Sympathomimetics (terbutaline, ephedrine)

Steroids (eg, betamethasone)

Sepsis (infection)

Stout (obesity)

Advanced gestation (>24 weeks)

accordance with glucose levels in the maternal bloodstream.[52] The higher the maternal BG, the more insulin the fetus produces. Overproduction of fetal insulin is associated with adverse outcomes, described previously. Evidence-based literature suggests that normal nonpregnant individuals exposed to transient glucose elevations show rapid reduction in lymphocytes, including all lymphocyte subsets.[55] Hyperglycemia is similarly associated with reduced T-cell populations for CD4 and CD8 subsets. These abnormalities are reversed when glucose is lowered.[55] It is wise to avoid hyperglycemia associated with such conditions as fever, infection, betamimetics, or betamethasone administration. During these periods of "stress" all insulin doses generally need to be doubled.

The most common stress during pregnancy is preterm labor often requiring tocolysis. Use of betamimetics, such as terbutaline, should be avoided and either magnesium sulfate or nifedipine should be used if necessary. If delivery seems imminent before 35 weeks, betamethasone may be indicated to accelerate fetal lung maturation. Within about 4 hours after the first injection of 12 mg of betamethasone, hyperglycemia ensues. One method of avoiding hyperglycemia associated with betamethasone treatment is illustrated in **Table 7**.

For women with hyperglycemia in pregnancy, BG should be checked more frequently during betamethasone treatment. Women should check premeal and postmeal BG, at bedtime, and at 3 AM for the first 3 to 5 days after beginning betamethasone two-dose therapy. For hyperglycemia in pregnancy, a premeal correction algorithm should be instituted in addition to doubling doses of insulin to avoid postmeal excursions out of target ranges (**Table 8**).

A premeal correction algorithm must be individualized. If the premeal glucose is elevated, "correction insulin" according to the algorithm table is needed to prevent postmeal hyperglycemia; this is not a sliding scale. An algorithm is directed at preventing hyperglycemia, not chasing it, which often results in "stacking" of insulin and a deleterious cycle of hyperglycemia and hypoglycemia.

For hyperglycemia in pregnancy, basal insulin may be needed temporarily. Neutral protamine Hagedorn insulin at 0.2 units per kg may be necessary every 8 to 12 hours for 3 to 5 days.

FETAL SURVEILLANCE AND TIMING OF DELIVERY

Well-controlled uncomplicated women with hyperglycemia during pregnancy may not require antenatal testing until 40 weeks and may await spontaneous labor.[56] Most are electively delivered by 41 weeks gestation. Women requiring medication with adequate control generally start weekly nonstress test and amniotic fluid index testing at 32 weeks gestation and twice weekly at 36 weeks gestation. A nonreactive nonstress test requires further testing, usually a biophysical profile and rarely a contraction

Table 7 Recommendation for increased insulin needs with betamethasone			
Day 1	**Day 2**	**Day 3**	**Day 4**
Double insulin dose (if basic dose is 10 units, then give 20 units)	Continue with increased dose; modify as needed for BG (+) doubled dose of 20 units	Decrease the previous day's increased dose by 50% and add to the basic dose (ie, 15 units)	Revert to pre-betamethasone insulin dose and regime (ie, 20 units)

Data from Kitzmiller J, Gavin L, Inturrisi M. Diabetes and pregnancy pocket guide. UCSF, 2002.

Table 8 Premeal correction algorithm		
If Premeal BG is	**Correct the Basic Dose by**	**And**
<70 mg/dL	2 units less	Eat right away, inject insulin after the meal
70–99 mg/dL	Give basic dose	Inject, eat carbohydrates right away
100–129 mg/dL	1 unit more	Inject, eat right away
130–159 mg/dL	2 units more	Inject, check BG in 15 min, eat when <110
160–189 mg/dL	3 units more	Inject, check BG in 15 min, eat when <110
>190 mg/dL	Add 4 units, call doctor, check ketones	May need to wait up to 1 h

Adapted with permission from the California Department of Public Health, California Diabetes and Pregnancy Program Sweet Success Guidelines for Care 2006 and the "Diabetes and Pregnancy Pocket Guide for Professionals" 2008 by the California Diabetes and Pregnancy Program. Funding for the development of the original materials was provided by the Federal Title V block grant from the California Maternal, Child and Adolescent Health Division.

stress test. Delivery before 39 weeks carries a risk of delivering an infant with immature lungs; therefore, most physicians opt for amniocentesis and lung maturity studies before elective induction of labor or cesarean delivery before 39 weeks. If the lung indices are immature and the gestational age is less than 35 weeks, betamethasone should be considered. Poor metabolic control or history of stillbirth is also an indication for amniocentesis and scheduled delivery before 39 weeks. Suspected LGA as an indication for delivery is controversial and contributes to the high cesarean section rate in women with diabetes.[54]

INTRAPARTUM RISKS

Intrapartum risks include prolonged labor, shoulder dystocia, operative delivery, poor metabolic control resulting in fetal hypoxia and neonatal hyperinsulinemia and reactive hypoglycemia, and birth injuries to the mother and newborn. A plan of care should be coordinated by the outpatient diabetes team well in advance of delivery so that the woman, her partner, and the delivery team is well informed and everyone understands the same plan. The plan must be clearly communicated in written and oral form. One approach is for the diabetes team to send a plan of care with the patient and to the labor delivery unit on or before the 36th week gestation.

Dystocias

A greater risk for labor abnormalities (dystocias) is unknown for women with diabetes. Arrest disorders were described in 9%, 19.4%, and 23.9% of women with diabetes in three reports compared with 6% to 8% in nondiabetic women with newborns of similar birth weights (3000–4500 g).[57,58] Risk for shoulder dystocia increases with increasing birth weight in both diabetic and nondiabetic women, varying from 8% to 23% across the 4000- to 4500-g range.[59] In one study fetal LGA predicted shoulder dystocia in 84% of the cases.[60] Because of wider shoulder width and central adiposity in infants of diabetic mothers in addition to increased obesity in diabetic mothers, the risk of shoulder dystocia maybe greater than in nondiabetic women even at birth weights of 3000–3900 g.[57,59,60] Birth trauma was found in 20% to 40% of the cases of shoulder dystocia, including fracture of the clavicle or humerus, facial palsy, or brachial plexus palsy.[59,60] Women with labor complicated by shoulder dystocias also incurred injuries, such as third- and fourth-degree perineal lacerations.[61]

Another approach to reduce the risks associated with dystocias is to induce labor before LGA becomes too severe or to electively perform a cesarean at 39 weeks gestation.[62] The ACOG clinical practice guideline does not endorse induction before 40 weeks (in nondiabetic pregnancies) because accurate determination of fetal size is difficult to determine.[63] The ADA recommendation is to induce labor or perform a cesarean delivery on an individualized basis when the estimated fetal weight is between 4000 and 4500 g. Primary cesarean is recommended in most cases when the estimated fetal weight is greater than 4499 g.[64] Labor induction protocols do not differ for women with diabetes versus no diabetes. However, continuous electronic fetal heart rate monitoring is advised.[64] There are no contraindications to epidural anesthesia, although the use of betamimetics for hypotension may raise the maternal BG for several hours.

Cesarean delivery raises the risk for infection, both uterine (endometritis) and wound infection, if BG is not meticulously controlled peripartum. The risk for deep vein thrombus after cesarean delivery is five times higher than that after a vaginal birth. Obesity increases these risks and women with diabetes are more likely to be obese. Prevention generally includes use of pneumonic pressure stockings intraoperatively and postoperatively until the woman is fully ambulatory. Heparin prophylaxis has no advantage over stockings in this setting and may cause heparin-induced thrombocytopenia.[65]

Intrapartum Insulin Management

The goals of intrapartum insulin management are to maintain maternal normoglycemia (BG 70–110 mg/dL) to optimize fetal tolerance of labor and prevent neonatal hypoglycemia. In the largest published experience with 233 insulin-treated pregnant women, the lowest risk of neonatal hypoglycemia occurred when intrapartum maternal glucose was maintained at less than 100 mg/dL. Intrapartum hyperglycemia had more effect on neonatal hypoglycemia than did antepartum glucose levels.[66]

Women with hyperglycemia in pregnancy generally do not require insulin during labor because the uterine muscle contractions of the labor process increase insulin sensitivity and reduce insulin needs. Even women with hyperglycemia in pregnancy may not require insulin during labor if carbohydrate intake (intravenous and oral) is restricted. To determine the need for insulin the BG should be followed closely as described in the section on monitoring.[63]

When intrapartum insulin is needed it is optimally delivered by intravenous drip (**Table 9**). The usual dose of intermediate-acting subcutaneous insulin is given at bedtime the night before induction of labor but the morning dose is withheld.[63]

POSTPARTUM RISKS

The most immediate risk postpartum is the risk for neonatal hypoglycemia. BG cutoffs for neonatal hypoglycemia vary slightly but on average the value of 45 mg/dL or less is consistent with the need for intervention. This risk, however, can also be attenuated by early (within the first hour of life) and often (every 2 hours) breastfeeding. The healthy newborn should be dried off and kept warm (preferably skin-to-skin with the mother) and placed at breast as soon after birth as possible. Acquisition of colostrum by the newborn may stimulate hepatic gluconeogenesis to help stabilize the newborn's BG. The newborn will have heel-stick glucose levels checked beginning around 30 minutes after birth. Various protocols exist to monitor the newborn's glucose until stable. Breastfeeding provides numerous health benefits to women with diabetes

Table 9			
Intrapartum intravenous insulin algorithm for hyperglycemia in pregnancy			
Capillary BG	**1 Unit Insulin = 1 mL**	**Intravenous Fluids**	**BG Checks**
<70 mg/dL	0	D5 0.5 NS at 200 mL/h	Every 15 min until >70 x2
70–110 mg/dL	0	D5 0.5 NS at 100 mL/h	Every 1–2 h
111–130 mg/dL	1	NS or LR at 100 mL/h	Every 30 min
131–150 mg/dL	2	NS or LR at 100 mL/h	until <110
151–170 mg/dL	3	NS or LR at 100 mL/h	Then every 1 hour
171–190 mg/dL	4	NS at 150/h	while on
>190 mg/dL	Check urine ketones call doctor for insulin dose	NS at 150/h	intravenous insulin drip

Abbreviations: D5, 5% dextrose; LR, lactated Ringers solution; NS, normal saline.
    Data from Palmer D, Inturrisi M. Insulin infusion therapy in the intrapartum period. J Perinat Neonat Nurs 1992;6(1):B14–25.

and offspring. Among those benefits is improved glucose use and reduced lipid levels in the mother.[67] A relationship has also been shown between breastfeeding and reduction of type 2 diabetes in Pima Indian children.[68] Infants of women with mild to severe glucose intolerance are at risk for infant and childhood obesity.[69,70] Breastfed infants tend to be leaner than formula-fed infants.[71] Lactation removes glucose from the maternal blood to create lactase for the breast milk, thus lowering maternal BG independent of the action of insulin.

Contraception for Women with a History of Hyperglycemia in Pregnancy

The use of progestin-only oral contraceptives almost tripled the conversion to type 2 diabetes in the 2 years after hyperglycemia in pregnancy in a study of Latina women who were breastfeeding compared with equivalent use of low-dose combination pills.[72] Because the underlying mechanism for conversion to type 2 diabetes in Hispanic women is the same for most other women (impaired β cell function and insulin resistance), the recommendation is that progesterone-only birth control be avoided when possible in previous hyperglycemia in pregnancy. Low-dose combination pills can be used safely in breastfeeding women with previous hyperglycemia in pregnancy.[72]

The interaction of medroxyprogesterone acetate (Depo-Provera) with breastfeeding is similar to that of progestin-only contraception with breastfeeding, adversely effecting diabetes risk.[72] Thus, medroxyprogesterone acetate should be used with caution in breastfeeding women and those with elevated triglyceride levels (≥150 mg/dL). Close attention should be paid to weight gain, which also has been demonstrated to increase the risk of subsequent diabetes.[72]

Progesterone does increase insulin resistance and lowers low-density lipoprotein and raises high-density lipoprotein. The lowest dose and potency of progestin should be used to minimize adverse effects on lipids and glucose control. The intrauterine device is metabolically neutral and highly efficacious. This is a good choice for most women with diabetes. The guidelines for use follow the same guidelines as healthy parous women, such as low risk for sexually transmitted disease and pelvic inflammatory disease.

Reducing Future Risk for T2DM in Hyperglycemia in Pregnancy

Hyperglycemia in pregnancy is not just a pregnancy problem. Approximately 55% of women with diagnosed hyperglycemia in pregnancy have overt T2DM, and another

20% to 30% have prediabetes.[73] Independent antepartum predictors of conversion from hyperglycemia in pregnancy to T2DM include low insulin sensitivity (elevated postmeal requiring insulin); high basal glucose production (elevated fasting BG requiring insulin); and abnormal 1-hour value on the OGTT.[74] Postpartum predictors of conversion from hyperglycemia in pregnancy to T2DM include obesity, pregnancy weight gain, high-fat diet, inactivity, and progesterone contraception.[74]

A woman who had hyperglycemia in pregnancy but has a negative test for preexisting diabetes should be counseled on the increased risk for developing hyperglycemia in pregnancy in future pregnancies. Women with a history of hyperglycemia in pregnancy have an increased risk for presenting with undiagnosed diabetes at the first prenatal visit in subsequent pregnancies. Counseling should include discussing the lifetime risk for developing T2DM and dyslipidemias. Because approximately one-third of women with a history of hyperglycemia in pregnancy have abnormal lipid profiles, lipid testing is recommended 1-year postpartum and annually thereafter. The 2-hour adult OGTT more accurately identifies this population than the fasting plasma glucose test.[75] The current recommendation is to obtain a 2-hour 75-g OGTT at 6 to 8 weeks postpartum and at 1 year. If within normal limits, then obtain fasting or hemoglobin A_{1C} yearly and OGTT every 3 years.

SUMMARY

Women who had hyperglycemia in pregnancy and have prediabetes on the OGTT should be referred for management that includes nutrition and exercise counseling and possibly treatment with metformin to prevent the conversion to T2DM. Women with prediabetes need to be tested for overt diabetes every year thereafter.

Women who have a history of hyperglycemia in pregnancy and have a subsequent positive test for T2DM should be referred for appropriate follow-up with a healthcare provider familiar with diabetes care. Women should be counseled on the importance of preconception care and also advised of the long-term complications associated with poor glycemic control. Attention should be given to attainment and maintenance of appropriate weight.

Hyperglycemia in pregnancy is an opportunity for women at risk for complications during pregnancy and beyond to change their life course to improve outcomes for themselves and their offspring. Providers of diabetes care during pregnancy complicated by hyperglycemia in pregnancy have the unique opportunity to make a significant difference.

REFERENCES

1. Expert Committee on the Diagnosis and Classification of Diabetes Mellitus. Report of the Expert Committee on the Diagnosis and Classification of Diabetes Mellitus. Diabetes Care 1997;20:1183–97.
2. International Association of Diabetes and Pregnancy Study Groups Consensus Panel. International associations of diabetes and pregnancy study groups recommendations on the diagnosis and classification of hyperglycemia in pregnancy. Diabetes Care 2010;33(3):676–82.
3. National Center for Health Statistics, National Diabetes Fact Sheet. Centers for Disease Control and Prevention; 2011. Available at: http://www.cdc.gov/diabetes/pubs/pdf/ndfs_2011.pdf. Accessed September 6, 2011.
4. Kim C, Newton KM, Knopp RH. Gestational diabetes and the incidence of type 2 diabetes: a systematic review. Diabetes Care 2002;25:1862–8.

5. Crowther CA, Hiller JE, Moss JR, et al. Effect of treatment of gestational diabetes mellitus on pregnancy outcomes from the Australian Carbohydrate Intolerance Study in Pregnant Women (ACHOIS) Trial. N Engl J Med 2005;352:24.

6. Landon MB, Spong CY, Thom E, et al. A multicenter, randomized trial of treatment for mild gestational diabetes. N Engl J Med 2009;361(14):1339–48.

7. American Diabetes Association. Diagnosis and classification of diabetes mellitus. Diabetes Care 2010;33(Suppl 1):S62–9.

8. American College of Obstetricians and Gynecologists (ACOG) Practice Bulletin 30, Gestational diabetes. Obstet Gynecol 2001;98(3):525–38.

9. U. S. Preventive Services Task Force (USPSTF). Screening for gestational diabetes mellitus: recommendations and rationale. Obstet Gynecol 2003;101(2):93–5.

10. Carpenter MW, Coustan DR. Criteria for screening tests for gestational diabetes. Am J Obstet Gynecol 1982;144:768–73.

11. American Diabetes Association Standards of Medical Care. Diabetes Care 2010; 33:S11–6.

12. The HAPO Study Cooperative Research Group. Hyperglycemia and adverse pregnancy outcomes. N Engl J Med 2008;358:1991–2002.

13. Reece EA, Coustan DR, Gabbe SG, editors. Diabetes mellitus in women. 3rd edition. Philadelphia: Lippincott Williams & Wilkins; 2004.

14. Lain KY, Catalano PM. Metabolic changes in pregnancy. Clin Obstet Gynecol 2007;50(4):938–48.

15. American Dietetic Association. Medical nutrition therapy evidence based guides for practice. Nutrition Practice Guidelines for Gestational Diabetes Mellitus; 2001.

16. Institute of Medicine. Dietary reference intakes for energy, carbohydrate, fiber, fat, fatty acids, cholesterol, protein, and amino acids. Food and Nutrition Board. Washington, DC: National Academy Press; 2002.

17. Position of the American Dietetic Association: use of nutritive and nonnutritive sweeteners. J Am Diet Assoc 1998;98:580–7.

18. Institute of Medicine Report Brief. Weight Gain during Pregnancy Reexamining the Guidelines 2009. Available at: http://www.iom.edu/~/media/Files/Report%20Files/2009/Weight-Gain-During-Pregnancy-Reexamining-the-Guidelines/Report%20Brief%20-%20Weight%20Gain%20During%20Pregnancy.pdf. Accessed September 3, 2011.

19. Scotland NE, Cheng YW, Hopkins LM, et al. Gestational weight gain and adverse neonatal outcome among term infants. Obstet Gynecol 2006;108(3 Pt 1):635–43.

20. Hedderson M, Weiss N, Sacks D, et al. Pregnancy weight gain and risk of neonatal complications. Macrosomia, hypoglycemia, and hyperbilirubinemia. Obstet Gynecol 2006;108:1153–66.

21. Cedergren MI. Optimal gestational weight gain for body mass index categories. Obstet Gynecol 2007;110(4):759–64.

22. Gunderson EP, Selvin S, Abrams B. The relative importance of gestational gain and maternal characteristics associated with the risk of becoming overweight after pregnancy. Int J Obes Relat Metab Disord 2000;24(12):1660–8.

23. Weight Control Information Network. Overweight and obesity. Available at: http://win.niddk.nih.gov/index.htm. Accessed September 1, 2011.

24. American College of Obstetricians and Gynecologists. ACOG Committee Opinion No. 315. Obesity in pregnancy. Obstet Gynecol 2005;106:671–5.

25. Shaw G, Velie E, Schaffer D. Risk of neural tube defect-affected pregnancies among obese women. JAMA 1996;275:1093–6.

26. Watkins M, Rasmussen S, Honein L, et al. Maternal obesity and risk for birth defects. Pediatrics 2003;111:1152–8.

27. Lashen H, Fear K, Sturdee D. Obesity is associated with increased risk of first trimester and recurrent miscarriage: matched case-control study. Hum Reprod 2004;19:1644–66.
28. Stephansson O, Dickman P, Johansson A, et al. Maternal weight, pregnancy weight gain and the risk of antepartum stillbirth. Am J Obstet Gynecol 2001; 184:463–9.
29. Kristensen J, Vestergaard M, Wisborg K, et al. Pre-pregnancy weight and the risk of stillbirth and neonatal death. Br J Obstet Gynaecol 2005;112:403–8.
30. Rasmussen K, Kjolhede C. Prepregnant overweight and obesity diminish the prolactin response to suckling in the first week postpartum. Pediatrics 2004; 113(5):465–71.
31. Kiel D, Dodson E, Artal R, et al. Gestational weight gain and pregnancy outcomes in obese women. Obstet Gynecol 2007;110(4):752–8.
32. Langer O, Yogev Y, Xenakis E, et al. Overweight and obese in gestational diabetes: the impact on pregnancy outcome. Am J Obstet Gynecol 2005;192:1768–76.
33. Cheng YW, Chung JH, Kurbisch-Block I, et al. Gestational weight gain and gestational diabetes mellitus perinatal outcomes. Obstet Gynecol 2008;12(5): 1015–22.
34. Sheine E, Menes T, Silverberg D, et al. Pregnancy outcome of patients with gestational diabetes mellitus following bariatric surgery. Am J Obstet Gynecol 2006; 194:431–5.
35. Woodward C. Pregnancy following bariatric surgery. J Perinat Neonatal Nurs 2004;18(4):329–40.
36. Artal R, O'Toole M, White S. Guidelines of the American College of Obstetricians and Gynecologists for exercise during pregnancy and the postpartum period. Br J Sports Med 2003;37:6–12.
37. Revelli A, Durando A, Massobrio M. Exercise and pregnancy: a review of maternal and fetal effects. Obstet Gynecol Surv 1992;47(6):355–67.
38. Clap J. Effects of diet and exercise of insulin resistance during pregnancy. Metab Syndr Relat Disord 2006;4(2):84–90.
39. Jovanovic-Peterson L, Peterson C. Is exercise safe or useful for gestational diabetic women? Diabetes 1991;(40):179–81.
40. American Diabetes Association. Physical activity, exercise and type 2 diabetes. Diabetes Care 2004;27(10):2518–39.
41. Yogev Y, Ben-Haroush A, Chen R, et al. Diurnal glycemic profile in obese and normal weight nondiabetic pregnant women. Am J Obstet Gynecol 2004;191: 949–53.
42. Bühling KJ, Winkel T, Wolf C, et al. Optimal timing for postprandial glucose measurement in pregnant women with diabetes and a non-diabetic pregnant population evaluated by the Continuous Glucose Monitoring System (CGMS). J Perinat Med 2005;33(2):125–31.
43. Ben-Haroush A, Yogev Y, Chen R, et al. The postprandial glucose profile in the diabetic pregnancy. Am J Obstet Gynecol 2004;191(2):576–81.
44. Hawkins JS, Casey BM, Lo JY, et al. Weekly compared with daily blood glucose monitoring in women with diet-treated gestational diabetes. Obstet Gynecol 2000;113(6):1307–13.
45. California Diabetes and Pregnancy Program Data Report 2009. Available at: http://www.cdph.ca.gov/programs/cdapp/Pages/SweetSuccessDataReport.aspx. Accessed September 6, 2011.
46. Langer O. Is normoglycemia the correct threshold to prevent complications in the pregnant diabetic patient? Diabetes Rev 1996;4(1):2–10.

47. Holemans K, Aerts L, Van Assche FA. Lifetime consequences of abnormal fetal pancreatic development. J Physiol 2003;547(1):11–20.
48. Langer O, Conway D, Berkus M, et al. A comparison of glyburide and insulin in women with gestational diabetes mellitus. N Engl J Med 2000;343:1134–8.
49. Rowan J, Hague W, Gao W, et al, MiG Trial Investigators. Metformin versus insulin for the treatment of gestational diabetes. N Engl J Med 2008;358(19):2003–215.
50. Moore TR. Glyburide for the treatment of gestational diabetes. A critical appraisal. Diabetes 2007;30(Suppl 2):S209–13.
51. Coetzee EJ, Ekpebegh CO, van der Merwe L, et al. 10-year retrospective analysis of pregnancy outcome in pregestational type 2 diabetes: comparison of insulin and oral glucose-lowering agents. Diabet Med 2007;24(3):253–8.
52. Pedersen J. The pregnant diabetic and her newborn. Baltimore (MD): Williams and Wilkins; 1977.
53. Cryer PE, Davis SN, Shamon H. Hypoglycemia in diabetes. Diabetes Care 2003; 26:1902–12.
54. Landon M, Gabbe S. Fetal surveillance in the pregnancy complicated by diabetes mellitus. Clin Obstet Gynecol 1991;34(3):535–43.
55. Clement S, Braithwaite SS, Magee MF, et al. Management of diabetes and hyperglycemia in hospitals. Diabetes Care 2004;27(2):553–81.
56. Kjos SL. Insulin-requiring diabetes in pregnancy: a randomized trial of active induction of labor and expectant management. Am J Obstet Gynecol 1993; 169:611–5.
57. Acker DB, Sachs BP, Friedman EA. Risk factors for shoulder dystocia. Obstet Gynecol 1985;66(6):762–8.
58. McFarland M, Hod M, Piper JM, et al. Are labor abnormalities more common in shoulder dystocia? Am J Obstet Gynecol 1995;173:1211–4.
59. Nesbitt TS, Gilbert WM, Herrchen B. Shoulder dystocia and associated risk factors with macrosomic infants born in California. Am J Obstet Gynecol 1998; 179(2):476–80.
60. Langer O, Berkus M, Huff R, et al. Shoulder dystocia: should the fetus weighing >/=4000gm be delivered by cesarean section? Am J Obstet Gynecol 1991;165: 831–7.
61. Ray JG, Vermeulen MJ, Shapiro JL, et al. Maternal and neonatal outcomes in pregestational and gestational diabetes mellitus, and the influence of maternal obesity and weight gain: the DEPOSIT* study. QJM 2001;94(7):347–56 An International Journal of Medicine.
62. Lurie S, Insler V, Hagay ZJ. Induction of labor at 38 to 39 weeks of gestation reduces the incidence of shoulder dystocia in gestational diabetic patients Class A2. Am J Perinatol 1996;13:293–6.
63. American College of Obstetricians and Gynecologists (ACOG) Practice Bulletin 60, Pregestational Diabetes Mellitus. Obstet Gynecol 2005;105(3):525–38.
64. Kitzmiller JL, Block JM, Brown FM, et al. Management of preexisting diabetes and pregnancy. Alexandria (VA): American Diabetes Association; 2008.
65. Gates S, Brocklehurst P, Davis LJ. Prophylaxis for venous thromboembolic disease in pregnancy and the early postnatal period. Cochrane Database Syst Rev 2002;2:CD001689.
66. Taylor R, Lee C, Kyne-Grzebalski D, et al. Clinical outcomes of pregnancy in women with type 1 diabetes. Obstet Gynecol 2002;99(4):537–41.
67. Kjos SL, Henry O, Lee RM, et al. The effect of lactation on glucose and lipid metabolism in women with recent gestational diabetes. Obstet Gynecol 1993; 82(3):451–5.

68. Pettitt DJ. Breastfeeding and incidence of non-insulin-dependent diabetes mellitus in Pima Indians. Lancet 1997;350:166–8.
69. Plagemann A, Harder T, Franke K, et al. Long-term impact of neonatal breastfeeding on body weight and glucose tolerance in children of diabetic mothers. Diabetes Care 2002;25(1):16–22.
70. Hillier TA, Pedula KL, Schmidt MM, et al. Childhood obesity and metabolic imprinting: the ongoing effects of maternal hyperglycemia. Diabetes Care 2007;30:2287–92.
71. Dewey K, Heinig M, Nommsen L. Breast-fed infants are leaner than formula-fed infants at 1 y of age: the DARLING study. Am J Clin Nutr 1993;57(2):140–5.
72. Kjos SL, Peters RK, Xiang A, et al. Contraception and the risk of type 2 diabetes mellitus in Latina women with prior gestational diabetes mellitus. JAMA 1998; 280(6):533–8.
73. Kitzmiller JL, Dang-Kilduff L, Taslimi MM. Gestational diabetes after delivery. Short-term management and long-term risks. Diabetes Care 2007;30(Suppl 2): S225–35.
74. Kjos SL, Buchanan TA, Greenspoon JS, et al. Gestational diabetes mellitus: the prevalence of glucose intolerance and diabetes mellitus in the first two months postpartum. Am J Obstet Gynecol 1990;163:93–8.
75. Metzger BE, Buchanan TA, Coustan DR, et al. Summary and recommendations of the fifth international workshop-conference on gestational diabetes mellitus. Diabetes Care 2007;30:3154.
76. WHO Expert Consultation. Appropriate body-mass index for Asian populations and its implications for policy and intervention strategies. Lancet 2004;363(9403): 157–63.

Pregnancy Management of Women with Pregestational Diabetes

Elisabeth R. Mathiesen, MD, DMSc[a],*, Lene Ringholm, MD, PhD[a],
Peter Damm, MD, DMSc[b]

KEYWORDS

- Pregestational diabetes • Pregnancy • Insulin analogues
- Antihypertensive treatment • Prepregnancy
- Preconceptional counseling

Pregnancy in women with pregestational diabetes is complicated by increased risk of adverse outcomes for mother and infant. Obtaining and maintaining optimal glycemic control before and during pregnancy is crucial for optimizing outcomes. In addition, indications for antihypertensive treatment need to be clear.

DIABETES AND ADVERSE FETAL, NEONATAL, AND MATERNAL OUTCOMES

Large observational studies have shown an increased risk of adverse outcomes in diabetic pregnancy, including fetal and neonatal death (death occurring between 22 gestational weeks and 28 days after delivery), congenital malformations, macrosomia, preterm delivery, preeclampsia, operative delivery, and maternal mortality.[1–11] In the data from the Confidential Enquiry into Maternal and Child Health (CEMACH) in the United Kingdom, diabetes was associated with a marked and significantly increased risk of death of the child during pregnancy or soon after delivery, compared with corresponding national rates in the general population.[3,8] Approximately 80% of these losses were stillbirths, 80% of these babies being structurally normal. These figures are consistent with observations of a fourfold to fivefold increase in perinatal mortality[2,5,8,10] and a fourfold to sixfold increase in stillbirth in pregnancies in diabetic mothers compared with the background population.[2,8,10]

It is also clear from the CEMACH study[3] and other studies that type 1 and type 2 diabetes confer a similar risk of perinatal mortality. Until recently, type 2 diabetes

Financial disclosures: the authors have nothing to disclose.
[a] Department of Endocrinology, Section 2132, Center for Pregnant Women with Diabetes, Rigshospitalet, University of Copenhagen, Blegdamsvej 9, DK 2100 Copenhagen Ø, Denmark
[b] Department of Obstetrics, Section 4033, Center for Pregnant Women with Diabetes, Rigshospitalet, University of Copenhagen, Blegdamsvej 9, DK 2100 Copenhagen Ø, Denmark
* Corresponding author.
E-mail address: em@rh.dk

Endocrinol Metab Clin N Am 40 (2011) 727–738
doi:10.1016/j.ecl.2011.08.005
0889-8529/11/$ – see front matter © 2011 Elsevier Inc. All rights reserved.

was uncommon in women of childbearing age. However, type 2 diabetes is being diagnosed at an increasingly young age and was present in about one-quarter of all diabetic pregnancies in the CEMACH study.[3]

ROLE OF PRECONCEPTIONAL COUNSELING

Intensive management of glycemic control before, as well as during, pregnancy delivers significant health benefits to pregnant diabetic women and their offspring. Preferably, this management should be a collaborative effort between an obstetrician, endocrinologist, dietician, and nurse educator before and during pregnancy. A recent study in 290 women with type 1 diabetes evaluated the impact of preconceptional care on glycemic control and outcome of pregnancy.[12] The rate of congenital malformations was about threefold lower in the preconceptional care group relative to the group starting care during pregnancy (1.8% vs 6.1%, respectively). Supplementation with folic acid before pregnancy and up to 12 gestational weeks may reduce the incidence of malformations in pregnant women with diabetes.[13] There is no consensus regarding the dose of folic acid; at least 400 µg per day is recommended, but some countries recommend 5 mg per day.[14] However, few women attend preconceptional counseling sessions, and poor glycemic control remains common among diabetic women.[3] In the CEMACH study, only 35% of women with pregestational diabetes received preconceptional counseling, only 37% had a measurement of long-term glycemic control as measured by hemoglobin A_{1c} (HbA_{1c}) within the 6 months before pregnancy, and less than 39% were taking folic acid before conception.[3] Overall, the risk of an adverse pregnancy outcome is halved with each percentage point HbA_{1c} reduction achieved before pregnancy.[15] This information may be useful as a motivating factor to achieve glycemic goals, and to reassure patients that all improvements in blood glucose are helpful, irrespective of the final value achieved. To improve the pregnancy outcome and the health of the newborn, the planning of pregnancy with HbA_{1c} less than 7.0% (51 IFCC units)[16] and supplementation with folic acid of at least 400 µg before pregnancy[14] is recommended. A HbA_{1c} less than 6.0% (42 IFCC) is desirable if it can be reached without risk of severe hypoglycemia (National Institute for Clinical Excellence [NICE] guidelines).[17] Insulin treatment in combination with diet and self-monitoring of the glucose levels are the cornerstones in optimizing the glycemic control in pregestational diabetes.

USE OF METFORMIN DURING PREGNANCY

Metformin is usually the drug of choice in nonpregnant patients with type 2 diabetes and many women are becoming pregnant while on metformin. First trimester use of metformin in either polycystic ovarian syndrome or diabetes does not seem to be associated with an increased risk of major malformations if correction for maternal glycemic levels is performed.[18] In many centers, metformin is therefore believed to be safe to use in the pregnancy planning phase. When pregnancy is established, the women can be shifted from metformin to insulin treatment immediately or metformin could be continued until 8 to 12 gestational weeks when the organogenesis and risk of early fetal loss have ended.[18]

SCREENING FOR LATE DIABETIC COMPLICATIONS

Screening for late diabetic complications such as diabetic retinopathy and diabetic nephropathy before pregnancy is of utmost importance. If sight-threatening retinopathy (ie, active proliferative diabetic retinopathy or significant diabetic macular edema) is present, it is advisable to postpone pregnancy until these conditions are properly treated and have remained in a stable phase for at least 6 months.[19,20] Diabetic nephropathy with significant loss of kidney function (serum creatinine >200 μmol/L) may lead to end-stage renal failure during pregnancy[21] and coronary heart disease is generally a contraindication for pregnancy, except in very well-controlled cases. Appropriate antihypertensive treatments with drugs that are approved for pregnancy are important.[22,23]

Thyroid dysfunction is prevalent among women with diabetes[24] and subclinical hypothyroidism may lead to cerebral dysfunction of the offspring.[25] Testing the thyroid stimulating hormone value and appropriate treatment of possible hyperfunction or hypofunction is therefore recommended before and during pregnancy.[26]

Safe contraception is an important part of preconception care.[27]

LIFESTYLE INTERVENTIONS DURING PREGNANCY

Diet and exercise are important lifestyle determinants for health. During pregnancy, minor modifications to the diet are required to cover the energy cost. Exercise patterns also need to be modified to accommodate the physiologic and anatomic changes that occur with increasing gestation. Although not reviewed separately here, patients should be encouraged to optimize both diet and physical activity (30 minutes per day) as far as possible during pregnancy. Observational studies in healthy women indicate that leisure time physical activity before and/or during pregnancy reduce the rate of preeclampsia and preterm delivery and improve physical fitness and emotional well-being.[28]

The overall aim in designing a diet for pregnant women with pregestational diabetes is to avoid single large meals and foods with a large percentage of simple carbohydrates. In particular, a small amount of carbohydrate at breakfast is advisable to control postprandial blood glucose at this time. At breakfast, 10 to 20 g of carbohydrate, corresponding to 10% of the daily carbohydrate intake, is often used.[29] Teaching women carbohydrate counting might be helpful.[30]

For obese women with type 2 diabetes, dietetic advice should aim at minimizing excess weight gain during pregnancy. Simple adjustments to dietary intake, including carbohydrates with a low glycemic index, can help to reduce postprandial hyperglycemia.

MATERNAL WEIGHT GAIN

The recently published Institute of Medicine (IOM) guidelines for weight gain during pregnancy recommend a gestational weight gain of 12.5 to 17.5 kg in normal-weight women. For obese women, a weight gain of 5.5 to 10 kg in pregnancy is recommended.[31] To obtain such a weight gain during pregnancy, the authors find it useful to advise normal-weight women to gain less than 5 kg in the first 20 weeks of pregnancy.

ORAL HYPOGLYCEMIC AGENTS DURING PREGNANCY

According to the NICE guidelines,[17] metformin can be useful during pregnancy for improved glucose control in insulin-resistant states and for women who refuse to use insulin therapy. However, metformin freely crosses the placenta and the long-term safety of metformin for the offspring has not been shown sufficiently.[18] At present there is no consensus worldwide about whether it is safe to use metformin in pregnancy.

Glyburide (glibenclamide) does not seem to be teratogenic, nor does it pass the placenta to a substantial extent. In women with type 2 diabetes, there is some concern regarding increased perinatal mortality with continued use of glyburide throughout pregnancy, and women should be switched to insulin during pregnancy. There is little experience with the use of other oral hypoglycemic agents and they are not recommended for use in pregnancy.[32]

INSULIN USE IN PREGNANCY

Insulin has been considered the gold standard for the management of diabetes during pregnancy because of its established efficacy in maintaining good glycemic control and its inability to cross the placenta.[33] The most basic preparation is soluble human insulin, which is short acting. This type of insulin is useful for multiple-dose regimens, insulin pumps, and continuous infusion during labor or medical emergencies. Longer-acting insulins, such as neutral protamine Hagedorn (NPH) have been developed to allow for less-frequent dosing and has been used in diabetic pregnancy for several decades.

The short-acting insulin analogue insulin aspart has been tested in a large randomized trial including 322 pregnant women with type 1 diabetes, showing that insulin aspart was at least as well tolerated and effective as human insulin when used as meal-time insulin in a basal-bolus regimen together with NPH insulin in pregnant women with type 1 diabetes. In addition, this insulin analogue may offer new clinical benefits in better postprandial glucose control and a trend toward reduction of preterm delivery compared with treatment with regular human insulin.[34,35] The effect of the insulin analogue lispro compared with regular insulin has been tested retrospectively in an Italian multicenter study.[7] In women treated with insulin lispro, there was a significantly greater reduction in HbA$_{1c}$ during the first trimester and the rate of congenital malformations was similar in the offspring of the 2 groups of women treated with insulin lispro or regular insulin. These findings suggest that insulin lispro could be useful for the treatment of hyperglycemia in type 1 diabetic pregnant women. The use of the fast-acting insulin analogues aspart and lispro are reviewed elsewhere[36] and are now accepted for use in pregnancy in the United States and in Europe. Until now, the authorities in the United States and Europe have not approved the use of long-acting insulin analogues in pregnancy, but these insulins are now widely used off-label in pregnancy. However, observational data with the use of the long-acting insulin analogues glargine and detemir in pregnancy do exist and no adverse effects have been observed,[37–39] but the published series are still few and small. An ongoing large randomized study investigating the effect of using insulin detemir in comparison with human insulin NPH, both in combination with insulin aspart, has included almost 300 pregnant women. The results are expected in 2011.

An alternative method of insulin administration is continuous subcutaneous insulin infusion (insulin pump), which, in theory, can lead to improved glycemic control with a lower prevalence of severe hypoglycemia.[40] However, until now this approach has been disappointing during pregnancy, with cohort studies and randomized control trials reporting only minor benefits, if any, compared with conventional therapy.[41]

The goal of insulin therapy during pregnancy is to attain glucose profiles similar to those of nondiabetic pregnant women. The NICE guidelines suggest the following goals: fasting values of 3.5 to 5.9 mmol/L (63–106 mg/dL) and 1-hour postprandial values of less than 7.8 mmol/L (140 mg/dL).[17] The American Diabetes Association (ADA) guidelines are close to these values, specifying fasting values of 3.4 to 5.5 mmol/L (60–99 mg/dL), 1-hour postprandial values of 5.5 to 7.1 mmol/L (100–129 mg/dL), and a 2-hour postprandial value of less than or equal to 6.7 mmol/L (129 mg/dL).[42] The editors recommend a fasting glucose less than 90 mg/dL and 1-hour, postprandial glucose less than 120 mg/dL. The challenge is to achieve a level of blood glucose sufficient to prevent adverse outcomes of pregnancy while avoiding hypoglycemia. Estimation of the number of episodes of severe hypoglycemia the year before pregnancy and the women's self-estimated hypoglycemia awareness is important before pregnancy and in early pregnancy. Based on this information, the individual risk of severe hypoglycemia can be estimated[43] and taken into account when the individual treatment regimen is tailored.

Simulating the glucose profiles of nondiabetic pregnant women necessitates meticulous blood glucose monitoring. The recording of blood glucose levels on a daily basis has a positive effect on glycemic control.[44] Both preprandial and postprandial glucose affect HbA_{1c} levels. The relative contribution of each is unclear,[45] although data from patients with type 2 diabetes suggest an increased contribution of fasting glycemia as overall hyperglycemia becomes more severe.[46] Continuous glucose monitoring may be superior to intermittent self-monitoring of plasma glucose in pregnancy.[47] In healthy pregnant women, a decline of the upper normal level of HbA_{1c} from 6.3% to 5.7% (45 and 39 IFCC, respectively) in early pregnancy and to 5.6% (38 IFCC) in the third trimester of pregnancy has been shown,[48] and can probably be ascribed to a decrease in fasting blood glucose[49] and a decreased expected erythrocyte lifespan in pregnancy.[50] In pregnant women with pregestational diabetes, it is helpful to monitor HbA_{1c} every 2 weeks, aiming at a goal close to the late pregnancy upper normal range of 5.6% (38 IFCC).[48] ADA recommends an HbA_{1c} value less than 6% (42 IFCC) in the second and third trimesters.[42]

In women with type 1 diabetes, there might be a need for reduction in insulin dose in early pregnancy (10–16 gestational weeks).[51] From 16 gestational weeks onwards, the weekly increase in daily insulin dose is approximately 2 IU insulin, leading to an almost doubling of insulin dose before delivery.[52]

HYPOGLYCEMIA

The risk of hypoglycemia remains a barrier to achieving tight glycemic control with insulin therapy. Hypoglycemic coma,[53] traffic accidents[54] and death[55] from severe hypoglycemia in pregnancy are significant problems. Severe hypoglycemia occurs most frequently in the first trimester, where the incidence is 5 times higher compared with the year preceding pregnancy.[43] Several studies have reported a peak of severe hypoglycemic events between 8 and 16 gestational weeks.[43,54,56] The risk of hypoglycemia during diabetic pregnancy may increase because the fetus continues to draw glucose across the placenta from the maternal bloodstream during periods of fasting. In accordance, the risk of hypoglycemia is highest between meals and during sleep. Surprisingly the presence of pregnancy-induced nausea and vomiting was not associated with a higher risk of severe hypoglycemia.[43] Risk factors for these episodes include a history of severe hypoglycemia before pregnancy, impaired hypoglycemia awareness, longer duration of diabetes, HbA_{1c} less than or equal to 6.5% at first pregnancy visit, and a higher total daily insulin dose.[43,53] Experimental data link hypoglycemia in early pregnancy with congenital abnormalities[57,58] and growth retardation,[59] although data in humans are lacking. The use of insulin analogues[33] and insulin pumps[40] may reduce the risk of severe hypoglycemia. Case reports indicate that continuous glucose monitoring is useful in preventing severe hypoglycemia in pregnant women with hypoglycemia unawareness.[60]

DIABETIC RETINOPATHY

Long-term optimal glycemic control decreases the risk of progression of diabetic retinopathy. Seemingly paradoxically, intensification of insulin therapy with an abrupt improvement in glycemic control has been associated with a temporary worsening of retinopathy.[61–63]

Pregnancy-induced deterioration of retinopathy may occur in type 1 diabetes.[20,64] Women with moderate or severe retinopathy have the highest risk of progression to sight-threatening retinopathy. Poor glycemic control and hypertension at first pregnancy visit increase the risk of progression.[20] For this reason, careful investigation of the retina before and during pregnancy is necessary. Additional laser treatment can be given before or during pregnancy.

HYPERTENSION, MICROALBUMINURIA, AND DIABETIC NEPHROPATHY

New-onset hypertension or preeclampsia are common and potentially serious complications of pregnancy. Hypertension may occur in 15% to 30% of diabetic women, compared with about 10% of the background population.[22,23,65] Several observational studies have linked the development of new-onset hypertension in pregnancy with hyperinsulinemia and insulin resistance.[66–69] Hypertension in type 1 diabetes is usually associated with diabetic nephropathy and sodium retention, and the presence of nephropathy increases the risk of hypertension during pregnancy.[70,71] Insulin is well known to promote weight gain, which may, in principle, tend to increase blood pressure. However, alterations in blood pressure or exacerbation of hypertension do not seem to be associated with the use of exogenous insulin to a clinically significant extent.

The development of nephropathy in patients with diabetes heralds an increased risk of mortality not only from end-stage renal failure but also from cardiovascular causes.[72] In nonpregnant patients with type 1 diabetes, poor glycemic control and hypertension accelerate the loss of renal function,[73] and improved glycemic control and antihypertensive treatment, mainly with drugs that block the renin-angiotensin system, slows the progression of renal disease.[73–75] Presence of microalbuminuria or overt diabetic nephropathy in early pregnancy is associated with increased risk of preterm delivery, mainly caused by preeclampsia.[22] Blockers of the renin-angiotensin system are contraindicated during pregnancy, mainly because of increased risk of malformations and fetal renal dysfunction.[76,77] One observational study has shown that early and intensive antihypertensive treatment in these women might improve the pregnancy outcome.[23] Methyldopa, labetalol, and nifedipine are approved for use in pregnancy and were the antihypertensive drugs that were mainly used in that study.[23]

Careful control of blood pressure and urinary albumin excretion before and during pregnancy is therefore necessary. Any possible treatment with blockers of the renin-angiotensin system should be changed to drugs approved for use in pregnancy, before pregnancy, or, at the latest, when pregnancy is confirmed. Tight antihypertensive treatment before and during pregnancy in preexisting microalbuminuria and diabetic nephropathy is recommended, aiming at blood pressure less than 135/85 mm Hg and urinary albumin excretion less than 300 mg/24 h.[23]

DISEASES AND DRUGS OFTEN USED IN DIABETES

The presence of active proliferative retinopathy, severe diabetic nephropathy with reduced glomerular filtration rate to 30% to 40% or less, or severe coronary heart disease may imply a seriously increased maternal risk leading to a recommendation of discontinuation of pregnancy.

Cholesterol-lowering agents are often given to diabetic patients but are not recommended for use in pregnancy.[78] Aspirin may reduce the risk of cardiovascular complications, but may also reduce the risk of preeclampsia and can be used during pregnancy.[78] Antithyroid drugs can be used if necessary (see article elsewhere in this issue). The possible use of antidepressive drugs during pregnancy should be discussed with a psychiatrist.

OBSTETRIC SURVEILLANCE

Extraobstetric ultrasound examinations are made until 20 gestational weeks to screen for congenital malformations. Later in pregnancy, the growth of the fetus is followed by regular ultrasound assessments. Antenatal surveillance tests, including ultrasound examinations of the fetal growth rate, kick-counting, and nonstress testing of fetal cardiac function, are widely used to identify pregnancies at high risk of stillbirth.[79]

Many centers use antenatal nonstress testing 1 to 2 times weekly from 32 to 34 weeks. Labor is often induced at 38 to 40 weeks and, in most centers, more than 50% deliver by cesarean section.[42]

INSULIN TREATMENT DURING DELIVERY

Tight glycemic control during delivery is necessary to reduce the excess fetal oxygen need that high glucose supplies demand. In addition, plasma glucose values exceeding 7 mmol/L (126 mg/dL) increase the newborn's risk of neonatal hypoglycemia. The goal for glucose values was therefore set to 4 to 7 mmol/L (72–126 mg/dL),[17] which can be achieved using supplements of small subcutaneous doses of fast-acting insulin during delivery or by insulin given intravenously. An intravenous glucose infusion is also often given to prevent catabolism and hypoglycemia.[80]

MATERNAL AND OFFSPRING TREATMENT AFTER DELIVERY

The neonate has an increased risk of morbidity such as neonatal hypoglycemia, respiratory distress, and jaundice. Early oral feedings every third hour during the first 24 hours can be given to avoid hypoglycemia, and close observation of the newborn is necessary. This observation can take place at a specialized maternity ward in most cases.[81]

The mother's need for insulin declines immediately after delivery to approximately 60% of the dose before pregnancy. There is also a concomitant increased risk of severe maternal hypoglycemia. The need for insulin gradually increases in the next weeks. In women who are breastfeeding, the need for insulin is still approximately 10% lower than the dose before pregnancy, with wide individual variations.[82]

PROVISION OF PREGNANCY CARE

A multidisciplinary team including endocrinologists, obstetricians, nurse educations, registered dieticians, midwives, and ophthalmologists is needed to manage the pregnant diabetic woman and her infant. A substantial number of deliveries of pregnant diabetic women each year is warranted to secure a routine in the care. Centralization of the pregnancy care for these high-risk pregnancies is therefore recommended. At our center, the pregnant women are provided with oral and written instructions for the goals of glycemic control during pregnancy and the expected pregnancy-induced changes in insulin needs.

SUMMARY

In women with pregestational diabetes, tight glycemic control before and during pregnancy is crucial, and the prevalence of severe hypoglycemia during pregnancy needs to be reduced. Fast-acting insulin analogues are regarded as safe to use in pregnancy and studies on long-acting insulin analogues are in progress. Supplementation with folic acid may reduce the risk of malformations. Screening for diabetic retinopathy, diabetic nephropathy, and thyroid dysfunction is important. Indications for antihypertensive treatment and treatment of thyroid dysfunction need to be clear before and during pregnancy.

REFERENCES

1. Boulot P, Chabbert-Buffet N, d'Ercole C, et al. French multicentric survey of outcome of pregnancy in women with pregestational diabetes. Diabetes Care 2003;26:2990–3.
2. Casson IF, Clarke CA, Howard CV, et al. Outcomes of pregnancy in insulin dependent diabetic women: results of a five year population cohort study. BMJ 1997; 315:275–8.
3. Confidential Enquiery into Maternal and Child Health. Confidential Enquiry into Maternal and Child Health: pregnancy in women with type 1 and type 2 diabetes in 2002-3 in England, Wales, and Northern Ireland. London: CEMACH; 2005.
4. Evers IM, de Valk HW, Visser GH. Risk of complications of pregnancy in women with type 1 diabetes: nationwide prospective study in the Netherlands. BMJ 2004; 328:915.
5. Hawthorne G, Robson S, Ryall EA, et al. Prospective population based survey of outcome of pregnancy in diabetic women: results of the Northern Diabetic Pregnancy Audit, 1994. BMJ 1997;315:279–81.
6. Jensen DM, Damm P, Moelsted-Pedersen L, et al. Outcomes in type 1 diabetic pregnancies: a nationwide, population-based study. Diabetes Care 2004;27:2819–23.
7. Lapolla A, Dalfra MG, Spezia R, et al. Outcome of pregnancy in type 1 diabetic patients treated with insulin lispro or regular insulin: an Italian experience. Acta Diabetol 2008;45:61–6.
8. Macintosh MC, Fleming KM, Bailey JA, et al. Perinatal mortality and congenital anomalies in babies of women with type 1 or type 2 diabetes in England, Wales, and Northern Ireland: population based study. BMJ 2006;333:177.
9. Penney GC, Mair G, Pearson DW. Outcomes of pregnancies in women with type 1 diabetes in Scotland: a national population-based study. BJOG 2003;110:315–8.
10. Platt MJ, Stanisstreet M, Casson IF, et al. St Vincent's Declaration 10 years on: outcomes of diabetic pregnancies. Diabet Med 2002;19:216–20.
11. Yang J, Cummings EA, O'Connell C, et al. Fetal and neonatal outcomes of diabetic pregnancies. Obstet Gynecol 2006;108:644–50.
12. Temple RC, Aldridge VJ, Murphy HR. Prepregnancy care and pregnancy outcomes in women with type 1 diabetes. Diabetes Care 2006;29:1744–9.
13. Wilson RD, Davies G, Desilets V, et al. The use of folic acid for the prevention of neural tube defects and other congenital anomalies. J Obstet Gynaecol Can 2003;25:959–73.
14. Capel I, Corcoy R. What dose of folic acid should be used for pregnant diabetic women? Diabetes Care 2007;30:e63.
15. Inkster ME, Fahey TP, Donnan PT, et al. Poor glycated haemoglobin control and adverse pregnancy outcomes in type 1 and type 2 diabetes mellitus: systematic review of observational studies. BMC Pregnancy Childbirth 2006;6:30.
16. Jensen DM, Korsholm L, Ovesen P, et al. Peri-conceptional A1C and risk of serious adverse pregnancy outcome in 933 women with type 1 diabetes. Diabetes Care 2009;32:1046–8.

17. National Institute of Health and Clinical Excellence. Diabetes in pregnancy. Management of diabetes and its complications from pre-conception to the post natal period. Available at: www.nice.org.uk/CG063. Accessed February 1, 2011. Nice Clinical guideline. 2008.

18. Simmons D. Metformin treatment for type 2 diabetes in pregnancy? Best Pract Res Clin Endocrinol Metab 2010;24:625–34.

19. Rasmussen KL, Laugesen CS, Ringholm L, et al. Progression of diabetic retinopathy during pregnancy in women with type 2 diabetes. Diabetologia 2010;53:1076–83.

20. Vestgaard M, Ringholm L, Laugesen CS, et al. Pregnancy-induced sight-threatening diabetic retinopathy in women with type 1 diabetes. Diabet Med 2010;27:431–5.

21. Purdy LP, Hantsch CE, Molitch ME, et al. Effect of pregnancy on renal function in patients with moderate-to-severe diabetic renal insufficiency. Diabetes Care 1996;19:1067–74.

22. Nielsen LR, Muller C, Damm P, et al. Reduced prevalence of early preterm delivery in women with type 1 diabetes and microalbuminuria–possible effect of early anti-hypertensive treatment during pregnancy. Diabet Med 2006;23:426–31.

23. Nielsen LR, Damm P, Mathiesen ER. Improved pregnancy outcome in type 1 diabetic women with microalbuminuria or diabetic nephropathy: effect of intensified antihypertensive therapy? Diabetes Care 2009;32:38–44.

24. Vestgaard M, Nielsen LR, Rasmussen AK, et al. Thyroid peroxidase antibodies in pregnant women with type 1 diabetes: impact on thyroid function, metabolic control and pregnancy outcome. Acta Obstet Gynecol Scand 2008;87:1336–42.

25. Haddow JE, Palomaki GE, Allan WC, et al. Maternal thyroid deficiency during pregnancy and subsequent neuropsychological development of the child. N Engl J Med 1999;341:549–55.

26. Abalovich M, Amino N, Barbour LA, et al. Management of thyroid dysfunction during pregnancy and postpartum: an Endocrine Society Clinical Practice Guideline. J Clin Endocrinol Metab 2007;92:S1–47.

27. Damm P, Mathiesen E, Clausen TD, et al. Contraception for women with diabetes mellitus. Metab Syndr Relat Disord 2005;3:244–9.

28. Hegaard HK, Pedersen BK, Nielsen BB, et al. Leisure time physical activity during pregnancy and impact on gestational diabetes mellitus, pre-eclampsia, preterm delivery and birth weight: a review. Acta Obstet Gynecol Scand 2007;86:1290–6.

29. Jovanovic L. Achieving euglycaemia in women with gestational diabetes mellitus: current options for screening, diagnosis and treatment. Drugs 2004;64:1401–17.

30. Leontos C. Implementing the American Diabetes Association's nutrition recommendations. J Am Osteopath Assoc 2003;103:S17–20.

31. Rasmussen KM, Yaktine AL. Weight gain during pregnancy: reexamining the guidelines. Institute of Medicine (US) and National Research Council (US) Committee to Reexamine IOM Pregnancy Weight Guidelines. The National Academies Collection: Reports funded by National Institutes of Health. Washington, DC: National Academies Press; 2009.

32. Feig DS. Oral hypoglycaemic agents in pregnancy. In: A practical manual of diabetes in pregnancy. Oxford (United Kingdom): Blackwell Publishing; 2010. p. 109–17.

33. Homko CJ, Sivan E, Reece AE. Is there a role for oral antihyperglycemics in gestational diabetes and type 2 diabetes during pregnancy? Treat Endocrinol 2004;3:133–9.

34. Hod M, Damm P, Kaaja R, et al. Fetal and perinatal outcomes in type 1 diabetes pregnancy: a randomized study comparing insulin aspart with human insulin in 322 subjects. Am J Obstet Gynecol 2008;198:186–7.
35. Mathiesen ER, Kinsley B, Amiel SA, et al. Maternal glycemic control and hypoglycemia in type 1 diabetic pregnancy: a randomized trial of insulin aspart versus human insulin in 322 pregnant women. Diabetes Care 2007;30:771–6.
36. Mathiesen ER, Vaz JA. Insulin treatment in diabetic pregnancy. Diabetes Metab Res Rev 2008;24(Suppl 2):S3–20.
37. Gallen IW, Jaap A, Roland JM, et al. Survey of glargine use in 115 pregnant women with type 1 diabetes. Diabet Med 2008;25:165–9.
38. Lapolla A, Di CG, Bruttomesso D, et al. Use of insulin detemir in pregnancy: a report on 10 type 1 diabetic women. Diabet Med 2009;26:1181–2.
39. Poyhonen-Alho M, Ronnemaa T, Saltevo J, et al. Use of insulin glargine during pregnancy. Acta Obstet Gynecol Scand 2007;86(10):1171–4.
40. Gabbe SG, Carpenter LB, Garrison EA. New strategies for glucose control in patients with type 1 and type 2 diabetes mellitus in pregnancy. Clin Obstet Gynecol 2007;50:1014–24.
41. McCance D, Holmes VA. Insulin regimens in pregnancy. In: A practical manual of diabetes in pregnancy. Oxford (United Kingdom): Blackwell Publishing; 2010. p. 99–109.
42. Kitzmiller JL, Jovanovic L, Brown F, et al, editors. Managing preexisting diabetes and pregnancy: technical reviews and consensus recommendations for care. Alexandria (VA): American Diabetes Association; 2008. p. 561–601.
43. Nielsen LR, Pedersen-Bjergaard U, Thorsteinsson B, et al. Hypoglycemia in pregnant women with type 1 diabetes: predictors and role of metabolic control. Diabetes Care 2008;31:9–14.
44. Kerssen A, de Valk HW, Visser GH. Do HbA1c levels and the self-monitoring of blood glucose levels adequately reflect glycaemic control during pregnancy in women with type 1 diabetes mellitus? Diabetologia 2006;49:25–8.
45. Schrot RJ. Targeting plasma glucose: preprandial versus postprandial. Clin Diabetes 2004;22:169–72.
46. Monnier L, Lapinski H, Colette C. Contributions of fasting and postprandial plasma glucose increments to the overall diurnal hyperglycemia of type 2 diabetic patients: variations with increasing levels of HbA(1c). Diabetes Care 2003;26:881–5.
47. Murphy HR, Rayman G, Lewis K, et al. Effectiveness of continuous glucose monitoring in pregnant women with diabetes: randomised clinical trial. BMJ 2008;337: a1680.
48. Nielsen LR, Ekbom P, Damm P, et al. HbA1c levels are significantly lower in early and late pregnancy. Diabetes Care 2004;27:1200–1.
49. Mills JL, Jovanovic L, Knopp R, et al. Physiological reduction in fasting plasma glucose concentration in the first trimester of normal pregnancy: the Diabetes in Early Pregnancy Study. Metabolism 1998;47:1140–4.
50. Lurie S, Danon D. Life span of erythrocytes in late pregnancy. Obstet Gynecol 1992;80:123–6.
51. Jovanovic L, Knopp RH, Brown Z, et al. Declining insulin requirement in the late first trimester of diabetic pregnancy. Diabetes Care 2001;24:1130–6.
52. Garcia-Patterson A, Gich I, Amini SB, et al. Insulin requirements throughout pregnancy in women with type 1 diabetes mellitus: three changes of direction. Diabetologia 2010;53:446–51.
53. Evers IM, ter Braak EW, de Valk HW, et al. Risk indicators predictive for severe hypoglycemia during the first trimester of type 1 diabetic pregnancy. Diabetes Care 2002;25:554–9.

54. Kimmerle R, Heinemann L, Delecki A, et al. Severe hypoglycemia incidence and predisposing factors in 85 pregnancies of type I diabetic women. Diabetes Care 1992;15:1034–7.
55. Leinonen PJ, Hiilesmaa VK, Kaaja RJ, et al. Maternal mortality in type 1 diabetes. Diabetes Care 2001;24:1501–2.
56. Rosenn BM, Miodovnik M, Holcberg G, et al. Hypoglycemia: the price of intensive insulin therapy for pregnant women with insulin-dependent diabetes mellitus. Obstet Gynecol 1995;85:417–22.
57. Buchanan TA, Schemmer JK, Freinkel N. Embryotoxic effects of brief maternal insulin-hypoglycemia during organogenesis in the rat. J Clin Invest 1986;78:643–9.
58. Kawaguchi M, Tanigawa K, Tanaka O, et al. Embryonic growth impaired by maternal hypoglycemia during early organogenesis in normal and diabetic rats. Acta Diabetol 1994;31:141–6.
59. Smoak IW, Sadler TW. Embryopathic effects of short-term exposure to hypoglycemia in mouse embryos in vitro2. Am J Obstet Gynecol 1990;163:619–24.
60. Worm D, Nielsen LR, Mathiesen ER, et al. Continuous glucose monitoring system with an alarm: a tool to reduce hypoglycemic episodes in pregnancy with diabetes. Diabetes Care 2006;29:2759–60.
61. Blood glucose control and the evolution of diabetic retinopathy and albuminuria. A preliminary multicenter trial. The Kroc Collaborative Study Group. N Engl J Med 1984;311:365–72.
62. The effect of intensive treatment of diabetes on the development and progression of long-term complications in insulin-dependent diabetes mellitus. The Diabetes Control and Complications Trial Research Group. N Engl J Med 1993;329:977–86.
63. Lawson PM, Champion MC, Canny C, et al. Continuous subcutaneous insulin infusion (CSII) does not prevent progression of proliferative and preproliferative retinopathy. Br J Ophthalmol 1982;66:762–6.
64. Chew EY, Mills JL, Metzger BE, et al. Metabolic control and progression of retinopathy. The Diabetes in Early Pregnancy Study. National Institute of Child Health and Human Development Diabetes in Early Pregnancy Study. Diabetes Care 1995;18:631–7.
65. National Institute of Health Publication no.00–3029. National High Blood Pressure Education Program. 2000. Available at: http://www.nhlbi.nih-gov/health/prof/heart/hbp/hbp-preg.htm. Accessed February 1, 2011.
66. Bartha JL, Romero-Carmona R, Torrejon-Cardoso R, et al. Insulin, insulin-like growth factor-1, and insulin resistance in women with pregnancy-induced hypertension. Am J Obstet Gynecol 2002;187:735–40.
67. Seely EW, Solomon CG. Insulin resistance and its potential role in pregnancy-induced hypertension. J Clin Endocrinol Metab 2003;88:2393–8.
68. Sierra-Laguado J, Garcia RG, Celedon J, et al. Determination of insulin resistance using the homeostatic model assessment (HOMA) and its relation with the risk of developing pregnancy-induced hypertension. Am J Hypertens 2007;20:437–42.
69. Solomon CG, Seely EW. Brief review: hypertension in pregnancy: a manifestation of the insulin resistance syndrome? Hypertension 2001;37:232–9.
70. Ferriss JB. The causes of raised blood pressure in insulin-dependent and non-insulin-dependent diabetes. J Hum Hypertens 1991;5:245–54.
71. Leguizamon GF, Zeff NP, Fernandez A. Hypertension and the pregnancy complicated by diabetes. Curr Diab Rep 2006;6:297–304.

72. Jensen T, Deckert T. Diabetic retinopathy, nephropathy and neuropathy. Generalized vascular damage in insulin-dependent diabetic patients. Horm Metab Res Suppl 1992;26:68–70.

73. Aoki TT, Grecu EO, Gollapudi GM, et al. Effect of intensive insulin therapy on progression of overt nephropathy in patients with type 1 diabetes mellitus. Endocr Pract 1999;5:174–8.

74. Kawazu S, Tomono S, Shimizu M, et al. The relationship between early diabetic nephropathy and control of plasma glucose in non-insulin-dependent diabetes mellitus. The effect of glycemic control on the development and progression of diabetic nephropathy in an 8-year follow-up study. J Diabetes Complications 1994;8:13–7.

75. Mulec H, Blohme G, Grande B, et al. The effect of metabolic control on rate of decline in renal function in insulin-dependent diabetes mellitus with overt diabetic nephropathy. Nephrol Dial Transplant 1998;13:651–5.

76. Cooper WO, Hernandez-Diaz S, Arbogast PG, et al. Major congenital malformations after first-trimester exposure to ACE inhibitors. N Engl J Med 2006;354:2443–51.

77. Shotan A, Widerhorn J, Hurst A, et al. Risks of angiotensin-converting enzyme inhibition during pregnancy: experimental and clinical evidence, potential mechanisms, and recommendations for use. Am J Med 1994;96:451–6.

78. Mathiesen ER, Damm P. Pregnancy - pharmacological problems. In: Mogensen CE, editor. Pharmacotherapy of diabetes: new developments. New York: Springer; 2009. p. 249–55.

79. Mathiesen ER, Ringholm L, Damm P. Stillbirth in diabetic pregnancies. Best Pract Res Clin Obstet Gynaecol 2011;25:105–11.

80. Jovanovic L. Glucose and insulin requirements during labor and delivery: the case for normoglycemia in pregnancies complicated by diabetes. Endocr Pract 2004;10(Suppl 2):40–5.

81. Stage E, Mathiesen ER, Emmersen PB, et al. Diabetic mothers and their newborn infants - rooming-in and neonatal morbidity. Acta Paediatr 2010;99:997–9.

82. Stage E, Norgard H, Damm P, et al. Long-term breast-feeding in women with type 1 diabetes. Diabetes Care 2006;29:771–4.

Thyroid Disorders in Pregnancy

Dorota A. Krajewski, MD[a], Kenneth D. Burman, MD[b,c],*

KEYWORDS

- Pregnancy • Thyroid dysfunction • Maternal hypothyroidism
- Gestational thyrotoxicosis • Graves' disease
- Postpartum thyroiditis • Fetal neurodevelopment
- Thyroid cancer

THYROID PHYSIOLOGY IN NORMAL PREGNANCY

Pregnancy is a time of complex hormonal changes. Maternal and fetal thyroid hormone profiles differ throughout gestation (**Fig. 1**). In women with normal thyroid function there is an increase in thyroxine (T4) and triiodothyronine (T3) production, which results in inhibition of thyroid-stimulating hormone (TSH) in the first trimester of pregnancy, due to a high human chorionic gonadotropin (hCG) level that stimulates the TSH receptor.[1,2] A large plasma volume and thus an altered distribution of thyroid hormone, increased thyroid hormone metabolism, increased renal clearance of iodide, and higher levels of hepatic production of thyroxine-binding globulin (TBG) in the hyperestrogenic state are responsible for higher thyroxine requirements in pregnancy.[1]

In the pregnant woman, elevated TBG and concomitant increases in total T4 and T3 levels plateau at 12 to 14 weeks of pregnancy, and free T4 measurements slowly decrease.[3] This hormonal milieu ensures a proper amount of thyroid hormone delivery to the fetus at a critical time of neurologic development and when the fetal thyroid is only beginning to develop. Levels of total T4, free T4, and total T3 gradually increase in the fetus between the second and third trimester, reflecting the rising contribution of the fetal thyroid (see **Fig. 1**). Type 3 deiodinase is expressed in high amounts in the placenta, and presumably protects the fetus from toxic levels of thyroid hormone by

Disclosures: Dr Burman is Former Chair of the FDA Endocrine Advisory Committee, Contributor to Medscape and UpToDate, Deputy Editor of the *Journal of Clinical Endocrinology and Metabolism*, and participates in Pfizer and Exelixis Clinical Thyroid Cancer Trials.

[a] Section of Endocrinology, Department of Medicine, Washington Hospital Center and Georgetown University Hospital, 4000 Reservoir Road, NW, Building D, Suite 232, Washington, DC 20007, USA

[b] Section of Endocrinology, Department of Medicine, Washington Hospital Center, Room 2A72, 110 Irving Street, NW, Washington, DC 20010, USA

[c] Department of Medicine, Georgetown University Hospital, 4000 Reservoir Road, NW, Building D, Suite 232, Washington, DC 20007, USA

* Corresponding author. Section of Endocrinology, Department of Medicine, Washington Hospital Center, Room 2A72, 110 Irving Street, NW, Washington, DC 20010.

E-mail address: Kenneth.D.Burman@Medstar.net

Endocrinol Metab Clin N Am 40 (2011) 739–763
doi:10.1016/j.ecl.2011.08.004
0889-8529/11/$ – see front matter © 2011 Elsevier Inc. All rights reserved.

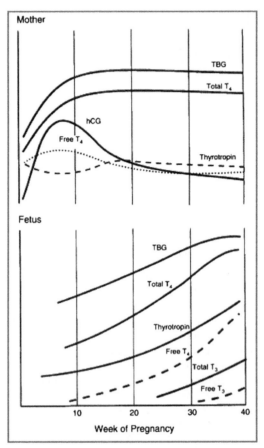

Fig. 1. Relative changes in maternal and fetal thyroid function during pregnancy. hCG, human chorionic gonadotropin; TBG, thyroxin-binding globulin. (*Adapted from* Burrow GN, Fisher DA, Larsen PR. Maternal and fetal thyroid function. N Engl J Med 1994;331(16):1072; with permission.)

converting T4 to biologically inactive reverse T3 in the periphery.[4,5] The presence of a uteroplacental barrier to the transfer of thyroid hormone from the mother to the fetus is yet another physiologic mechanism in place to keep the fetus euthyroid.[1]

In 1976 Burman and colleagues[6] compared thyroid hormone levels in human amniotic fluid and fetal cord serum, as well as maternal serum, with those in euthyroid nonpregnant controls. The investigators found that amniotic fluid concentrations of T3, T4, and TBG were significantly lower than reverse T3, 3,3'-T2, and dialyzable T3 and T4. Other studies have subsequently confirmed that levels of total T4 in coelomic and amniotic fluid are in fact 100 times lower than in the maternal serum whereas T3 levels are 30 times lower than T4 concentrations, and thus barely detectable. However, free T4 levels in the fetus are comparable with maternal concentrations, due to a significantly smaller amount of T4 binding proteins in the fetus.[1,5,7] A study in neonates with congenital hypothyroidism secondary to thyroid agenesis or a defect in thyroid hormone organification showed significant amounts of T4 (35–70 nmol/L or 2.72–5.44 μg/dL) in fetal cord serum, providing indirect evidence that maternal-fetal transfer of thyroxine is substantial.[8] Women with hypothyroidism are reliant on exogenous levothyroxine rather than endogenous thyroid gland secretion, and require higher doses of levothyroxine throughout pregnancy.[2,9,10]

THYROID HORMONE–DEPENDENT FETAL NEURODEVELOPMENT

During embryogenesis, thyroid hormone is of critical importance in the normal development of the human central nervous system.[11] Several studies in rodents have demonstrated potential molecular pathways in which thyroid hormone regulates expression of genes responsible for neuronal migration and growth in the cerebral cortex[12] and hippocampus,[13] alters levels of neurotransmitters,[14] and results in neuronal loss when thyroid hormone is lacking.[15] Furthermore, maternal hypothyroxinemia, or a low serum free T4, has been shown to be associated with abnormal neuronal migration and behavioral abnormalities in rats, including a lower threshold for seizure activity induced by audio stimuli.[11] Although the fetal thyroid in humans is histologically developed and can synthesize thyroid hormone by the 10th to 12th week of gestation,[16] thyroid maturation takes longer, and it is not until midgestation that substantial amounts of thyroid hormone are produced by the fetal thyroid gland.[1,8] Maternal hypothyroidism during the first trimester can thus have deleterious effects on fetal neurodevelopment, which is largely dependent on maternal thyroxine.[11] **Fig. 2** depicts stages of fetal neurodevelopment during pregnancy. Epidemiologic and prospective evidence suggests that early-gestation maternal hypothyroidism can result in mental and motor delay in children when assessed at 1 and 2 years of age,[17,18] and in some cases may even lead to profound mental retardation and cretinism.[1]

HYPOTHYROIDISM

The National Health and Nutrition Examination Survey (NHANES 1999–2002) indicates that 3.1% of women of reproductive age in the United States may have hypothyroidism.[19] The prevalence of overt hypothyroidism in pregnancy is estimated to be between 0.3% and 1.5% in different studies.[18,20,21] The frequency of subclinical hypothyroidism, clinically defined as an elevated TSH but a normal free T4, which tends to be asymptomatic, is higher. Klein and colleagues[20] found that 49 of 2000 (2.5%) pregnant women had a TSH greater than 6 μU/mL. Of these women, 6 also had a low free T4. More recently, in 2007 Vaidya and colleagues[21] also documented a prevalence of 2.6% for TSH above 4.2 μU/mL in a group of 1560 pregnant women at 9 weeks of gestation. With approximately 4 million live births per year in the United States as reported by the Centers for Disease Control and Prevention, this prevalence translates into approximately 100,000 to 200,000 fetuses each year having developed in utero while the mother was hypothyroid.

Thyroid autoimmunity is an important marker for subsequent development of hypothyroidism. Serum antithyroid peroxidase antibody (TPO-Ab) and antithyroglobulin antibody (Tg-Ab) positivity in pregnancy is approximately 8% and as high as 20%, and confers a fivefold to eightfold increased relative risk of developing maternal thyroid dysfunction.[21–24] It has been postulated that women with a TSH greater than 2.0 μU/mL and high titer of TPO-Abs are more likely to develop hypothyroidism.[24,25] The measurement of antibody levels may be helpful in determining the frequency of monitoring thyroid function during the remainder of gestation.

Pregnancy Complications in Hypothyroidism

Abnormal thyroid function during pregnancy is clinically significant for the mother and fetus, and may have long-term implications for the growing child as well as the mother's future health. Data from the Northern Finland Birth Cohort over 20 years of

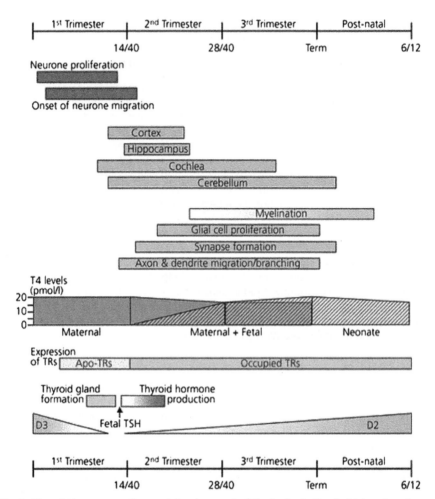

Fig. 2. Thyroid hormone action and development of the brain. In the first trimester of pregnancy, early neuronal proliferation and migration is dependent on maternal thyroxine (T4). In fetal tissues, inactivating type 3 deiodinase (D3) enzyme expression falls and development of the thyroid gland begins, in the first trimester. As the fetal hypothalamic-pituitary axis develops, a surge in thyroid-stimulating hormone (TSH) secretion results in the onset of fetal thyroid hormone production, expression of the activating type 2 iodothyronine deiodinase enzyme (D2), and increasing occupation of thyroid hormone receptors (TRs) by 3,5,3′-l-triiodothyronine (T3). In the second and third trimesters, the brain continues to develop relying increasingly on T4 produced by both the fetus and the mother. Postnatal development is entirely dependent on neonatal thyroid hormone production. Apo-TR, unliganded unoccupied thyroid hormone receptor. (*Adapted from* Williams GR. Neurodevelopmental and neurophysiological actions of thyroid hormone. J Neuroendocrinol 2008;20(6):785; with permission.)

follow-up showed that overt hypothyroidism in pregnancy was associated with maternal thyroid dysfunction and the development of diabetes mellitus later in life.[26] Overt hypothyroidism is also associated with multiple adverse effects in pregnancy (**Table 1**). The rate of miscarriage was 17% in women with positive thyroid antibodies compared with 8.4% in autoantibody-negative women. This difference was not

Table 1
Adverse effects of overt hypothyroidism in pregnancy on the mother and fetus

Maternal Complications	Fetal Complications
Hypertension/preeclampsia	Preterm delivery
Placental abruption	Low fetal birth weight
Increased miscarriage rate	Increased perinatal morbidity
Risk of cesarean section	Increased fetal and perinatal mortality
Postpartum hemorrhage	Neuropsychologic and cognitive impairment

explained by thyroid hormone levels, maternal age, or previous obstetric history.[23] An elegant study by Negro and colleagues[24] showed that when euthyroid pregnant women with TPO-Ab positivity were treated with levothyroxine (low dose 0.5–1.0 μg/kg/d) to normalize serum TSH, the rate of miscarriage was similar to antibody-negative women (3.5% vs 2.4%), whereas untreated TPO-Ab–positive pregnant women had a significantly higher TSH and a higher miscarriage rate of 13.8%. A TSH level above 6 μU/mL was associated with a fourfold increase in fetal death in one population-based study of more than 9000 pregnant women, but other complications including abruptio placentae, pregnancy-induced hypertension, low Apgar score, and cesarean section were comparable with those in euthyroid women.[27] Casey and colleagues[28] analyzed a cohort of more than 17,000 women and found that pregnancy in those with subclinical hypothyroidism was 3 times more likely to be complicated by placental abruption and had twice the risk of preterm delivery. Other literature finds no difference in obstetric outcomes in euthyroid when compared with levothyroxine-treated women.[22] A recent study of a large cohort of TPO-Ab–negative pregnant women showed that those with a TSH of 2.5 μU/mL or less in the first trimester had a lower rate of spontaneous pregnancy loss (3.6%) than women with a TSH between 2.5 and 5 μU/mL (6.1%).[29] This observation suggests that the upper limit of normal for TSH in the first trimester of pregnancy should be 2.5 μU/mL.

In addition to adverse effects on pregnancy outcomes, maternal hypothyroidism has been associated with impaired neuropsychological development in the child. Lower average IQ scores have been reported in children aged 7 to 9 years without congenital hypothyroidism but born to mothers with an elevated TSH (mean 13.2 ± 0.3 μU/mL) and low free T4 (mean 0.71 ± 0.1 ng/dL) during the second trimester.[30] Children from women who were treated with levothyroxine, in contrast to those that were not treated, did not have a lower IQ when tested at 7 to 9 years of age. However, this study must be interpreted in the context of its small sample size, single TSH value measured, the unknown significance of a 4-point to 7-point lowering of IQ, lack of information on the children's developmental milestones before the age of 7, and lack of statistical significance in children of mothers with subclinical hypothyroidism.

Hypothyroidism and Iodine Requirements in Pregnancy

The most common cause of maternal hypothyroidism worldwide is iodine deficiency, but in developed countries autoimmune thyroid disease or Hashimoto's thyroiditis is more prevalent.[21,22] Iodine is a critical substrate for the thyroid to synthesize and secrete thyroid hormone,[31,32] and is either trapped by the thyroid gland or excreted in the urine. The World Health Organization recommends that pregnant and lactating women have an iodine intake of 250 μg per day, which is 100 μg above that recommended for nonpregnant adults, to compensate for increased thyroxine requirements, renal iodine losses, and fetal iodine requirements in pregnancy.[33] The American

Thyroid Association (ATA) recommends that all prenatal vitamins and supplements contain at least 150 µg of iodine.[34] Further details are given in the article by Leung and colleagues elsewhere in this issue on iodine nutrition in pregnancy and lactation.

Diagnosis and Screening of Hypothyroidism in Pregnancy

Screening for thyroid disease in pregnancy has been a matter of debate. Current guidelines by the ATA, the American Association of Clinical Endocrinologists, and the Endocrine Society recommend targeted case-finding in pregnant women with a personal history of thyroid disease, a positive family history, type 1 diabetes mellitus or other autoimmune disorders, infertility, history of miscarriage or preterm delivery, and clinical signs or symptoms of thyroid disease that would classify them as high risk.[15,21,35,36] However, Vaidya and colleagues[21] advocate that up to one-third of hypothyroid women (TSH >4.2 µU/mL) will be missed with case-finding alone based on a study of 1560 consecutive pregnancies, and that universal screening for thyroid disorders would be more prudent. By contrast, in a group of 4562 women, the number of adverse obstetric and neonatal outcomes were similar regardless of whether they were in the universal screening group (n = 1559) or case-finding group (n = 1545).[37] In this study, women classified as at low risk for thyroid disease who were randomized to universal screening benefited from treatment of abnormal TSH, with a statistically significant reduction noted in risk of adverse events. In the high-risk women, there was no difference in adverse outcomes between the case-finding and the universal screening groups. The number needed to screen in the low-risk group to find one hypothyroid or hyperthyroid woman was 36, but 60 women would have to be screened to prevent one woman from having an adverse event.[37] Most recently, preliminary results from the prospective Controlled Antenatal Thyroid Screening (CATS) study of more than 22,000 pregnant women suggest a benefit of hypothyroidism screening and treatment in gestation. Of 700 children whose IQ was tested at 3 years of age, thus far 15.6% who were not screened for hypothyroidism in utero had an IQ of less than 85, compared with only 9.2% of those children born to mothers who had been diagnosed with hypothyroidism and treated with levothyroxine before birth. However, data are still being collected and analyzed prior to any specific conclusions being reached.[38] More frequent thyroid testing may be necessary during gestation to identify women who develop thyroid insufficiency later in pregnancy, especially if they are TPO-Ab positive.[22] In a cohort of 220 pregnant women, Moleti and colleagues[22] reported that more than 40% of hypothyroidism was diagnosed during the second and third trimester.

Thyroid function testing in pregnancy is affected by a multitude of physiologic and exogenous factors that can influence interpretation of laboratory results. Thyrotropin is suppressed early in gestation as high levels of hCG stimulate T4 and T3 secretion, which in turn lowers TSH and subsequently lowers free thyroxine (free T4) and T3 as well, as already discussed.[1,2] Assay-dependent variation in free T4 levels has been reported secondary to fluctuating levels of TBG and hypoalbuminemia during pregnancy.[39] Serum free T4 measurements in pregnant women were lower than in nonpregnant women, with many maternal free T4 levels below the normal range, whereas total T4 was significantly higher.[39] Trimester-specific ranges for more accurate assessment of thyroid function tests should be used with the understanding that TSH levels can be affected to varying degrees by TPO-Ab positivity, hyperemesis gravidarum, twin pregnancies, and iodine status.[40–42] **Fig. 3** depicts the median TSH values and the 2.5th to 97.5th TSH percentiles for each trimester of pregnancy in women without TPO-Abs, confirming the downward shift of serum TSH during pregnancy, especially in the first trimester (see **Fig. 3**).

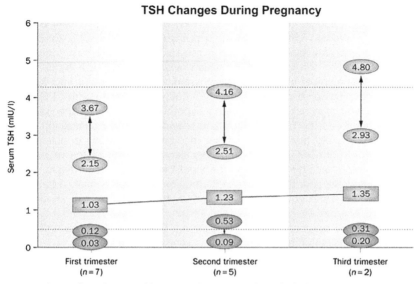

Fig. 3. Median values (*rectangle*) versus the range of 2.5th (*ellipse, bottom*) and 97.5th (*ellipse, top*) percentiles for each trimester of pregnancy taken from 8 studies of trimester-specific TSH reference intervals, reported between 2004 and 2009, for women without thyroid peroxidase autoantibodies from iodine-sufficient populations. The dotted horizontal lines show the typical nonpregnant reference range (0.4–4.1 µU/mL). (*From* Glinoer D, Spencer CA. Serum TSH determinations in pregnancy: how, when and why? Nat Rev Endocrinol 2010;6(9):527; with permission.)

Management of Hypothyroidism in Pregnancy

According to the Endocrine Society guidelines on management of thyroid dysfunction in pregnancy and postpartum,[36] in women with a prior history of hypothyroidism the preconception and first-trimester TSH level should not exceed 2.5 µU/mL. In the second and third trimesters, a TSH of less than 3.0 µU/mL is desirable. Alexander and colleagues[10] showed that levothyroxine requirements increase as early as the eighth week of gestation, by a mean dose increase of 47% to maintain thyrotropin at prepregnancy values, and this effect persisted throughout gestation. A pregnant woman receiving an established, stable dose of levothyroxine will likely need a 30% to 50% dose augmentation by the fourth through sixth week of gestation. The THERAPY trial set out to test the efficacy of preventing maternal hypothyroidism by having women increase their levothyroxine dose by either an additional 2 or 3 tablets per week as soon as pregnancy was confirmed. All women achieved a TSH level below 5 µU/mL during the first trimester with dose augmentation, whether they were in the groups taking either 2 or 3 additional levothyroxine tablets per week. With the regimen of 2 additional levothyroxine tablets per week, 2 women with a history of thyroid cancer needed a further increase in levothyroxine dose and 32% of women (8 of 25) had a suppressed TSH level below 0.5 µU/mL. In the group receiving 3 additional levothyroxine tablets per week, only one woman required further levothyroxine dose escalation; however, TSH suppression occurred in 65% of subjects (15 of 23).[9] The etiology of hypothyroidism may play an important role in the magnitude of levothyroxine requirements during pregnancy. Patients with Graves' disease and goiter treated with ablative radioiodine (I-131) or thyroidectomy required larger doses of levothyroxine during pregnancy compared with patients with primary hypothyroidism;

however, thyroid cancer patients had smaller dose adjustments throughout gestation, which may be attributed to their higher levothyroxine doses at baseline for TSH suppression.[43] Women with subclinical hypothyroidism, according to Endocrine Society guidelines, should be treated with levothyroxine based on the potential benefit of reduced obstetric complications for which evidence is fair. It has not yet been proven that treatment of subclinical hypothyroidism in the mother improves long-term neurologic outcome in her offspring.[36] Euthyroid women with TPO-Abs are believed to be at high risk for developing hypothyroidism later in pregnancy, and should be monitored for TSH elevation and receive prenatal counseling; however, treatment with thyroid hormone is not yet recommended in this population. After delivery, thyroid hormone requirements may decrease back to the prepregnancy baseline, therefore levothyroxine dosing should be adjusted accordingly. Maternal weight changes may alter the levothyroxine requirement after delivery. Monitoring of thyroid function tests in pregnant women with hypothyroidism should occur frequently, as often as every 2 to 4 weeks throughout midgestation and 4 to 8 weeks in the second half of pregnancy, as this time interval has been shown to identify 90% of abnormal TSH values that resulted in levothyroxine dose adjustment.[9]

HYPERTHYROIDISM

Gestational hyperthyroidism is much less common than gestational hypothyroidism, with a prevalence rate of about 0.2%.[2,38,44] The differential diagnosis of thyrotoxicosis in pregnancy is similar to that of nonpregnant women: autoimmune thyroid disease (eg, Graves' disease, hashitoxicosis), toxic adenoma or goiter, transient thyroiditis (eg, subacute thyroiditis, silent thyroiditis), iodine-induced hyperthyroidism and, rarely, a pituitary adenoma secreting TSH or thyroid hormone resistance. Additional consideration of hCG-mediated hyperthyroidism including gestational transient thyrotoxicosis (GTT) and its association with hyperemesis gravidarum becomes very important. Postpartum thyroiditis is also unique to the pregnant cohort within several months of delivery.

Graves' Disease in Pregnancy

The most common cause of hyperthyroidism in pregnancy, as in all women of reproductive age, is autoimmune Graves' disease with circulating TSH receptor antibodies (TRAbs) stimulating the thyroid gland and TSH receptor, resulting in unabated thyroid hormone synthesis and secretion.[2] Graves' disease may be challenging to diagnose in the hypermetabolic state of pregnancy because of similar symptoms in both conditions.[2,39,45] Features suggestive of Graves' hyperthyroidism in normal pregnancy include a diffuse goiter, which is usually larger with Graves' disease than in normal pregnancy, evidence of ophthalmopathy, TRAb or thyroid-stimulating immunoglobulin (TSI) positivity, and a family history of autoimmune thyroid disease.[2] The extent of elevation of thyroid function tests typically is higher in Graves' disease than in hyperemesis gravidarum. The immune-tolerant state of pregnancy is associated over time with a decrease in TRAb titers, thus the hyperthyroidism secondary to Graves' disease may subside in severity as gestation progresses.[2] However, exacerbations of hyperthyroidism are reported to occur early in pregnancy corresponding to a peak in hCG at 10 to 12 weeks, and these women are at an additional risk of Graves' disease recurrence postpartum.[46] Rotondi and colleagues[47] showed that women with Graves' disease in remission after treatment with methimazole (MMI) prior to pregnancy were more likely to have a relapse 4 to 8 months postpartum than women in remission who did not get pregnant (84% vs 56%, $P<.05$).

Gestational Transient Thyrotoxicosis

GTT differs from Graves' disease in that it is a self-limited, nonautoimmune form of hyperthyroidism with negative TRAbs.[2] Indeed, it is related to the elevation of hCG, which can then cross-react with the TSH receptor and induce thyroidal iodothyronine secretion. According to one European study, as many as 2.4% of women may be affected by GTT during pregnancy.[2,41,48] Women with this entity have a TSH that is in the low to normal range for pregnancy or is frequently undetectable, elevated free T4 and free T3 levels, and prolonged abnormally high concentrations of hCG in the first and second trimesters, occasionally higher than 100,000 U/L.[48] These patients present with symptoms of hyperthyroidism in about 50% of cases, and the emesis or symptoms from thyrotoxicosis may be severe enough to require hospitalization. It is thought that the homology between the β subunit of the hCG and TSH molecules and both of their receptors is responsible for the thyrotropic effect of elevated hCG.[2,49] Some investigators postulate that more biologically active isoforms of hCG exist, which may explain why some women with GTT do not have impressive elevation of hCG.[50] Most women do not require treatment with antithyroid drugs; however, β-blockers and supportive measures may become necessary in some cases.[48] Most β-blockers are classified as pregnancy category C, meaning that they were not studied in pregnant humans but appear to cause harm to the fetus in animal studies (eg, carvedilol, esmolol, metoprolol, nadolol, nebivolol, propranolol, timolol).[51] Acebutolol, pindolol, and sotalol are category B (inadequately studied in humans but appear to cause no harm in animal studies), but atenolol is category D and has been shown to cause harm to the fetus in pregnant women.[51] β-blocker use especially late in pregnancy presents risks to the fetus including low heart rate, hypoglycemia,[52] respiratory distress, and low birth weight; therefore, risks and benefits of treatment must be considered before initiating therapy.[51] Hyperemesis gravidarum, characterized by excessive nausea and vomiting, which causes a greater than 5% weight loss, dehydration, and ketonuria in early pregnancy, is a milder form of GTT in that women have subclinical or very mild overt hyperthyroidism in one-third to two-thirds of cases.[53] In a study by Goodwin and colleagues[54] TSH was suppressed to below 0.2 μU/mL in 60% of women with hyperemesis compared with only 9% of pregnant women without symptoms, and hCG, estradiol, and free T4 levels were higher in the hyperemesis group and positively correlated with the severity of emesis. Choriocarcinoma and hydatidiform mole are rare causes of hCG-mediated hyperthyroidism that resolve with chemotherapy and/or surgical removal, and are beyond the scope of this review.

Pregnancy Complications of Hyperthyroidism

Maternal hyperthyroidism increases the risk of pregnancy complications in both the mother and the fetus. Preeclampsia,[55] congestive heart failure,[56] placental abruption and cesarean delivery,[57] and even thyrotoxic periodic paralysis[58] have been reported to occur more frequently in pregnant women with uncontrolled hyperthyroidism in comparison with euthyroid pregnant women. Fetal risks of maternal thyrotoxicosis include spontaneous abortion,[59] premature labor and low birth weight,[55] stillbirth,[56] and congenital abnormalities.[60] To delineate the effects of hyperthyroidism on the fetus, Refetoff and colleagues[59] studied pregnant women with thyroid hormone resistance due to a thyroid hormone receptor β gene mutation. In this study population, the mothers were euthyroid with detectable TSH despite having elevated free T4 and T3 levels, and without autoantibodies allowing for the direct effects of excess thyroid hormone, rather than the possible effects of thyroid antibodies on the fetus, to be assessed. The investigators reported a much higher miscarriage rate in mothers carrying the thyroid hormone receptor β mutation (23.7%) compared with unaffected first-degree relatives (8.8%) and the general population (8.1%). Furthermore, women with thyroid hormone resistance had higher than expected numbers of affected offspring (20 affected vs 11 unaffected neonates), suggesting that the miscarriages may have involved predominantly unaffected fetuses. The neonates were not shown to have a T3 receptor mutation. Of interest, unaffected infants born to affected mothers had lower birth weights in the setting of exposure to excess thyroid hormone, whereas unaffected infants of only affected fathers had normal birth weights, likely due to their gestational environment from a euthyroid mother. The frequency of adverse events such as preterm delivery, stillbirth, preeclampsia, and perinatal loss, reported with other forms of maternal hyperthyroidism, were not increased in women with resistance to thyroid hormone. Of note, Casey and colleagues[61] did not identify any adverse pregnancy outcomes in 433 women with subclinical hyperthyroidism, arguing that diagnosis and treatment of a low TSH is unwarranted if free T4 is in the normal range.

Negative effects on neurodevelopment in hypothyroidism have previously been discussed, and seem to be more detrimental but also more extensively studied than the effects of hyperthyroidism. In rats, excess thyroid hormone resulted in increased fetal brain weight, decreased glial fibrillary acidic protein expression, and increased neurofilament 68, suggesting accelerated neuronal differentiation.[62] Excess T3 inhibits embryonic neural stem cell proliferation in mice.[63] The significance of these animal studies in humans is unknown.

Treatment of Hyperthyroidism in Pregnancy

Treatment of hyperthyroidism in nonpregnant patients, specifically Graves' hyperthyroidism and toxic goiter in adults, includes the use of antithyroid drugs (ATDs), thyroid ablation with I-131, or thyroidectomy. Each treatment modality poses special consideration in pregnancy, but radioactive iodine administration for diagnostic scans and treatment is absolutely contraindicated in pregnant patients and in women considering becoming pregnant in the near future, secondary to adverse effects on the fetus and the fetal thyroid gland. Nonetheless, there are several reports of inadvertently administering radioactive iodide to pregnant women, and these reports give important clinical information regarding the possible consequences. A case report of inadvertent exposure to 19.8 millicuries (mCi) of I-131 in the first few days of gestation notes no significant harm to the fetus other than transient neonatal thyrotoxicosis at birth, attributed to maternal TRAb rather than the radioactive iodine itself, which resolved within 6 months of clinical observation without treatment.[64] The consequences of I-131 exposure after the 10th week of gestation, when the fetal thyroid is developed and able to trap and concentrate iodine, include fetal/neonatal hypothyroidism, subsequent cognitive impairment, and even fetal death if the dose of radiation is high enough.[65,66] When 3700 megabecquerel (MBq) or approximately 100 mCi of I-131 was inadvertently administered to a pregnant woman for ablation of multifocal papillary thyroid carcinoma, a whole body scan showed avid uptake in the fetal thyroid and amniotic fluid, as shown in **Fig. 4**. A theoretical risk of radiation-induced childhood malignancy exists as well, and an increased risk of thyroid carcinoma has been reported in children of mothers in the Ukraine who were exposed in utero to I-131 fallout during the Chernobyl nuclear accident in April 1986.[67] Radioactive iodine is thus absolutely contraindicated in all stages of pregnancy, which precludes the use of diagnostic radioactive iodine uptake and scans as well as I-123 whole-body scans in thyroid cancer management and, of course, also precludes the use of I-131 therapy for hyperthyroidism or thyroid cancer treatment. The American College of Radiology (ACR)

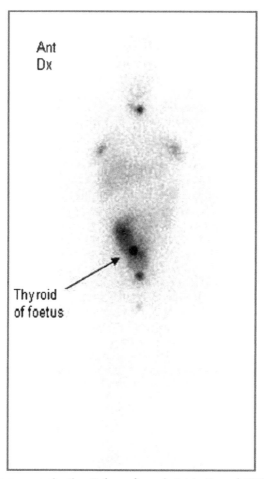

Fig. 4. Gamma camera examination 6 days after administration of 3700 MBq or approximately 100 mCi of iodine-131 for treatment of thyroid cancer. Note small uptake in the thyroid bed, uptake in mammary glands, and uptake in the fetal thyroid and fetal body/amniotic fluid. (*Adapted from* Berg G, Jacobsson L, Nystrom E, et al. Consequences of inadvertent radio-iodine treatment of Graves' disease and thyroid cancer in undiagnosed pregnancy. Can we rely on routine pregnancy testing? Acta Oncol 2008;47(1):146; with permission.)

strongly recommends confirmation that a woman of childbearing potential is not pregnant, using clinical history and testing of serum hCG concentration, before any diagnostic or therapeutic radioactive iodine use.[68,69] When unintended exposure to I-131 occurs in a pregnant woman, it is imperative that a multidisciplinary approach is undertaken to determine fetal age at the time of exposure, and to estimate the amount of radiation absorbed by the fetus to anticipate the magnitude of potential consequences such as fetal thyroid ablation and spontaneous abortion.[65] Fetal thyroid ultrasonography to assess the possibility of thyroid hypoplasia or fetal goiter and cordocentesis for fetal thyroid hormone measurements may be helpful in evaluating the status of the fetal thyroid and for treatment considerations.[69] Information regarding risks of possible fetal radiation exposure should be shared with the patient so that she can make an informed decision.

Antithyroid Drug Use in Pregnancy

Treatment of hyperthyroidism with antithyroid medications, namely propylthiouracil (PTU) and methimazole (MMI) in the United States, and the MMI analogue carbimazole in the United Kingdom, has been the standard of care for approximately 5 decades. These drugs are effective in blocking thyroid hormone synthesis, and it is now known that they all cross the placenta to a varying degree.[60,70,71] Over the last decade, MMI has gained in popularity and has become the first-line treatment because of better patient adherence, better control of severe hyperthyroidism, and less toxicity in the nonpregnant state.[72] During pregnancy, medical treatment is preferred despite class D classification of thionamides by the Food and Drug Administration (FDA),[72] because radioactive iodine cannot be used and surgery is typically reserved for severe thyrotoxicosis that has failed medical therapy.[36] PTU had been the drug of choice during pregnancy to avoid MMI-associated scalp defects of aplasia cutis or choanal/esophageal atresia, to treat thyroid storm because of enhanced conversion of T4 to T3, and for use in those patients intolerant to MMI.[36,72] Recently, however, PTU use has been closely reexamined by several organizations including the ATA and the FDA. To date there are 33 and 14 published reports of severe liver failure in adults and children, respectively, attributed to PTU, leading to liver transplantation and death in some cases.[73–75] The FDA Adverse Events Reporting System identified at least 2 mothers with liver injury during pregnancy and 2 fetuses with hepatitis from PTU treatment of their mother.[73] In their recent editorial in the *Journal of Clinical Endocrinology and Metabolism*, Cooper and Rivkees[73] caution that based on the current birth rate, the prevalence of hyperthyroidism in pregnancy, and current PTU use, an estimated 4 women per year are at risk of liver failure during pregnancy from their treatment. Although MMI is a well-known cause of elevated transaminases, it typically induces cholestasis, which is usually reversible with drug discontinuation.[72] In comparison with PTU-related liver transplants reported between 1990 and 2007, none were seen with MMI.[73] Updated guidelines from the ATA and American Association of Clinical Endocrinologists are expected in 2011 to delineate a limited therapeutic window for PTU during the first trimester of pregnancy, in the treatment of thyroid storm, and in patients with minor reactions to MMI who refuse radioactive iodine therapy or surgery; otherwise MMI should be used in every patient who chooses antithyroid drug therapy for Graves' disease.[76]

Effects on the Fetus from Maternal Hyperthyroidism and its Treatment

Significant effects on both the mother and the fetus can result from treatment of maternal Graves' disease, including birth defects from ATDs, inadequate treatment of the mother, overtreatment, transplacental passage of maternal antibodies, and fetal thyroid problems. A case-control study in 2008 showed an increased odds ratio (17.75; 95% confidence interval [CI] 3.49–121.40) of choanal atresia in children with prenatal exposure to hyperthyroidism treated with MMI, although it could not delineate whether the causal factor was the hyperthyroid state or its treatment.[77] A more recent case-affected control analysis of prenatal exposure to antithyroid agents in 127 neonates suggested an increased incidence of situs inversus, kidney agenesis, and cardiac outflow tract defects with PTU as well as choanal atresia, omphalocele, and situs inversus with MMI exposure.[78] MMI has also been associated with aplasia cutis, a scalp defect that has not been reported with PTU.[79] Although the number of cases is small and the defects are rare, it appears that both medications have a small increased risk of inducing birth defects. However, inadequately treated Graves' disease in the mother may lead to fetal thyroid underdevelopment and low birth weight in the neonate. As a result, thyroid hormone supplementation at birth may become necessary secondary to excess thyroid hormone exposure in utero, which interferes with maturation of the fetal thyroid axis and alters the fetal pituitary set point for TSH secretion.[80,81] It appears that on rare occasions, PTU at appropriate doses to the mother can cause fetal hypothyroidism, although it is possible that the mothers were overtreated. There is not always a direct relationship between maternal and fetal thyroid function. In a prospective observational controlled cohort study, 7 of 74 fetuses exposed to PTU at a dose of 150 to 300 mg per day developed hypothyroidism, and 9 of 87 developed hyperthyroidism.[82] Fetal goiter occurred in 4 of the hypothyroid and 2 of the hyperthyroid fetuses, indicating that the presence of a goiter cannot reliably distinguish between the two states. The series of 77 women with Graves' hyperthyroidism treated with thionamides throughout pregnancy reported by Momotani and colleagues[83] showed no significant difference in fetal thyroid hormone levels obtained by cordocentesis at delivery after exposure to MMI as compared with PTU. Low free T4 was documented in 6% to 7% of fetuses exposed to either thionamide, but 21% of fetuses on PTU had a high TSH compared with only 14% of those exposed to MMI, although this difference was not statistically significant.[83] Cordocentesis performed in the third trimester can be used in selected cases to measure thyroid hormone levels in the fetus if the diagnosis cannot be ascertained from clinical data and potential management would change.[36,84] However, this procedure may be dangerous, and a multidisciplinary approach should be taken when cordocentesis is being considered. Fetal ultrasonography aimed at the thyroid gland is recommended by some investigators at week 32 in women with Graves' disease and positive TRAb/TSI to best detect and treat fetal thyroid abnormalities.[85] It is known that transplacental passage of maternal thyroid antibodies occurs, and that it may cause fetal/neonatal hypothyroidism if they are blocking antibodies and fetal/neonatal hyperthyroidism (1%–2% of offspring) if they are stimulating antibodies.[81,86] Thyrotoxicosis and primary hyperthyroidism in the neonate is usually transient, and remits with clearance of maternal TRAbs in the first 3 to 6 months of life.[81,87] Treatment antepartum is targeted at medication adjustment in the mother; postpartum short-term levothyroxine administration to the hypothyroid neonate is recommended, and the hyperthyroidism should only be treated with antithyroid agents if the neonate has clinically severe thyrotoxicosis.[82] Exposure in utero to ATDs has not been shown to affect children's intellectual development at a later age provided that the child was euthyroid and without goiter at birth.[88]

Management of Hyperthyroidism in Pregnancy

Management of hyperthyroidism in pregnancy should focus on the mother as well as the fetus, and largely depends on the maternal thyroid status and her history.[89] The assessment and treatment of these patients requires a multidisciplinary approach between primary care physicians, endocrinologists, obstetricians, and pediatricians. When the mother is euthyroid after ATD treatment of Graves' disease but has not been definitively treated, she is at risk of recurrence, especially postpartum, and her thyroid function should be monitored during pregnancy and after delivery.[47] If the mother has had thyroid ablation or surgery she may still be TRAb positive, and antibodies may cause fetal hyperthyroidism via passage through the placenta.[75,89,90] According to the 2007 Endocrine Society guidelines, TRAb titers should be measured before pregnancy or at the end of the second trimester in all pregnant women with current or a history of Graves' disease to assess the risk of neonatal hyperthyroidism in the fetus.[36,41] If titers are high, further assessment with fetal ultrasonography is necessary to look for growth restriction, hydrops, goiter, and cardiac failure in addition to clinical monitoring of the fetus for hyperthyroidism.[36] Evaluation for thyroid dysfunction must take place at birth in all newborns of mothers with Graves' disease. Further, fetal thyroid evaluation should occur closely in the first several weeks after pregnancy, as the fetus can manifest thyroid abnormalities within the first several weeks of life that were not present at birth. For example, Zakarija and colleagues[91] reported late onset of hyperthyroidism in an infant 45 days after delivery whose mother with Graves' disease likely had thyrotropin-binding inhibitor antibodies that initially prevented the effect of her thyroid-stimulating antibodies. Antithyroid drug therapy should be initiated for overt hyperthyroidism secondary to Graves' disease or hyperfunctioning thyroid nodules in pregnancy.[36] The goal of therapy is to use the lowest dose of medication to maintain maternal free T4 in the upper nonpregnant reference range, as this minimizes the risk of hypothyroidism to the fetus.[92] In 2009 the ATA affirmed that PTU is no longer considered first-line medical therapy for thyrotoxicosis, with the possible exceptions of during the first trimester of pregnancy and in those with moderate adverse effects to MMI.[93] In 2010, the FDA also announced a black-box warning regarding PTU and liver failure. This guideline implies a major change in management in the second and third trimesters of pregnancy of switching from PTU to MMI if antithyroid drug therapy is still needed. Updated guidelines from the ATA and American Association of Clinical Endocrinologists are expected in 2011 to delineate a limited therapeutic window for PTU during the first trimester of pregnancy, in the treatment of thyroid storm, and in patients with minor reactions to MMI who refuse radioactive iodine therapy or surgery. In all other cases, MMI should be used in every patient who chooses antithyroid drug therapy for Graves' disease.[76] Subtotal thyroidectomy can usually be performed in the second trimester of pregnancy, in situations whereby hyperthyroidism is uncontrolled with ATDs, treatment requires persistently high doses of antithyroid medication (generally thought to be more than approximately 300 mg of PTU daily), or if the mother has a serious adverse effect to medical therapy.[36] To avoid the complications of untreated hyperthyroidism and the risks associated with its treatment in pregnancy, definitive therapy with I-131 ablation must be considered in all women of childbearing age with Graves' disease prior to pregnancy, with the understanding that TRAb titers may remain positive in the mother for many years.[94] Women who receive I-131 therapy for Graves' disease should wait at least 6 months before becoming pregnant, although this is an empiric recommendation. These patients should become hypothyroid within 2 to 3 months, and it may subsequently take 1 to 2 months to restore euthyroidism with exogenous levothyroxine.

Lactation and Treatment of Thyroid Dysfunction

Breastfeeding is considered safe in mothers with hypothyroidism and hyperthyroidism taking thyroid medications. Although MMI and PTU both appear in human milk, it is at very small concentrations.[95] Only a mean total of 0.025% of the administered dose of PTU was actually excreted in breast milk over a 4-hour period.[96] MMI concentration in breast milk is 5 to 6 times higher than PTU concentration, with a mean milk/serum ratio of 0.98 and 0.14% of the oral dose being excreted after 8 hours.[97] In 88 thyrotoxic and lactating mothers treated with a daily dose of 5 to 20 mg of MMI it was shown that their babies' thyroid function and intellectual development was normal after up to 74 months of follow-up.[98] Similarly, PTU doses of 300 to 750 mg daily for 3 to 9 months did not significantly affect thyroid function in infants.[99] However, these studies are relatively small, with limited follow-up and testing. The decision whether to breastfeed while taking antithyroid agents is an individual decision that should be discussed by the patient and her physician.

Postpartum Thyroid Dysfunction

Postpartum thyroid dysfunction (PPTD) classically manifests as an autoimmune destructive thyroiditis (PPT) with a period of thyrotoxicosis, hypothyroidism, or both, followed by recovery in the first year after delivery.[100] It is frequent and occurs in about 8% of women worldwide, and is strongly associated with TPO-Ab positivity.[100] PPTD occurs most frequently at about the fourth month after delivery, although it can take place any time between 1 and 12 months postpartum. The pathophysiology is probably related to an exacerbation of underlying autoimmune thyroiditis that was quiescent during the immunosuppressed state of pregnancy, which then flares with immune rebound following delivery.[100–102] Up to 50% of pregnant women with TPO-Abs will develop PPTD, and of these about 20% may develop permanent hypothyroidism over the next several years.[44,87,102,103] Risk factors for subsequent and permanent hypothyroidism include a postpartum peak TSH greater than 20 μU/mL, a high titer of TPO-Abs, hypoechogenicity on thyroid ultrasonography, and a hypothyroid phase of PPTD.[88,103] Women with postpartum thyroid dysfunction in their first pregnancy have been shown to have a 70% rate of recurrence after a subsequent delivery.[104] In one study, 26.7% of women with postpartum thyroiditis (8 of 30) also had positive serum pituitary antibodies compared with 4.7% of healthy controls (1 of 21).[105] Whether these women have an increased predilection for autoimmune hypophysitis is not known. The 25% prevalence of PPTD in women with type 1 diabetes mellitus further stresses the importance of autoimmunity in this entity.[106] Postpartum depression has been linked to TPO-Ab positivity, but evidence is inconclusive.[107] The hypothyroid phase of PPTD should be considered for treatment with levothyroxine at replacement doses given the clinical context, especially when TSH is 10 μU/mL or greater; some investigators suggest indefinite treatment because of the high likelihood of permanent hypothyroidism.[100,103] However, other investigators would attempt to stop the medication after approximately 6 to 12 months of treatment to determine if the hypothyroidism is permanent and then, if normal, perform periodic monitoring. In a prospective, randomized, placebo-controlled study, 200 μg per day of selenium supplementation was shown to reduce the incidence of PPTD (28.6% vs 48.6%, $P<.01$) as well as hypothyroidism (11.7% vs 20.3%, $P<.01$) in women with positive TPO-Abs.[102] Despite the demonstration that selenium has some efficacy it is not routinely prescribed for this purpose, as more clinical evidence is needed to establish whether selenium supplementation can prevent thyroid dysfunction. The Endocrine Society recommends screening for PPTD by measuring TSH at 3 and 6 months postpartum in all women with TPO-Abs and type 1 diabetes mellitus, as well as annually in those with a history of PPTD in prior pregnancy.[36] Mothers who experience depression in the postpartum period should also be screened for hypothyroidism, and treated accordingly.

THYROID NODULES IN PREGNANCY

Thyroid nodules are a common clinical finding in the general population, ranging in prevalence between 4% and 7% by palpation and from 20% to 76% by radiologic detection; however, only 1 in 20 nodules will harbor malignancy.[93,108–110] A recent report of a Chinese cohort of pregnant women found a 15% incidence of thyroid nodules (34 of 221 women) which, with the exception of 2 nodules, all significantly enlarged in volume throughout gestation. New thyroid nodules developed in 25 or 11% of women; however, thyroid malignancy did not occur.[111] As in nonpregnant individuals, when a thyroid nodule is discovered during pregnancy it is important to assess possible compressive symptoms, rapidity of nodule growth, a history of head or neck radiation, and whether there is a family history of thyroid malignancy, each of which indicate a higher suspicion for thyroid cancer.[109–111] Ultrasonography of the thyroid should be performed if a thyroid nodule is diagnosed by physical examination or another imaging modality, to confirm the number of nodules present and to establish the presence of suspicious characteristics such as hypoechogenicity, microcalcifications, irregular margins, and intranodular vascularity.[112] Fine-needle aspiration is a reliable, safe procedure and should be performed in all solid thyroid nodules greater than or equal to 10 mm in size to establish a diagnosis, regardless of the gestational age of the fetus.[36,95,113,114] Current guidelines by the ATA, American Association of Clinical Endocrinologists, Associazione Medici Endocrinologi, and European Thyroid Association recommend fine-needle aspiration of lesions as small as 5 mm if suspicious ultrasound features are present or if a patient has a family history of thyroid malignancy, as thyroid cancer prevalence is similar in nodules both smaller and larger than 10 mm.[110,112–115] Further management depends on the fine-needle aspiration result; benign lesions may be followed for growth over time with possible repeat aspiration, unsatisfactory samples require a repeat fine-needle aspiration, and thyroid surgery is recommended for cases of malignancy.[95,110,116] It is not clear whether these guidelines are directly relevant to the pregnant population, but it seems reasonable at present to also apply them to pregnant women. Follicular and Hürthle cell neoplasms present a clinical challenge because a definite cytologic diagnosis cannot be made, therefore there is a degree of uncertainty as to their malignant potential.[117] In addition, a physiologic increase in thyroid follicular epithelium in pregnancy may result in a false-positive diagnosis of follicular neoplasm, so surgical decisions should be seriously considered and, when appropriate, postponed to the postpartum period.[110] Treatment with exogenous levothyroxine is used in patients with known differentiated thyroid cancer to suppress TSH. Thyroid hormone suppression, although having some efficacy in reducing thyroid nodule volume[118] and new nodule growth,[119] is not recommended for use, especially in pregnant women, because of limited efficacy[118] and adverse cardiovascular[35] and bone density effects.[120] In pregnancy, the timing of thyroid surgery requires assessment of risks and benefits (see the next section). Radioactive iodine use for scintigraphy and radioactive iodine treatment is contraindicated in pregnancy, and should not be used within several months of a patient desiring to become pregnant or in breastfeeding or lactating women.[110] The ACR stresses that breastfeeding should be discontinued before radioactive iodine therapy and should not be resumed until subsequent pregnancy. Furthermore, lactating women should not undergo treatment, even if not breastfeeding, for at least 3 months after lactation ceases because a significant amount of I-131 trapping occurs in the lactating breast, resulting in a radiation dose to the patient's breasts.[68]

THYROID CANCER

Although thyroid cancer is infrequent in the general population, it is the most likely malignancy to occur in women of reproductive age between 15 and 44 years, with a prevalence of 3.6 to 14 per 100,000 live births.[121–123] It is controversial whether pregnancy accelerates progression of thyroid cancer. Some studies report increased thyroid nodule growth throughout gestation,[124] with a higher incidence of thyroid cancer,[125] a weak association between thyroid cancer and parity,[126] and endogenous estrogen as well as the presence of estrogen-binding activity in neoplastic thyroid tissue.[127] However, the prognosis of differentiated thyroid carcinoma (DTC) is excellent in young individuals younger than 40 years,[98,128,129] and survival in pregnant women may not differ from their nonpregnant, age-matched counterparts with similar cancer.[122,124] A sample of 29 women with DTC diagnosed and treated prior to pregnancy were followed throughout gestation on levothyroxine suppression until 12 to 84 months after delivery, without a significant effect on the disease-free period.[123] Moosa and Mazzaferri[122] reported similar long-term outcomes in 61 women with a diagnosis of DTC in pregnancy, in comparison with 528 female, age-matched, nonpregnant controls with DTC at a median follow-up of 22.4 and 19.5 years, respectively. The most common presentation in pregnancy was a single, asymptomatic thyroid nodule with a mean size of 2.1 cm; only 13% (n = 4) of women had local tumor invasion at surgery, but 41% (n = 25) had metastatic lymph nodes and 2% (n = 1) had distant metastases at presentation. Most of the pregnant women (77%, n = 47) underwent thyroidectomy after delivery, and 30% (n = 18) had thyroid remnant ablation with radioactive I-131; the control group treatment also consisted of surgery and I-131 treatment in selected patients, without statistical differences compared with the pregnant cohort. The time from discovery of the thyroid nodule to treatment was 12.7 months (95% CI 7.9–17.4) in pregnant women compared with 10.8 months (95% CI 8.8–12.7) in the control group. Cancer recurred in 15% (n = 9) of pregnant women as compared with 23% (n = 115) of nonpregnant controls, distant site metastasis was found in 2% versus 3% in the respective groups, and no cancer deaths occurred in pregnancy, yet 1% (n = 6) of women in the control group died of thyroid cancer. The investigators concluded that in most pregnant women diagnostic studies and treatment of thyroid cancer may be delayed until after delivery, especially if the cancer is well differentiated and there is no evidence of advanced disease.[36,105,122] Although thyroidectomy is generally a safe procedure, it is not without its risks; pregnant patients have been reported to have a twofold higher rate of endocrine and general complications after thyroid surgery when compared with nonpregnant individuals.[130] Thyroid surgery, when indicated, should be performed in the second trimester if the diagnosis of thyroid cancer occurs early in pregnancy, the disease is advanced, or there is rapid growth, although the decision to operate during pregnancy should be individualized.[36,114,131] Surgery should be performed by an experienced team. However, there are data to suggest that delaying treatment for more than 1 year, which can occur if the mother chooses to postpone diagnostic scans and radioactive iodine therapy in favor of breastfeeding, may increase mortality due to thyroid cancer from 4% to 10%.[124,129] Levothyroxine treatment is recommended in women with previously treated thyroid carcinoma and in women who have a positive or suspicious fine-needle aspirate for malignancy but who delay surgery until postpartum.[36] The degree of TSH suppression is controversial, as it should also be noted that the normal TSH reference range during pregnancy is altered, generally being approximately 0.1 to 2.5 μU/mL in the first trimester and approximately 0.1 to 3.0 μU/mL in the second and third trimester.[132] Although controversial, the TSH should probably be in the range of 0.1 to 0.5 μU/mL during pregnancy in patients with a positive or suspicious thyroid fine-needle aspirate who are not going to undergo thyroidectomy during pregnancy.

SUMMARY

Normal thyroid function is essential in pregnancy to avoid complications in gestation and to ensure delivery, to the best extent possible, of a healthy baby. Women with hypothyroidism and/or thyroid antibodies are at increased risk of miscarriage. Low thyroid hormone levels during pregnancy can have detrimental effects on the development of the fetal central nervous system, and predispose to preterm delivery and spontaneous pregnancy loss. An iodine intake of at least 250 μg per day is recommended in pregnant and lactating women. Screening for thyroid dysfunction should be performed in women who are at high risk for thyroid disease. Interpretation of thyroid function testing ought to use trimester-specific ranges. Treatment of hypothyroidism should target a TSH of 2.5 μU/mL or less in the first trimester and less than 3.0 μU/mL in the second and third trimesters. It is important to anticipate that levothyroxine requirements will increase, especially early in gestation, and decrease after delivery. Monitoring of thyroid function may be as frequent as every 2 to 4 weeks until midgestation and 4 to 8 weeks in the second half of pregnancy. Hyperthyroidism in pregnancy is much less common than hypothyroidism. It is important to distinguish Graves' disease from gestational transient thyrotoxicosis, as the latter may be self-limiting. ATDs, specifically PTU, are recommended for treatment of hyperthyroidism in the first 12 weeks of pregnancy to avoid congenital defects associated with MMI; however, because of an increased risk of liver failure with PTU, MMI should be used after the first trimester. Radioactive iodine is contraindicated in pregnancy, because of the adverse complication of neonatal hypothyroidism and subsequent cognitive impairment as well as fetal death. In addition, breastfeeding and lactating women should not receive I-131 treatment to avoid radiation exposure to the lactating breast, which traps iodine, for at least 3 months after lactation is discontinued. Thyroidectomy, if needed, should usually be performed in the second trimester of pregnancy. Fetal monitoring is imperative if the mother is receiving treatment for hyperthyroidism, and may include fetal thyroid ultrasonography and, rarely, cordocentesis for thyroid hormone measurements. Cautious adjustment of medication dosing to maintain maternal free T4 in the upper nonpregnant reference range is necessary. After delivery, neonates whose mothers have TRAb positivity are at risk of neonatal hyperthyroidism, and the mother may experience a recurrence of Graves' disease postpartum. Breastfeeding is considered safe during treatment with levothyroxine and antithyroid agents. Postpartum thyroiditis is strongly associated with TPO-Ab positivity and incurs a higher risk of permanent hypothyroidism in the mother. It is important to assess thyroid nodules in pregnancy with fine-needle aspiration of the thyroid. If a diagnosis of thyroid carcinoma is made in pregnancy the prognosis is usually good, and typically diagnostic studies and treatment may be delayed until after delivery as long as there are no compelling signs or symptoms to suggest an aggressive tumor. The decision to perform thyroidectomy in pregnancy should be individualized. Cautious treatment with levothyroxine to a goal TSH of 0.1 to 0.5 μU/mL is recommended for any pregnant woman with thyroid cancer or a fine-needle aspiration of the thyroid that is suspicious for malignancy.[1,8,100]

REFERENCES

1. Williams GR. Neurodevelopmental and neurophysiological actions of thyroid hormone. J Neuroendocrinol 2008;20(6):784–94.
2. Glinoer D. The regulation of thyroid function in pregnancy: pathways of endocrine adaptation from physiology to pathology. Endocr Rev 1997;18(3):404–33.
3. Burrow GN, Fisher DA, Larsen PR. Maternal and fetal thyroid function. N Engl J Med 1994;331(16):1072–8.
4. Celi F. Thyroid physiology and drugs affecting thyroid function. Paper presented at: A Review of Endocrinology: Diagnosis & Treatment. Bethesda (MD), October 12, 2010.
5. Calvo RM, Jauniaux E, Gulbis B, et al. Fetal tissues are exposed to biologically relevant free thyroxine concentrations during early phases of development. J Clin Endocrinol Metab 2002;87(4):1768–77.
6. Burman KD, Read J, Dimond RC, et al. Measurement of 3,3',5'-triiodothyroinine (reverse T3), 3,3'-L-diiodothyronine, T3 and T4 in human amniotic fluid and in cord and maternal serum. J Clin Endocrinol Metab 1976;43(6):1351–9.

7. Contempre B, Jauniaux E, Calvo R, et al. Detection of thyroid hormones in human embryonic cavities during the first trimester of pregnancy. J Clin Endocrinol Metab 1993;77(6):1719–22.
8. Vulsma T, Gons MH, de Vijlder JJ. Maternal-fetal transfer of thyroxine in congenital hypothyroidism due to a total organification defect or thyroid agenesis. N Engl J Med 1989;321(1):13–6.
9. Yassa L, Marqusee E, Fawcett R, et al. Thyroid Hormone Early Adjustment in Pregnancy (the THERAPY) trial. J Clin Endocrinol Metab 2010;95:3234–41.
10. Alexander EK, Marqusee E, Lawrence J, et al. Timing and magnitude of increases in levothyroxine requirements during pregnancy in women with hypothyroidism. N Engl J Med 2004;351(3):241–9.
11. Auso E, Lavado-Autric R, Cuevas E, et al. A moderate and transient deficiency of maternal thyroid function at the beginning of fetal neocorticogenesis alters neuronal migration. Endocrinology 2004;145(9):4037–47.
12. Morte B, Diez D, Auso E, et al. Thyroid hormone regulation of gene expression in the developing rat fetal cerebral cortex: prominent role of the Ca^{2+}/calmodulin-dependent protein kinase IV pathway. Endocrinology 2010;151(2):810–20.
13. Liu D, Teng W, Shan Z, et al. The effect of maternal subclinical hypothyroidism during pregnancy on brain development in rat offspring. Thyroid 2010;20(8):909–15.
14. Ahmed OM, Abd El-Tawab SM, Ahmed RG. Effects of experimentally induced maternal hypothyroidism and hyperthyroidism on the development of rat offspring: I. The development of the thyroid hormones-neurotransmitters and adenosinergic system interactions. Int J Dev Neurosci 2010;28(6):437–54.
15. Sinha RA, Pathak A, Kumar A, et al. Enhanced neuronal loss under perinatal hypothyroidism involves impaired neurotrophic signaling and increased proteolysis of p75(NTR). Mol Cell Neurosci 2009;40(3):354–64.
16. Fisher DA, Klein AH. Thyroid development and disorders of thyroid function in the newborn. N Engl J Med 1981;304(12):702–12.
17. Pop VJ, Brouwers EP, Vader HL, et al. Maternal hypothyroxinaemia during early pregnancy and subsequent child development: a 3-year follow-up study. Clin Endocrinol (Oxf) 2003;59(3):282–8.
18. Li Y, Shan Z, Teng W, et al. Abnormalities of maternal thyroid function during pregnancy affect neuropsychological development of their children at 25-30 months. Clin Endocrinol (Oxf) 2010;72(6):825–9.
19. Aoki Y, Belin RM, Clickner R, et al. Serum TSH and total T4 in the United States population and their association with participant characteristics: National Health and Nutrition Examination Survey (NHANES 1999-2002). Thyroid 2007;17(12):1211–23.
20. Klein RZ, Haddow JE, Faix JD, et al. Prevalence of thyroid deficiency in pregnant women. Clin Endocrinol (Oxf) 1991;35(1):41–6.
21. Vaidya B, Anthony S, Bilous M, et al. Detection of thyroid dysfunction in early pregnancy: universal screening or targeted high-risk case finding? J Clin Endocrinol Metab 2007;92(1):203–7.
22. Moleti M, Lo Presti VP, Mattina F, et al. Gestational thyroid function abnormalities in conditions of mild iodine deficiency: early screening versus continuous monitoring of maternal thyroid status. Eur J Endocrinol 2009;160(4):611–7.
23. Stagnaro-Green A, Roman SH, Cobin RH, et al. Detection of at-risk pregnancy by means of highly sensitive assays for thyroid autoantibodies. JAMA 1990;264(11):1422–5.
24. Negro R, Formoso G, Mangieri T, et al. Levothyroxine treatment in euthyroid pregnant women with autoimmune thyroid disease: effects on obstetrical complications. J Clin Endocrinol Metab 2006;91(7):2587–91.

25. Glinoer D, Riahi M, Grun JP, et al. Risk of subclinical hypothyroidism in pregnant women with asymptomatic autoimmune thyroid disorders. J Clin Endocrinol Metab 1994;79(1):197–204.

26. Mannisto T, Vaarasmaki M, Pouta A, et al. Thyroid dysfunction and autoantibodies during pregnancy as predictive factors of pregnancy complications and maternal morbidity in later life. J Clin Endocrinol Metab 2010;95(3): 1084–94.

27. Allan WC, Haddow JE, Palomaki GE, et al. Maternal thyroid deficiency and pregnancy complications: implications for population screening. J Med Screen 2000; 7(3):127–30.

28. Casey BM, Dashe JS, Wells CE, et al. Subclinical hypothyroidism and pregnancy outcomes. Obstet Gynecol 2005;105(2):239–45.

29. Negro R, Schwartz A, Gismondi R, et al. Increased pregnancy loss rate in thyroid antibody negative women with TSH levels between 2.5 and 5.0 in the first trimester of pregnancy. J Clin Endocrinol Metab 2010;95(9):E44–8.

30. Haddow JE, Palomaki GE, Allan WC, et al. Maternal thyroid deficiency during pregnancy and subsequent neuropsychological development of the child. N Engl J Med 1999;341(8):549–55.

31. Alvarez-Pedrerol M, Guxens M, Mendez M, et al. Iodine levels and thyroid hormones in healthy pregnant women and birth weight of their offspring. Eur J Endocrinol 2009;160(3):423–9.

32. de Escobar GM, Obregon MJ, del Rey FE. Maternal thyroid hormones early in pregnancy and fetal brain development. Best Pract Res Clin Endocrinol Metab 2004;18(2):225–48.

33. Andersson M, de Benoist B, Delange F, et al. Prevention and control of iodine deficiency in pregnant and lactating women and in children less than 2-years-old: conclusions and recommendations of the Technical Consultation. Public Health Nutr 2007;10(12A):1606–11.

34. Becker DV, Braverman LE, Delange F, et al. Iodine supplementation for pregnancy and lactation-United States and Canada: recommendations of the American Thyroid Association. Thyroid 2006;16(10):949–51.

35. Surks MI, Ortiz E, Daniels GH, et al. Subclinical thyroid disease: scientific review and guidelines for diagnosis and management. JAMA 2004;291(2):228–38.

36. Abalovich M, Amino N, Barbour LA, et al. Management of thyroid dysfunction during pregnancy and postpartum: an Endocrine Society Clinical Practice Guideline. J Clin Endocrinol Metab 2007;92(Suppl 8):S1–47.

37. Negro R, Schwartz A, Gismondi R, et al. Universal screening versus case finding for detection and treatment of thyroid hormonal dysfunction during pregnancy. J Clin Endocrinol Metab 2010;95(4):1699–707.

38. Lazarus J. Pregnancy and thyroid diseases. Paper presented at: The 14th International Thyroid Congress. Paris, September 11-16, 2010.

39. Roti E, Gardini E, Minelli R, et al. Thyroid function evaluation by different commercially available free thyroid hormone measurement kits in term pregnant women and their newborns. J Endocrinol Invest 1991;14(1):1–9.

40. Baloch Z, Carayon P, Conte-Devolx B, et al. Laboratory medicine practice guidelines. Laboratory support for the diagnosis and monitoring of thyroid disease. Thyroid 2003;13(1):3–126.

41. Mandel SJ, Spencer CA, Hollowell JG. Are detection and treatment of thyroid insufficiency in pregnancy feasible? Thyroid 2005;15(1):44–53.

42. Glinoer D, Spencer CA. Serum TSH determinations in pregnancy: how, when and why? Nat Rev Endocrinol 2010;6(9):526–9.

43. Loh JA, Wartofsky L, Jonklaas J, et al. The magnitude of increased levothyroxine requirements in hypothyroid pregnant women depends upon the etiology of the hypothyroidism. Thyroid 2009;19(3):269–75.
44. Lazarus JH, Premawardhana LD. Screening for thyroid disease in pregnancy. J Clin Pathol 2005;58(5):449–52.
45. Innerfield R, Hollander CS. Thyroidal complications of pregnancy. Med Clin North Am 1977;61(1):67–87.
46. Tamaki H, Itoh E, Kaneda T, et al. Crucial role of serum human chorionic gonadotropin for the aggravation of thyrotoxicosis in early pregnancy in Graves' disease. Thyroid 1993;3(3):189–93.
47. Rotondi M, Cappelli C, Pirali B, et al. The effect of pregnancy on subsequent relapse from Graves' disease after a successful course of antithyroid drug therapy. J Clin Endocrinol Metab 2008;93(10):3985–8.
48. Glinoer D. The thyroid in pregnancy: the European perspective. Thyroid Today 1995;18:1–11.
49. Kosugi S, Mori T. TSH receptor and LH receptor, 1995. Endocr J 1995;42(5): 587–606.
50. Tsuruta E, Tada H, Tamaki H, et al. Pathogenic role of asialo human chorionic gonadotropin in gestational thyrotoxicosis. J Clin Endocrinol Metab 1995; 80(2):350–5.
51. Monson K, Schoenstadt A. Beta blockers and pregnancy. eMedTV. Available at: http://senior-health.emedtv.com/beta-blockers/beta-blockers-and-pregnancy. html. Accessed October 31, 2010.
52. Davis RL, Eastman D, McPhillips H, et al. Risks of congenital malformations and perinatal events among infants exposed to calcium channel and beta-blockers during pregnancy. Pharmacoepidemiol Drug Saf 2011;20(2):138–45.
53. Hershman JM. Human chorionic gonadotropin and the thyroid: hyperemesis gravidarum and trophoblastic tumors. Thyroid 1999;9(7):653–7.
54. Goodwin TM, Montoro M, Mestman JH, et al. The role of chorionic gonadotropin in transient hyperthyroidism of hyperemesis gravidarum. J Clin Endocrinol Metab 1992;75(5):1333–7.
55. Luewan S, Chakkabut P, Tongsong T. Outcomes of pregnancy complicated with hyperthyroidism: a cohort study. Arch Gynecol Obstet 2011;283(2):243–7.
56. Davis LE, Lucas MJ, Hankins GD, et al. Thyrotoxicosis complicating pregnancy. Am J Obstet Gynecol 1989;160(1):63–70.
57. Pillar N, Levy A, Holcberg G, et al. Pregnancy and perinatal outcome in women with hyperthyroidism. Int J Gynaecol Obstet 2010;108(1):61–4.
58. Donovan L, Parkins VM, Mahalingham A. Thyrotoxic periodic paralysis in pregnancy with impaired glucose tolerance: a case report and discussion of management issues. Thyroid 2007;17(6):579–83.
59. Anselmo J, Cao D, Karrison T, et al. Fetal loss associated with excess thyroid hormone exposure. JAMA 2004;292(6):691–5.
60. Bánhidy F, Puhó EH, Czeizel AE. Possible association between hyperthyroidism in pregnant women and obstructive congenital abnormalities of urinary tract in their offspring—a population-based case-control study. J Matern Fetal Neonatal Med 2011;24(2):305–12.
61. Casey BM, Dashe JS, Wells CE, et al. Subclinical hyperthyroidism and pregnancy outcomes. Obstet Gynecol 2006;107(2 Pt 1):337–41.
62. Evans IM, Pickard MR, Sinha AK, et al. Influence of maternal hyperthyroidism in the rat on the expression of neuronal and astrocytic cytoskeletal proteins in fetal brain. J Endocrinol 2002;175(3):597–604.

63. Chen C, Zhou Z, Zhong M, et al. Excess thyroid hormone inhibits embryonic neural stem/progenitor cells proliferation and maintenance through STAT3 signalling pathway. Neurotox Res 2011;20(1):15–25.

64. Tran P, Desimone S, Barrett M, et al. I-131 treatment of graves' disease in an unsuspected first trimester pregnancy; the potential for adverse effects on the fetus and a review of the current guidelines for pregnancy screening. Int J Pediatr Endocrinol 2010;2010:858359.

65. Berg G, Jacobsson L, Nystrom E, et al. Consequences of inadvertent radioiodine treatment of Graves' disease and thyroid cancer in undiagnosed pregnancy. Can we rely on routine pregnancy testing? Acta Oncol 2008;47(1):145–9.

66. Stoffer SS, Hamburger JI. Inadvertent ^{131}I therapy for hyperthyroidism in the first trimester of pregnancy. J Nucl Med 1976;17(02):146–9.

67. Hatch M, Brenner A, Bogdanova T, et al. A screening study of thyroid cancer and other thyroid diseases among individuals exposed in utero to iodine-131 from Chernobyl fallout. J Clin Endocrinol Metab 2009;94(3):899–906.

68. Practice guideline for the performance of therapy with unsealed radiopharmaceutical sources. ACR; 2010. Available at: http://www.acr.org/SecondaryMainMenuCategories/quality_safety/guidelines/nuc_med/unsealed_radiopharmaceuticals.aspx. Accessed October 31, 2010.

69. Basbug M, Ozgun MT, Murat N, et al. Prenatal diagnosis of fetal hypothyroidism after maternal radioactive iodine exposure during pregnancy. J Clin Ultrasound 2010;38(9):506–8.

70. Gardner DF, Cruikshank DP, Hays PM, et al. Pharmacology of propylthiouracil (PTU) in pregnant hyperthyroid women: correlation of maternal PTU concentrations with cord serum thyroid function tests. J Clin Endocrinol Metab 1986;62(1):217–20.

71. Mortimer RH, Cannell GR, Addison RS, et al. Methimazole and propylthiouracil equally cross the perfused human term placental lobule. J Clin Endocrinol Metab 1997;82(9):3099–102.

72. Cooper DS. Antithyroid drugs. N Engl J Med 2005;352(9):905–17.

73. Cooper DS, Rivkees SA. Putting propylthiouracil in perspective. J Clin Endocrinol Metab 2009;94(6):1881–2.

74. Rivkees SA, Mattison DR. Propylthiouracil (PTU) hepatotoxicity in children and recommendations for discontinuation of use. Int J Pediatr Endocrinol 2009;2009:132041.

75. Russo MW, Galanko JA, Shrestha R, et al. Liver transplantation for acute liver failure from drug induced liver injury in the United States. Liver Transpl 2004;10(8):1018–23.

76. Burch HS. ATA-AACE Hyperthyroidism guidelines 2010. A review of endocrinology: diagnosis & treatment. Lecture at the Endocrinology Board Review Course. FAES (The Foundation for Advanced Education in the Sciences, Inc. at the National Institutes of Health and The George Washington University Medical Center). Bethesda (MD), October 12, 2010.

77. Barbero P, Valdez R, Rodriguez H, et al. Choanal atresia associated with maternal hyperthyroidism treated with methimazole: a case-control study. Am J Med Genet A 2008;146(18):2390–5.

78. Clementi M, Di Gianantonio E, Cassina M, et al. Treatment of hyperthyroidism in pregnancy and birth defects. J Clin Endocrinol Metab 2010;95(11):E337–41.

79. Mandel SJ, Brent GA, Larsen PR. Review of antithyroid drug use during pregnancy and report of a case of aplasia cutis. Thyroid 1994;4(1):129–33.

80. Kempers MJ, van Trotsenburg AS, van Rijn RR, et al. Loss of integrity of thyroid morphology and function in children born to mothers with inadequately treated Graves' disease. J Clin Endocrinol Metab 2007;92(8):2984–91.
81. Papendieck P, Chiesa A, Prieto L, et al. Thyroid disorders of neonates born to mothers with graves' disease. J Pediatr Endocrinol Metab 2009;22(6):547–53.
82. Rosenfeld H, Ornoy A, Shechtman S, et al. Pregnancy outcome, thyroid dysfunction and fetal goitre after in utero exposure to propylthiouracil: a controlled cohort study. Br J Clin Pharmacol 2009;68(4):609–17.
83. Momotani N, Noh JY, Ishikawa N, et al. Effects of propylthiouracil and methimazole on fetal thyroid status in mothers with Graves' hyperthyroidism. J Clin Endocrinol Metab 1997;82(11):3633–6.
84. Gruner C, Kollert A, Wildt L, et al. Intrauterine treatment of fetal goitrous hypothyroidism controlled by determination of thyroid-stimulating hormone in fetal serum. A case report and review of the literature. Fetal Diagn Ther 2001; 16(1):47–51.
85. Luton D, Le Gac I, Vuillard E, et al. Management of Graves' disease during pregnancy: the key role of fetal thyroid gland monitoring. J Clin Endocrinol Metab 2005;90(11):6093–8.
86. McKenzie JM, Zakarija M. Fetal and neonatal hyperthyroidism and hypothyroidism due to maternal TSH receptor antibodies. Thyroid 1992;2(2):155–9.
87. Connors MH, Styne DM. Transient neonatal 'athyreosis' resulting from thyrotropin-binding inhibitory immunoglobulins. Pediatrics 1986;78(2):287–90.
88. Eisenstein Z, Weiss M, Katz Y, et al. Intellectual capacity of subjects exposed to methimazole or propylthiouracil in utero. Eur J Pediatr 1992;151(8):558–9.
89. Laurberg P, Bournaud C, Karmisholt J, et al. Management of Graves' hyperthyroidism in pregnancy: focus on both maternal and foetal thyroid function, and caution against surgical thyroidectomy in pregnancy. Eur J Endocrinol 2009; 160(1):1–8.
90. Laurberg P, Nygaard B, Glinoer D, et al. Guidelines for TSH-receptor antibody measurements in pregnancy: results of an evidence-based symposium organized by the European Thyroid Association. Eur J Endocrinol 1998;139(6): 584–6.
91. Zakarija M, McKenzie JM, Munro DS. Immunoglobulin G inhibitor of thyroid-stimulating antibody is a cause of delay in the onset of neonatal Graves' disease. J Clin Invest 1983;72(4):1352–6.
92. Momotani N, Noh J, Oyanagi H, et al. Antithyroid drug therapy for Graves' disease during pregnancy. Optimal regimen for fetal thyroid status. N Engl J Med 1986;315(1):24–8.
93. Bahn RS, Burch HS, Cooper DS, et al. The Role of propylthiouracil in the management of Graves' disease in adults: report of a meeting jointly sponsored by the American Thyroid Association and the Food and Drug Administration. Thyroid 2009;19(7):673–4.
94. Laurberg P, Wallin G, Tallstedt L, et al. TSH-receptor autoimmunity in Graves' disease after therapy with anti-thyroid drugs, surgery, or radioiodine: a 5-year prospective randomized study. Eur J Endocrinol 2008;158(1):69–75.
95. Mandel SJ, Cooper DS. The use of antithyroid drugs in pregnancy and lactation. J Clin Endocrinol Metab 2001;86(6):2354–9.
96. Kampmann JP, Johansen K, Hansen JM, et al. Propylthiouracil in human milk. Revision of a dogma. Lancet 1980;1(8171):736–7.
97. Johansen K, Andersen AN, Kampmann JP, et al. Excretion of methimazole in human milk. Eur J Clin Pharmacol 1982;23(4):339–41.

98. Azizi F, Khoshniat M, Bahrainian M, et al. Thyroid function and intellectual development of infants nursed by mothers taking methimazole. J Clin Endocrinol Metab 2000;85(9):3233–8.

99. Momotani N, Yamashita R, Makino F, et al. Thyroid function in wholly breast-feeding infants whose mothers take high doses of propylthiouracil. Clin Endocrinol (Oxf) 2000;53(2):177–81.

100. Roti E, Uberti E. Post-partum thyroiditis—a clinical update. Eur J Endocrinol 2002;146(3):275–9.

101. Kokandi AA, Parkes AB, Premawardhana LD, et al. Association of postpartum thyroid dysfunction with antepartum hormonal and immunological changes. J Clin Endocrinol Metab 2003;88(3):1126–32.

102. Negro R, Greco G, Mangieri T, et al. The influence of selenium supplementation on postpartum thyroid status in pregnant women with thyroid peroxidase auto-antibodies. J Clin Endocrinol Metab 2007;92(4):1263–8.

103. Premawardhana LD, Parkes AB, Ammari F, et al. Postpartum thyroiditis and long-term thyroid status: prognostic influence of thyroid peroxidase antibodies and ultrasound echogenicity. J Clin Endocrinol Metab 2000;85(1):71–5.

104. Lazarus JH, Ammari F, Oretti R, et al. Clinical aspects of recurrent postpartum thyroiditis. Br J Gen Pract 1997;47(418):305–8.

105. Manetti L, Parkes AB, Lupi I, et al. Serum pituitary antibodies in normal pregnancy and in patients with postpartum thyroiditis: a nested case-control study. Eur J Endocrinol 2008;159(6):805–9.

106. Weetman AP. Insulin-dependent diabetes mellitus and postpartum thyroiditis: an important association. J Clin Endocrinol Metab 1994;79(1):7–9.

107. Kuijpens JL, Vader HL, Drexhage HA, et al. Thyroid peroxidase antibodies during gestation are a marker for subsequent depression postpartum. Eur J Endocrinol 2001;145(5):579–84.

108. Singer PA, Cooper DS, Daniels GH, et al. Treatment guidelines for patients with thyroid nodules and well-differentiated thyroid cancer. American Thyroid Association. Arch Intern Med 1996;156(19):2165–72.

109. Hegedus L. Clinical practice. The thyroid nodule. N Engl J Med 2004;351(17):1764–71.

110. Gharib H, Papini E, Paschke R, et al. American Association of Clinical Endocrinologists, Associazione Medici Endocrinologi, and European Thyroid Association medical guidelines for clinical practice for the diagnosis and management of thyroid nodules. Endocr Pract 2010;16(Suppl 1):1–43.

111. Kung AW, Chau MT, Lao TT, et al. The effect of pregnancy on thyroid nodule formation. J Clin Endocrinol Metab 2002;87(3):1010–4.

112. Papini E, Guglielmi R, Bianchini A, et al. Risk of malignancy in nonpalpable thyroid nodules: predictive value of ultrasound and color-Doppler features. J Clin Endocrinol Metab 2002;87(5):1941–6.

113. Burch HB. Evaluation and management of the solid thyroid nodule. Endocrinol Metab Clin North Am 1995;24(4):663–710.

114. Cooper DS, Doherty GM, Haugen BR, et al. Management guidelines for patients with thyroid nodules and differentiated thyroid cancer. Thyroid 2006;16(2):109–42.

115. Cooper DS, Doherty GM, Haugen BR, et al. Revised American Thyroid Association management guidelines for patients with thyroid nodules and differentiated thyroid cancer. Thyroid 2009;19(11):1167–214.

116. Cobin RH, Gharib H, Bergman DA, et al. AACE/AAES medical/surgical guidelines for clinical practice: management of thyroid carcinoma. American Association of Clinical Endocrinologists. American College of Endocrinology. Endocr Pract 2001;7(3):202–20.

117. Gharib H, Goellner JR, Zinsmeister AR, et al. Fine-needle aspiration biopsy of the thyroid. The problem of suspicious cytologic findings. Ann Intern Med 1984; 101(1):25–8.
118. Castro MR, Caraballo PJ, Morris JC. Effectiveness of thyroid hormone suppressive therapy in benign solitary thyroid nodules: a meta-analysis. J Clin Endocrinol Metab 2002;87(9):4154–9.
119. Papini E, Petrucci L, Guglielmi R, et al. Long-term changes in nodular goiter: a 5-year prospective randomized trial of levothyroxine suppressive therapy for benign cold thyroid nodules. J Clin Endocrinol Metab 1998;83(3):780–3.
120. Uzzan B, Campos J, Cucherat M, et al. Effects on bone mass of long term treatment with thyroid hormones: a meta-analysis. J Clin Endocrinol Metab 1996; 81(12):4278–89.
121. Donegan WL. Cancer and pregnancy. CA Cancer J Clin 1983;33(4):194–214.
122. Moosa M, Mazzaferri EL. Outcome of differentiated thyroid cancer diagnosed in pregnant women. J Clin Endocrinol Metab 1997;82(9):2862–6.
123. Zamperini P, Gibelli B, Gilardi D, et al. Pregnancy and thyroid cancer: ultrasound study of foetal thyroid. Acta Otorhinolaryngol Ital 2009;29(6):339–44.
124. Vini L, Hyer S, Pratt B, et al. Management of differentiated thyroid cancer diagnosed during pregnancy. Eur J Endocrinol 1999;140(5):404–6.
125. Rosen IB, Walfish PG. Pregnancy as a predisposing factor in thyroid neoplasia. Arch Surg 1986;121(11):1287–90.
126. Galanti MR, Lambe M, Ekbom A, et al. Parity and risk of thyroid cancer: a nested case-control study of a nationwide Swedish cohort. Cancer Causes Control 1995;6(1):37–44.
127. Imai Y, Yamakawa M, Matsuda M, et al. Endogenous sex hormone and estrogen binding activity in thyroid cancer. Histol Histopathol 1989;4(1):39–45.
128. Woolner LB, Beahrs OH, Black BM, et al. Classification and prognosis of thyroid carcinoma. A study of 885 cases observed in a thirty year period. Am J Surg 1961;102:354–87.
129. Mazzaferri EL, Jhiang SM. Differentiated thyroid cancer long-term impact of initial therapy. Trans Am Clin Climatol Assoc 1995;106:151–68 [discussion: 168–70].
130. Kuy S, Roman SA, Desai R, et al. Outcomes following thyroid and parathyroid surgery in pregnant women. Arch Surg 2009;144(5):399–406 [discussion: 406].
131. Choe W, McDougall IR. Thyroid cancer in pregnant women: diagnostic and therapeutic management. Thyroid 1994;4(4):433–5.
132. Panesar NS, Li CY, Rogers MS. Reference intervals for thyroid hormones in pregnant Chinese women. Ann Clin Biochem 2001;38(Pt 4):329–32.

Iodine Nutrition in Pregnancy and Lactation

Angela M. Leung, MD, MSc, Elizabeth N. Pearce, MD, MSc*,
Lewis E. Braverman, MD

KEYWORDS

• Iodine • Pregnancy • Lactation

IODINE PHYSIOLOGY DURING PREGNANCY

Beginning in early gestation, maternal thyroid hormone production normally increases by approximately 50% in response to increased levels of serum thyroxine-binding globulin (resulting from the increase in estrogen levels) and because of stimulation of thyrotropin (TSH) receptors by human chorionic gonadotropin.[1] The placenta is a rich source of the type 3 inner ring deiodinase, which enhances the degradation of thyroxine (T_4) to bioactive reverse triiodothyronine (T_3).[2] Thus, thyroid hormone demand increases, which requires an adequate iodine supply that is obtained primarily from the diet and/or as supplemental iodine (**Fig. 1**). In addition, fetal thyroid hormone production increases during the second half of pregnancy, further contributing to increased maternal iodine requirements because iodide readily crosses the placenta.

After oral ingestion, iodide is rapidly absorbed through the stomach and duodenum.[3] Iodide, in its pure form, is 100% bioavailable and fully absorbed. Plasma inorganic iodide is then transported through the circulation to be either taken up by the thyroid in varying amounts (5%–100% of absorbed iodine), depending on the iodine supply and the functional state of the thyroid,[3] or it is renally excreted. The normal thyroid gland contains approximately 15 g of iodine.[4] The inability to compensate for the increased iodine demand of pregnancy is associated with the development of maternal goiter due to TSH stimulation.[5]

The primary route of iodine excretion is through the kidney,[6] which accounts for more than 90% of ingested iodine.[3] Beginning in early pregnancy, the glomerular filtration rate of iodide increases by 30% to 50%,[1] thereby further decreasing the

All authors have nothing to disclose.

Section of Endocrinology, Diabetes, and Nutrition, Boston University School of Medicine, Boston, MA, USA

* Corresponding author. Section of Endocrinology, Diabetes, and Nutrition, Boston University School of Medicine, 88 East Newton Street, Evans 201, Boston, MA 02118.

E-mail address: elizabeth.pearce@bmc.org

doi:10.1016/j.ecl.2011.08.001
0889-8529/11/$ – see front matter © 2011 Elsevier Inc. All rights reserved.
endo.theclinics.com

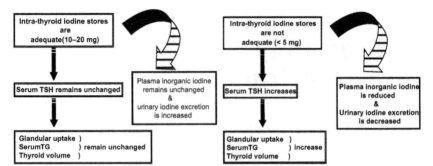

Fig. 1. Conceptual models of adequate (*left panel*) and inadequate (*right panel*) iodine nutrition and thyroid function. (*Adapted from* Glinoer D. The importance of iodine nutrition during pregnancy. Public Health Nutr 2007;10(12A):1543; with permission.)

circulating pool of plasma iodine.[7] Stilwell and colleagues[8] reported that median urinary iodine levels in Tasmania, a region of mild iodine deficiency, decline after the elevated excretion seen in early pregnancy. A comparison of pregnant women from various countries demonstrated that peak gestational urinary iodine levels vary, thus suggesting differences in renal excretion thresholds by regional dietary iodine intake.[9]

Because of increased thyroid hormone production, increased renal iodine losses, and fetal iodine requirements in pregnancy, dietary iodine requirements are higher in pregnant adults than in nonpregnant adults.[10] Guidelines for daily dietary iodine intake of pregnant women, based on several studies that assessed the effect of iodine supplementation on maternal thyroid volume,[11] indicate a higher iodine requirement in these women than that for nonpregnant nonlactating adolescents and adults (**Table 1**).

METHODS TO ASSESS IODINE SUFFICIENCY

There are several accepted methods used in the monitoring of population iodine sufficiency.[11] Median spot urinary iodine concentrations (as a biomarker for dietary iodine intake)[12] reflect iodine intake over the recent few days. Thresholds for median urinary iodine sufficiency have been identified for populations but not for individuals, given significant day-to-day variation of iodine intake.[13] As shown in **Table 2**, population iodine sufficiency is defined by median urinary iodine concentrations of 100 μg/L or more in nonpregnant women and children younger than 2 years and 150 μg/L or more in pregnant women.[14]

Table 1			
Guidelines for daily dietary iodine intake			
Institute	**Nonpregnant Nonlactating Adolescents and Adults (μg)**	**Pregnant Women (μg)**	**Lactating Women (μg)**
Institute of Medicine[48]	150	220	290
WHO, UNICEF, ICCIDD[15]	150	250	250
Endocrine Society[89]	—	250	250

Table 2
Thresholds for population iodine sufficiency based on median urinary iodine concentrations

	Pregnancy (μg/L)	Lactation (μg/L)	Children Younger Than 2 Y (μg/L)
Insufficient	<150	<100	<100
Adequate	≥150	≥100	≥100

Data from Li M, Eastman CJ. Neonatal TSH screening: is it a sensitive and reliable tool for monitoring iodine status in populations? Best Pract Res Clin Endocrinol Metab 2010;24(1):63–75.

Serum levels of TSH and thyroglobulin increase over weeks to months of iodine deficiency, although these concentrations often remain in the normal range and are thus not a good measure of mild iodine deficiency. The World Health Organization (WHO) guideline of using the upper limit (3%) of neonatal TSH values of more than 5 mIU/L has been regarded as one method to define population iodine sufficiency, although it has been suggested to be unreliable.[15] Goiter size, assessed by palpation or ultrasonography, is used to assess long-term iodine sufficiency. The WHO has established international reference ranges for serum thyroglobulin and thyroid gland volumes to be used in the monitoring of iodine deficiency in school-aged children.[16,17]

IMPORTANCE OF ADEQUATE IODINE NUTRITION

Consequences of iodine deficiency include endemic goiter, cretinism, intellectual impairments, growth retardation, neonatal hypothyroidism, and increased pregnancy loss and infant mortality,[18] many of which were recognized beginning in the 1970s by Pharoah and colleagues[19] in Papua New Guinea. Research since then has shown that thyroid hormone plays a particularly vital role in fetal and infant neurodevelopment in in utero and in early life because it is required for oligodendrocyte differentiation and myelin distribution.[20] Animal studies have demonstrated that low levels of thyroid hormone in early pregnancy up to midgestation, when the developing fetus is completely reliant on maternal thyroid hormone stores, impair radial migration of neurons to the cortex and hippocampus and result in behavior changes.[21]

Insufficient iodine levels during pregnancy and the immediate postpartum period result in neurologic and psychological deficits in children.[22,23] The prevalence of attention deficit and hyperactivity disorders is higher in the offspring of women living in iodine-deficient areas than those in iodine-replete regions.[24] Intelligence quotient (IQ) levels of children living in severely iodine-deficient areas are an average of 12.45 points lower than those living in iodine-sufficient areas and are improved with iodine supplementation.[25] In Spain, a region of mild iodine deficiency, children with urinary iodine levels more than 100 μg/L have significantly higher IQ levels than those with urinary iodine levels less than this threshold.[26] Although public health efforts have improved iodine nutrition over the past few decades, iodine deficiency affects more than 2.2 billion individuals (38% of the world's population)[27] and remains the leading cause of preventable mental retardation worldwide.[14]

IODINE SUPPLEMENTATION DURING PREGNANCY

Many studies have established the benefits of iodine supplementation during pregnancy in areas of severe iodine deficiency.[28] One of the earliest studies was a randomized controlled trial during the early 1970s in Papua New Guinea, in which pregnant women living in the remote highlands were administered injections of Lipiodol, a solution of iodinated poppy seed oil, and found to have decreased rates of fetal death and endemic cretinism for up to 5 years compared with untreated women.[19]

There have been 6 controlled trials to assess the effects of iodine supplementation during pregnancy in several moderately iodine-deficient European regions. In Italy, 18 iodine-untreated women had larger thyroid volumes than 17 women who received 120 to 180 µg/d of iodine beginning during the first trimester.[29] Investigators in Denmark reported that iodine-treated women have decreased maternal TSH levels compared with women who received no supplementation.[30,31] Among 180 pregnant women in Belgium, the infants of those who received 100 µg/d potassium iodide had decreased thyroid volumes.[32] Liesenkotter and colleagues[33] reported similar findings among the infants of 38 pregnant women in Germany who received 300 µg/d potassium iodide starting at 10 to 12 weeks' gestation. In contrast, Antonangeli and colleagues[34] reported that there were no differences in maternal thyroid function or thyroid gland size between 86 iodine-supplemented and iodine-unsupplemented women.

In a mildly iodine-deficient area of Italy, consumption of iodized salt in the 24 months preceding pregnancy, compared with initiation of iodized salt ingestion on becoming pregnant, decreased the risk of maternal thyroid dysfunction in women with negative thyroid antibody titers.[35] In the only 2 studies of iodine supplementation in mildly and moderately iodine-deficient women evaluating neurobehavioral outcomes, infants born to mothers who received iodine during pregnancy had improved psychological and neurocognitive measures compared with those born to nonsupplemented mothers. Berbel and colleagues[36] reported that children of women who were both mildly hypothyroxinemic from a mildly iodine-deficient region and supplemented with 200 µg potassium iodide per day beginning at 12 to 14 gestational weeks compared with women who received no supplementation had delayed neurocognitive performance at 18 months of age compared with children of women who received supplementation at 4 to 6 gestational weeks. Similarly, Velasco and colleagues[37] found that infants aged 3 to 18 months of mildly iodine-deficient mothers who received 300 µg potassium iodide per day during the first trimester had higher neuropsychological assessment scores than those of mothers who received no iodine supplementation.

CONSEQUENCES OF HYPOTHYROIDISM IN PREGNANCY

Maternal hypothyroidism, as characterized by elevated TSH levels, occurs in an estimated 2.5% of all pregnancies in the United States.[38] The fetal thyroid does not begin to concentrate iodine until 10 to 12 weeks of gestation and is not controlled by fetal pituitary TSH until approximately 20 weeks of gestation.[39] Before this, the fetus is reliant on maternal T_4 that crosses the placenta in very small quantities.[40]

Because thyroid hormone is required for normal neurodevelopment,[41] even mildly low maternal T_4 and/or elevated maternal serum TSH levels during pregnancy may result in cognitive delays in the offspring. Haddow and colleagues[42] reported that 7- to 9-year-old children whose pregnant mothers had untreated mild hypothyroidism have an average of 7 IQ points lower than those of matched euthyroid control mothers. Subclinical hypothyroidism and low free T_4 concentrations in women during pregnancy are independent predictors of impaired neurodevelopment in their children.[43–47] The most recent study supporting these data was the Dutch Generation R study of 3659 women and their infants, in which severe maternal hypothyroxinemia was associated with both expressive language delay and nonverbal cognitive delay in their infants at 30 months.[47]

IODINE PHYSIOLOGY DURING LACTATION

Thyroidal iodine turnover rate is more rapid in infants.[11] Thus, adequate breast milk iodine levels are particularly important for proper neurodevelopment in nursing infants. Iodine is secreted into breast milk at a concentration gradient 20 to 50 times that of plasma[48] through increased expression of the sodium/iodide symporter (NIS) present on lactating breast cells.[49] In iodine-sufficient areas, breast milk iodine concentrations are generally adequate to meet infants' iodine nutritional needs based on iodine balance studies.[50] Even compensatory mechanisms may not be adequate to meet the increased demands for thyroid hormone production and iodine intake for mothers living in iodine-deficient areas. In a recent study, the iodine needs for breastfed infants in iodine-deficient New Zealand remained inadequate even when their mothers were supplemented with 150 µg/d of iodine during the first 6 postpartum months.[51]

IODINE NUTRITION IN LACTATION

Because breastfed infants are reliant on maternal dietary iodine intake, recommendations for dietary iodine intake during lactation range from 250 to 290 µg/d, higher than the 150 µg/d recommended for nonpregnant and nonlactating adolescents and adults (see **Table 1**). These thresholds were determined based on a mean breast milk iodine concentration of 146 µg/L, as was measured in 37 women in the United States,[52] and the assumption that infants ingest an average of 0.78 L/d of breast milk during 0 to 6 months and 0.60 L/d during 6 to 12 months.[53]

Data regarding breast milk iodine levels in lactating women in the United States are extremely limited. Small studies (57 women in the largest sample)[54] have demonstrated that median breast milk iodine levels in women in the United States range from 35 to 155 µg/L.[52,54–57] Furthermore, breast milk iodine levels vary temporally, as was reported by Kirk and colleagues[56] in a study of 10 lactating women in the United States. Among 108 total samples, there was considerable variation of breast milk iodide levels (which comprises 89%–90% of breast milk iodine [S. Pino, BS, unpublished data, 2004]) within and between individuals over a 3-day period. Larger studies are needed to determine the iodine sufficiency of lactating women in the United States and their breastfed infants.

IODINE NUTRITION IN THE UNITED STATES

Since the 1920s, dietary iodine in the United States has been considered adequate. However, sources of iodine in the US diet have been difficult to identify because there are a wide variety of potential sources and a wide variation in the iodine content of some common foods and food iodine content is not listed on packaging. In the United States, population iodine deficiency has been eliminated by means of silent prophylaxis. Sources of dietary iodine include iodized salt (due to the addition of iodine to table salt as a public health measure), dairy foods (due to the iodophor cleansers of milk cans and teats), and bread dough (due to the use of iodate as bread conditioners in some bakeries).[58]

Results of the Total Diet Studies by the US Food and Drug Administration (FDA) have demonstrated that iodine is found mostly in grain products, milk, and cheese in the United States.[59] Most foods contain 3 to 75 µg of iodine per serving.[53] Based on the most recent US FDA's Total Diet Study, the estimated average daily iodine intake ranges from 138 to 353 µg per person.[60] A survey of more than 700 schoolchildren in the United States during the early 1970s using diet frequency diaries and urinary iodine levels found that milk, iodized salt, and iodated bread were the primary sources of iodine intake.[61] In addition, sources of iodine exposure may include use of iodine-rich medications (such as amiodarone), topical antiseptics, multivitamins, radiographic contrast agents, and water purification tablets.

According to data from the National Health and Nutrition Examination Survey (NHANES), the median urinary iodine concentration in adults in the United States decreased by more than 50% from the early 1970s to the late 1990s (**Fig. 2**).[62] Of particular concern in the NHANES data is that the prevalence of urinary iodine values less than 50 μg/L among women of childbearing age increased by almost 4-fold, from 4% to 15%, during this period. The most recent NHANES survey (2005–2008) demonstrated that 35.3% of pregnant women had urinary iodine levels less than 100 μg/L,[63] which suggests mild iodine sufficiency.[14] Reductions in the US dietary iodine level have been variously ascribed to a possible reduction in the iodine content of dairy products, the removal of iodate dough conditioners in commercially produced bread, new recommendations for reduced salt intake for blood pressure control, and the increasing use of noniodized salt in manufactured or premade convenience foods.[64]

A study of aggregate NHANES data from 2001 to 2006 showed that the included pregnant women in the United States were marginally iodine sufficient (N = 326; median urinary iodine = 153 μg/L) and lactating (N = 53; median urinary iodine = 115 μg/L) and nonpregnant nonlactating women (N = 1,437; median urinary iodine = 130 μg/L) were both iodine deficient.[60] We reported that the median urinary iodine concentration of a sample of 100 women in the Boston area in their first or second trimesters of pregnancy was 149 μg/L, including 9% with values less than 50 μg/L.[65]

PUBLIC HEALTH EFFORTS OF IODINE SUPPLEMENTATION

A public health approach to iodine supplementation in the United States has been advocated. The American Thyroid Association has recommended that women in North America receive dietary supplements containing 150 μg of iodine daily during pregnancy and lactation and that all prenatal vitamins contain 150 μg of iodine.[66] These recommendations have not yet been widely adopted. Only 20.3% of pregnant and 14.5% of lactating women in the United States take a supplement containing iodine, according to the NHANES data.[67] At present, 114 of 223 (51%) brands of prescription and nonprescription prenatal multivitamins marketed in the United States list iodine as a constituent, and many of those which contain iodine do not contain the labeled amount, especially when kelp is the iodine source.[68] The US Women, Infants, and Children Nutrition Program has recommended that all prenatal multivitamins administrated to women in its program contain 150 μg of iodine per daily serving beginning in 2010.

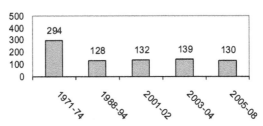

Fig. 2. US dietary iodine in women of childbearing age: NHANES data from 1971 to 2008. (*Data from* Refs.[62,63,88,89])

The major concerns regarding the global burden of iodine deficiency are related to goiter; neurocognitive impairments; and, in severe deficiency, hypothyroidism resulting in cretinism. In 1990, the United Nations World Summit for Children set forth the goal of eliminating iodine deficiency worldwide,[69] and considerable progress has since been achieved. This goal has largely been led by programs of universal salt iodization in various countries, in line with the recommendations by the WHO and the International Council for the Control of Iodine Deficiency Disorders[27,70] and use of oral potassium iodide drops or intramuscular iodized oil injections. Median urinary iodine concentrations of infants residing in iodine-sufficient countries range from 90 to 170 μg/L, which suggests optimal iodine nutrition by criteria as defined by the WHO.[14] Although these efforts have been successful in many countries, the WHO estimates that 2 billion people, including 285 million school-aged children, remain iodine deficient.[71]

The WHO has proposed that an iodine intake of 500 μg/d poses no excessive risk,[14] and the European Food Safety Agency and the US Institute of Medicine have recommended 600 μg/d and 1100 μg/d, respectively, as the tolerable upper limit for iodine per day.[53,72] Thus, although the overall US adult population remains iodine sufficient by WHO standards, a subset of pregnant and lactating women may have inadequate dietary iodine intake.

SUBSTANCES INTERFERING WITH IODINE USE

Competitive inhibitors of NIS, such as perchlorate, thiocyanate, and nitrate, can decrease the entry of iodine into the thyroid and lactating breast, thereby potentially exacerbating the effects of dietary iodine insufficiency. Low-level perchlorate exposure seems to be ubiquitous in the US, European, and South American population. Environmental perchlorate comes from a variety of sources, is extremely stable as an inorganic salt, and persists in low levels in soil and groundwater over long periods.[73] In the United States, perchlorate has been found in many substances, including tobacco, alfalfa, tomato, cow's milk,[55] cucumber, lettuce, soybeans, eggs, and multivitamins (including prenatal multivitamins).[74] Following the development of sensitive detection methods, perchlorate has been measured in the drinking water of communities around the United States.

When given in pharmacologic doses, perchlorate decreases the active transport of iodine into the thyroid and possibly breast milk by competitively inhibiting the NIS with 30 times its affinity for iodide.[75] Furthermore, recent studies in lactating mice have suggested that perchlorate is actively transported into breast milk,[76] thus potentially decreasing infants' thyroidal iodine uptake. In the NHANES 2001 to 2002 survey, perchlorate was detected in all 2820 spot urine samples (median urine perchlorate concentration, 3.6 μg/L) and was a significant negative predictor of total T_4 values and a positive predictor of TSH values in women, primarily those with urine iodine concentrations less than 100 μg/L.[77,78] However, these relationships were not seen in men,[78] a follow-up subset analysis of this dataset (which analyzed only women of childbearing age) using creatinine-adjusted urinary iodine values,[79] or a large European study assessing serum thyroid function tests of iodine-deficient pregnant women.[80] Recently, the US FDA reported in a Total Diet Study that infants and children have the highest estimated intakes of perchlorate by body weight.[81]

There are limited data regarding breast milk iodine[82] and perchlorate concentrations in women in the United States. We reported that the median breast milk iodine concentration in 57 women in Boston area was 155 μg/L,[54] similar to that of a 1984 study of 37 women (178 μg/L).[52] However, the median breast milk iodine levels in our study were far higher than those (33.5, 43.0, and 55.2 μg/L) observed recently by Kirk and colleagues[55,56] in 3 studies.[57] Kirk and colleagues[55] also measured perchlorate levels in the breast milk of 36 women from 18 states and found detectable levels in all the samples (range, 0.6–2.2 μg/L). Breast milk iodide and perchlorate levels were inversely correlated in the 6 samples with perchlorate concentrations of at least 10 μg/L, although there were no correlations between breast milk iodide and perchlorate in the full data set.[55] We reported no correlation between breast milk and colostrum iodine and perchlorate concentrations, even in those breast milk samples with perchlorate concentrations of 10 μg/L or more.[54,83]

Similarly, exposures to thiocyanate, a metabolite of cyanide that is produced as a byproduct of cigarette smoke, and nitrate, which is produced naturally and is present in many prepared foods, are able to decrease NIS activity, thereby decreasing iodine availability. Naturally goitrogenic foods include those that contain cyanogenic glucosides (which become metabolized to thiocyanate), such as cassava, millet, maize, sweet potatoes, lima beans, and cruciferous vegetables (which contain thiocyanates and isothiocyanates), such as cabbage, Brussels sprouts, cauliflower, broccoli, and horseradish.[18] However, the thiocyanate content of these foods is low, and their ingestion does not usually produce clinically significant sequelae unless severe iodine deficiency is present.

One recent study in Denmark concluded that cigarette smoking decreases breast milk iodine concentrations,[84] and we demonstrated the same effect in a small cohort of lactating women in Boston area.[54] Comparatively, perchlorate is a potent inhibitor of NIS; its effects are 15-fold greater than thiocyanate, 30-fold compared with iodide, and 240-fold compared with nitrate.[75] Nonetheless, because exposure to thiocyanate and nitrate is ubiquitous, the additive effects on iodide uptake may be important when assessing iodine availability.

The urinary levels of selenium and iodine in pregnant women are closely correlated.[85] Selenium is an important component of glutathione peroxidase and selonoproteins, which include the 3 thyroid hormone deiodinases. Thus, insufficient selenium may result in the accumulation of damaging peroxides in the thyroid and impair the peripheral deiodination process required to generate the active thyroid hormone, T_3, from T_4. Although selenium nutrition is generally adequate in humans, rare conditions resulting in selenium deficiency may be important in the pathogenesis of hypothyroidism.[86] A recent study by Negro and colleagues[87] reported that selenium supplementation of 200 μg/d during pregnancy and in the postpartum period reduced the prevalence of permanent maternal hypothyroidism (11.7%) compared with women who did not receive supplementation (20.3%) ($P<.01$). The findings of this study are very preliminary, and currently there are no recommendations for selenium supplementation during pregnancy and lactation.

SUMMARY

Adequate iodine nutrition during pregnancy and lactation is needed for thyroid hormone synthesis and normal neurodevelopment of the developing fetus in utero and in the breastfed infant. Iodine deficiency during pregnancy has been associated with impairments of infant neurologic and psychological outcomes. Studies of maternal iodine supplementation in severe iodine deficiency have demonstrated reductions in the rates of fetal death and endemic cretinism. Iodine supplementation in areas of moderate iodine deficiency has shown decreased maternal thyroid volumes and TSH levels and, in areas of mild iodine deficiency, improvements in infants' neurocognitive measures.

Although the overall adult population in the United States remains iodine sufficient in recent national surveys, a subset of pregnant and lactating women may have inadequate dietary iodine intake. A public health approach has been undertaken to achieve recommended median urinary iodine concentrations during pregnancy and lactation. Recent guidelines have recommended that women in the United States take a multivitamin containing 150 μg of iodine during pregnancy and lactation. Further studies are needed to assess the impact of environmental exposures to substances that may interfere with iodine use.

REFERENCES

1. Glinoer D. The importance of iodine nutrition during pregnancy. Public Health Nutr 2007;10(12A):1542–6.
2. Roti E, Fang SL, Emerson CH, et al. Placental inner ring iodothyronine deiodination: a mechanism for decreased passage of T4 and T3 from mother to fetus. Trans Assoc Am Physicians 1981;94:183–9.
3. Zimmermann MB, Jooste PL, Pandav CS. Iodine-deficiency disorders. Lancet 2008;372(9645):1251–62.
4. Fisher DA, Oddie TH. Thyroid iodine content and turnover in euthyroid subjects: validity of estimation of thyroid iodine accumulation from short-term clearance studies. J Clin Endocrinol Metab 1969;29(5):721–7.
5. Smyth PP, Hetherton AM, Smith DF, et al. Maternal iodine status and thyroid volume during pregnancy: correlation with neonatal iodine intake. J Clin Endocrinol Metab 1997;82(9):2840–3.
6. Wayne EJ, Koutras DA, Alexander WD. Excretion of iodine. In: Clinical aspects of iodine metabolism. Philadelphia: Oxford, Blackwell; 1964. p. 73–83.
7. Dafnis E, Sabatini S. The effect of pregnancy on renal function: physiology and pathophysiology. Am J Med Sci 1992;303(3):184–205.
8. Stilwell G, Reynolds PJ, Parameswaran V, et al. The influence of gestational stage on urinary iodine excretion in pregnancy. J Clin Endocrinol Metab 2008;93(5):1737–42.
9. Smyth PP. Variation in iodine handling during normal pregnancy. Thyroid 1999;9(7):637–42.
10. Glinoer D. Pregnancy and iodine. Thyroid 2001;11(5):471–81.
11. Zimmermann MB. Iodine deficiency. Endocr Rev 2009;30(4):376–408.
12. Vought RL, London WT. Iodine intake, excretion and thyroidal accumulation in healthy subjects. J Clin Endocrinol Metab 1967;27(7):913–9.
13. Rasmussen LB, Ovesen L, Christiansen E. Day-to-day and within-day variation in urinary iodine excretion. Eur J Clin Nutr 1999;53(5):401–7.
14. WHO, UNICEF, ICCIDD. Assessment of the iodine deficiency disorders and monitoring their elimination. Geneva (Switzerland): World Health Organization; 2007. WHO/NHD/01.1.
15. Li M, Eastman CJ. Neonatal TSH screening: is it a sensitive and reliable tool for monitoring iodine status in populations? Best Pract Res Clin Endocrinol Metab 2010;24(1):63–75.
16. Zimmermann MB, Hess SY, Molinari L, et al. New reference values for thyroid volume by ultrasound in iodine-sufficient schoolchildren: a World Health Organization/Nutrition for Health and Development Iodine Deficiency Study Group report. Am J Clin Nutr 2004;79(2):231–7.
17. Zimmermann MB, de Benoist B, Corigliano S, et al. Assessment of iodine status using dried blood spot thyroglobulin: development of reference material and

establishment of an international reference range in iodine-sufficient children. J Clin Endocrinol Metab 2006;91(12):4881–7.

18. Boyages SC. Clinical review 49: iodine deficiency disorders. J Clin Endocrinol Metab 1993;77(3):587–91.

19. Pharoah PO, Buttfield IH, Hetzel BS. Neurological damage to the fetus resulting from severe iodine deficiency during pregnancy. Lancet 1971;1(7694):308–10.

20. Younes-Rapozo V, Berendonk J, Savignon T, et al. Thyroid hormone deficiency changes the distribution of oligodendrocyte/myelin markers during oligodendroglial differentiation in vitro. Int J Dev Neurosci 2006;24(7):445–53.

21. de Escobar GM, Obregon MJ, del Rey FE. Iodine deficiency and brain development in the first half of pregnancy. Public Health Nutr 2007;10(12A):1554–70.

22. Cao XY, Jiang XM, Dou ZH, et al. Timing of vulnerability of the brain to iodine deficiency in endemic cretinism. N Engl J Med 1994;331(26):1739–44.

23. Zoeller RT, Rovet J. Timing of thyroid hormone action in the developing brain: clinical observations and experimental findings. J Neuroendocrinol 2004;16(10):809–18.

24. Vermiglio F, Lo Presti VP, Moleti M, et al. Attention deficit and hyperactivity disorders in the offspring of mothers exposed to mild-moderate iodine deficiency: a possible novel iodine deficiency disorder in developed countries. J Clin Endocrinol Metab 2004;89(12):6054–60.

25. Qian M, Wang D, Watkins WE, et al. The effects of iodine on intelligence in children: a meta-analysis of studies conducted in China. Asia Pac J Clin Nutr 2005;14(1):32–42.

26. Santiago-Fernandez P, Torres-Barahona R, Muela-Martinez JA, et al. Intelligence quotient and iodine intake: a cross-sectional study in children. J Clin Endocrinol Metab 2004;89(8):3851–7.

27. International Council for the Control of Iodine Deficiency Disorders (ICCIDD). Available at: http://www.iccidd.org. Accessed August 31, 2011.

28. Chen ZP, Hetzel BS. Cretinism revisited. Best Pract Res Clin Endocrinol Metab 2010;24(1):39–50.

29. Romano R, Jannini EA, Pepe M, et al. The effects of iodoprophylaxis on thyroid size during pregnancy. Am J Obstet Gynecol 1991;164(2):482–5.

30. Nohr SB, Laurberg P. Opposite variations in maternal and neonatal thyroid function induced by iodine supplementation during pregnancy. J Clin Endocrinol Metab 2000;85(2):623–7.

31. Pedersen KM, Laurberg P, Iversen E, et al. Amelioration of some pregnancy-associated variations in thyroid function by iodine supplementation. J Clin Endocrinol Metab 1993;77(4):1078–83.

32. Glinoer D, De Nayer P, Delange F, et al. A randomized trial for the treatment of mild iodine deficiency during pregnancy: maternal and neonatal effects. J Clin Endocrinol Metab 1995;80(1):258–69.

33. Liesenkotter KP, Gopel W, Bogner U, et al. Earliest prevention of endemic goiter by iodine supplementation during pregnancy. Eur J Endocrinol 1996;134(4):443–8.

34. Antonangeli L, Maccherini D, Cavaliere R, et al. Comparison of two different doses of iodide in the prevention of gestational goiter in marginal iodine deficiency: a longitudinal study. Eur J Endocrinol 2002;147(1):29–34.

35. Moleti M, Lo Presti VP, Campolo MC, et al. Iodine prophylaxis using iodized salt and risk of maternal thyroid failure in conditions of mild iodine deficiency. J Clin Endocrinol Metab 2008;93(7):2616–21.

36. Berbel P, Mestre JL, Santamaria A, et al. Delayed neurobehavioral development in children born to pregnant women with mild hypothyroxinemia during the first

month of gestation: the importance of early iodine supplementation. Thyroid 2009;19(5):511–9.

37. Velasco I, Gonzalez-Romero S, Soriguer F. Iodine and thyroid function during pregnancy. Epidemiology 2010;21(3):428–9.

38. Klein RZ, Haddow JE, Faix JD, et al. Prevalence of thyroid deficiency in pregnant women. Clin Endocrinol (Oxf) 1991;35(1):41–6.

39. Brown RS. Minireview: developmental regulation of thyrotropin receptor gene expression in the fetal and newborn thyroid. Endocrinology 2004;145(9):4058–61.

40. de Escobar GM, Obregon MJ, del Rey FE. Maternal thyroid hormones early in pregnancy and fetal brain development. Best Pract Res Clin Endocrinol Metab 2004;18(2):225–48.

41. Iskaros J, Pickard M, Evans I, et al. Thyroid hormone receptor gene expression in first trimester human fetal brain. J Clin Endocrinol Metab 2000;85(7):2620–3.

42. Haddow JE, Palomaki GE, Allan WC, et al. Maternal thyroid deficiency during pregnancy and subsequent neuropsychological development of the child. N Engl J Med 1999;341(8):549–55.

43. Pop VJ, Brouwers EP, Vader HL, et al. Maternal hypothyroxinaemia during early pregnancy and subsequent child development: a 3-year follow-up study. Clin Endocrinol (Oxf) 2003;59(3):282–8.

44. Choudhury N, Gorman KS. Subclinical prenatal iodine deficiency negatively affects infant development in northern China. J Nutr 2003;133(10):3162–5.

45. Kooistra L, Crawford S, van Baar AL, et al. Neonatal effects of maternal hypothyroxinemia during early pregnancy. Pediatrics 2006;117(1):161–7.

46. Li Y, Shan Z, Teng W, et al. Abnormalities of maternal thyroid function during pregnancy affect neuropsychological development of their children at 25-30 months. Clin Endocrinol (Oxf) 2010;72(6):825–9.

47. Henrichs J, Schenk JJ, Roza SJ, et al. Maternal psychological distress and fetal growth trajectories: the Generation R Study. Psychol Med 2010;40(4):633–43.

48. Eskandari S, Loo DD, Dai G, et al. Thyroid Na+/I− symporter. Mechanism, stoichiometry, and specificity. J Biol Chem 1997;272(43):27230–8.

49. Tazebay UH, Wapnir IL, Levy O, et al. The mammary gland iodide transporter is expressed during lactation and in breast cancer. Nat Med 2000;6(8):871–8.

50. Bruhn JC, Franke AA. Iodine in human milk. J Dairy Sci 1983;66(6):1396–8.

51. Mulrine HM, Skeaff SA, Ferguson EL, et al. Breast-milk iodine concentration declines over the first 6 mo postpartum in iodine-deficient women. Am J Clin Nutr 2010;92(4):849–56.

52. Gushurst CA, Mueller JA, Green JA, et al. Breast milk iodide: reassessment in the 1980s. Pediatrics 1984;73(3):354–7.

53. Food and Nutrition Board, Institute of Medicine. Dietary reference intakes. Washington, DC: National Academy Press; 2006.

54. Pearce EN, Leung AM, Blount BC, et al. Breast milk iodine and perchlorate concentrations in lactating Boston-area women. J Clin Endocrinol Metab 2007; 92(5):1673–7.

55. Kirk AB, Martinelango PK, Tian K, et al. Perchlorate and iodide in dairy and breast milk. Environ Sci Technol 2005;39(7):2011–7.

56. Kirk AB, Dyke JV, Martin CF, et al. Temporal patterns in perchlorate, thiocyanate, and iodide excretion in human milk. Environ Health Perspect 2007;115(2):182–6.

57. Dasgupta PK, Kirk AB, Dyke JV, et al. Intake of iodine and perchlorate and excretion in human milk. Environ Sci Technol 2008;42(21):8115–21.

58. Pearce EN, Pino S, He X, et al. Sources of dietary iodine: bread, cows' milk, and infant formula in the Boston area. J Clin Endocrinol Metab 2004;89(7):3421–4.

59. Pennington JA, Schoen SA. Contributions of food groups to estimated intakes of nutritional elements: results from the FDA total diet studies, 1982-1991. Int J Vitam Nutr Res 1996;66(4):342–9.

60. Perrine CG, Herrick K, Serdula MK, et al. Some subgroups of reproductive age women in the United States may be at risk for iodine deficiency. J Nutr 2010; 140(8):1489–94.

61. Kidd PS, Trowbridge FL, Goldsby JB, et al. Sources of dietary iodine. J Am Diet Assoc 1974;65(4):420–2.

62. Hollowell JG, Staehling NW, Hannon WH, et al. Iodine nutrition in the United States. Trends and public health implications: iodine excretion data from National Health and Nutrition Examination Surveys I and III (1971-1974 and 1988-1994). J Clin Endocrinol Metab 1998;83(10):3401–8.

63. Caldwell KL, Makhmudov A, Ely E, et al. Iodine status of the U.S. population, national health and nutrition examination survey, 2005-2006 and 2007-2008. Thyroid 2011;21(4):419–27.

64. Lee SY, Leung AM, He X, et al. Iodine content in fast foods: comparison between two fast-food chains in the United States. Endocr Pract 2010;16(6):1071–2.

65. Pearce EN, Bazrafshan HR, He X, et al. Dietary iodine in pregnant women from the Boston, Massachusetts area. Thyroid 2004;14(4):327–8.

66. Becker DV, Braverman LE, Delange F, et al. Iodine supplementation for pregnancy and lactation—United States and Canada: recommendations of the American Thyroid Association. Thyroid 2006;16(10):949–51.

67. Gregory CO, Serdula MK, Sullivan KM. Use of supplements with and without iodine in women of childbearing age in the United States. Thyroid 2009;19(9):1019–20.

68. Leung AM, Pearce EN, Braverman LE. Iodine content of prenatal multivitamins in the United States. N Engl J Med 2009;360(9):939–40.

69. World Declaration on the Survival, Protection and Development of Children. 1990. Available at: http://www.unicef.org/wsc/declare.htm. Accessed August 31, 2011.

70. Iodine and health: eliminating iodine deficiency disorders safely through salt iodization. Geneva: World Health Organization (WHO); 1994. Report No.: WHO/NUT/94.4.

71. Andersson M, Takkouche B, Egli I, et al. Current global iodine status and progress over the last decade towards the elimination of iodine deficiency. Bull World Health Organ 2005;83(7):518–25.

72. Opinion of the Scientific Committee on Food on the tolerable upper intake level of iodine. 2002. Available at: http://ec.europa.eu/food/fs/sc/scf/out146_en.pdf. Accessed August 31, 2011.

73. Dasgupta PK, Dyke JV, Kirk AB, et al. Perchlorate in the United States. Analysis of relative source contributions to the food chain. Environ Sci Technol 2006;40(21):6608–14.

74. Renner R. Perchlorate found in vitamins and elsewhere. Environ Sci Technol 2006;40(8):2498–9.

75. Tonacchera M, Pinchera A, Dimida A, et al. Relative potencies and additivity of perchlorate, thiocyanate, nitrate, and iodide on the inhibition of radioactive iodide uptake by the human sodium iodide symporter. Thyroid 2004;14(12):1012–9.

76. Dohan O, Portulano C, Basquin C, et al. The Na+/I− symporter (NIS) mediates electroneutral active transport of the environmental pollutant perchlorate. Proc Natl Acad Sci U S A 2007;104(51):20250–5.

77. Blount BC, Valentin-Blasini L, Osterloh JD, et al. Perchlorate exposure of the US population, 2001-2002. J Expo Sci Environ Epidemiol 2007;17(4):400–7.

78. Blount BC, Pirkle JL, Osterloh JD, et al. Urinary perchlorate and thyroid hormone levels in adolescent and adult men and women living in the United States. Environ Health Perspect 2006;114(12):1865–71.

79. Lamm SH, Hollowell JG, Engel A, et al. Perchlorate, thiocyanate, and low iodine association not seen with low creatinine-adjusted urine iodine among women of child-bearing age. Thyroid 2007;17:S51.

80. Pearce EN, Lazarus JH, Smyth PP, et al. Perchlorate and thiocyanate exposure and thyroid function in first-trimester pregnant women. J Clin Endocrinol Metab 2010;95(7):3207–15.

81. Murray CW, Egan SK, Kim H, et al. US Food and Drug Administration's Total Diet Study: dietary intake of perchlorate and iodine. J Expo Sci Environ Epidemiol 2008;18(6):571–80.

82. Azizi F, Smyth P. Breastfeeding and maternal and infant iodine nutrition. Clin Endocrinol (Oxf) 2009;70(5):803–9.

83. Leung AM, Pearce EN, Hamilton T, et al. Colostrum iodine and perchlorate concentrations in Boston-area women: a cross-sectional study. Clin Endocrinol (Oxf) 2009;70(2):326–30.

84. Laurberg P, Nohr SB, Pedersen KM, et al. Iodine nutrition in breast-fed infants is impaired by maternal smoking. J Clin Endocrinol Metab 2004;89(1):181–7.

85. Szybinski Z, Walas S, Zagrodzki P, et al. Iodine, selenium, and other trace elements in urine of pregnant women. Biol Trace Elem Res 2010;138(1–3):28–41.

86. Gartner R. Selenium and thyroid hormone axis in critical ill states: an overview of conflicting view points. J Trace Elem Med Biol 2009;23(2):71–4.

87. Negro R, Greco G, Mangieri T, et al. The influence of selenium supplementation on postpartum thyroid status in pregnant women with thyroid peroxidase autoantibodies. J Clin Endocrinol Metab 2007;92(4):1263–8.

88. Caldwell KL, Jones R, Hollowell JG. Urinary iodine concentration: United States National Health and Nutrition Examination Survey 2001-2002. Thyroid 2005;15(7):692–9.

89. Caldwell KL, Miller GA, Wang RY, et al. Iodine status of the U.S. population, National Health and Nutrition Examination Survey 2003-2004. Thyroid 2008;18(11):1207–14.

Adrenal Disorders in Pregnancy

Dima Abdelmannan, MD, FRCP, David C. Aron, MD, MS*

KEYWORDS

- Adrenal tumor • Cushing syndrome • Hyperaldosteronism
- Pheochromocytoma • Addison disease • Pregnancy

Like other conditions, adrenal disorders may become manifest in the course of pregnancy in three basic ways: (1) clearly developing de novo during the pregnancy (eg, adrenal hemorrhage), (2) present but undiagnosed before pregnancy, and (3) diagnosed and treated before pregnancy, so that the issue is continued management. Naturally, the distinction between the first two can only occasionally be made with certainty. Finally, adrenal disorders may present as hormonal hypofunction or hyperfunction (eg, glucocorticoids, mineralocorticoids, androgens, and catecholamines) or with mass effects or other nonendocrine effects (eg, unilateral adrenal hemorrhage causing shock).

HYPOTHALAMUS-PITUITARY-GLUCOCORTICOID AXIS IN PREGNANCY

Pregnancy presents special problems in the evaluation of the hypothalamic-pituitary-adrenal (HPA) axis in addition to the usual considerations, including episodic secretion of hormones, circadian rhythm, negative feedback, total versus free cortisol in serum, and characteristics of the tests themselves.[1,2] In general, pregnancy constitutes a general state of HPA axis activation resulting in a state of physiologic hypercortisolism, yet lacking specific clinical manifestations of hypercortisolism.[3–8] Hepatic production of corticosteroid-binding globulin (CBG) increases twofold to threefold, reaching the highest levels during the latter part of pregnancy. The peak of this estrogen-mediated effect is typically reached by the third trimester and is maintained until delivery. Total plasma cortisol levels are elevated because plasma assays generally measure total plasma cortisol levels, which mainly represent the bound fraction and depend on cortisol-binding globulin levels. However, not only do total plasma cortisol levels increase during pregnancy, but plasma-free cortisol levels also rise.

The views expressed are those of the authors and do not represent the views of the Department of Veterans Affairs or any other federal agency.

Division of Clinical and Molecular Endocrinology, Department of Medicine, Louis Stokes Cleveland Department of Veterans Affairs Medical Center, Case Western Reserve University School of Medicine, 10701 East Boulevard, Cleveland, OH 44106, USA

* Corresponding author. Louis Stokes Department of Veterans Affairs Medical Center, Education Office 14 (W), 10701 East Boulevard, Cleveland, OH 44106.

E-mail address: david.aron@va.gov

Endocrinol Metab Clin N Am 40 (2011) 779–794
doi:10.1016/j.ecl.2011.09.001
0889-8529/11/$ – see front matter © 2011 Published by Elsevier Inc.

Thus, total plasma-cortisol levels and urinary-free cortisol excretion may overlap those found in Cushing syndrome. However, in contrast to Cushing syndrome, the normal diurnal variation of plasma cortisol is maintained.[9] Dexamethasone suppressibility as judged by standard criteria may be impaired because of the relatively high levels of bound cortisol. In addition, dexamethasone suppressibility of plasma-free cortisol levels decreases as pregnancy advances. As pregnancy progresses, plasma corticotropin levels rise (**Fig. 1**). Why this occurs in the setting of increased plasma free cortisol is not clear. There is also decreased suppression of the HPA axis by exogenous glucocorticoids that may persist for as long as 5 weeks postpartum.[5] Plasma corticotropin-releasing hormone (CRH) levels rise during pregnancy, reaching very high levels at term, and abruptly falling after delivery.[10] CRH is secreted from the placental unit. In contrast to the usual negative feedback that cortisol has on hypothalamic CRH production, there is increased production in placental CRH in response to cortisol.[11] Placental CRH drives corticotropin in a noncircadian fashion. It has been proposed that CRH is a biologic clock that times labor and delivery and may have effects on maturation of the fetal adrenal, fetal-placental unit circulation, and a paracrine effect on the placenta. A high affinity binding protein for placental CRH blunts the corticotropin-releasing activity of CRH.[12] Up until about 33 weeks of gestation, 90% to 95% of fetal cortisol derives from maternal sources. After that, fetal adrenal cortisol

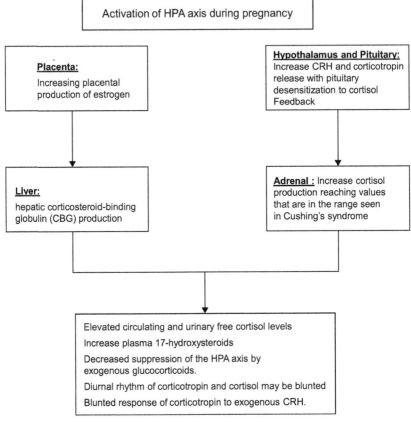

Fig. 1. Activation of the HPA axis during pregnancy.

production increases and maternal contribution decreases. Placental 11β-hydroxys-teroid dehydrogenase 2 (11β-HSD2), which converts cortisol to its inactive 11-keto metabolite cortisone, protects the fetus from excessive hydrocortisone. Plasma cortisol levels generally do not rise to the point at which they overwhelm 11β-HSD2.

RENIN-ANGIOTENSIN-ALDOSTERONE AXIS IN PREGNANCY

The renin-angiotensin-aldosterone axis undergoes major changes during preg-nancy.[13] Extrarenal renin secretion by the ovaries and maternal decidua produce an early increase in renin levels. Angiotensinogen synthesis by the liver is increased by the increased estrogen levels. Angiotensin II levels rise and stimulate the zona glomer-ulosa so that aldosterone levels increase. However, much of the increased mineralo-corticoid activity relates to the greatly increased production of deoxycorticosterone (DOC). During pregnancy, much of this DOC is produced from progesterone and at an extra-adrenal site. However, progesterone itself has natriuretic activity; it is a competitive inhibitor of aldosterone in the distal tubule. Therefore, the physiologic effects of increased aldosterone are attenuated in pregnancy. In addition, vascular refractoriness to the pressor effects angiotensin II develops. In short, the situation reflects a complex series of interactions and interdependencies that result in blood volume expansion during pregnancy.

ADRENAL INSUFFICIENCY

In the developed world, autoimmune Addison disease (AAD) accounts for most cases of primary adrenal insufficiency.[14] AAD tends to affect young and middle-aged women, so it is not surprising that women with treated AAD who become pregnant require special management considerations. Although there are few clinical data, Arlt and Allolio[15] sug-gested increasing cortisol replacement doses by 50% in the last trimester based on the physiologic increase in CBG. This would be analogous to increasing the dose of levothyroxine during pregnancy to compensate for increased levels of thyroxine-binding globulin.[16] Some additional support for this approach is provided by the finding of twofold to fivefold increased cortisol responsiveness to corticotropin in pregnancy.[17] Progesterone alters mineralocorticoid action but, because plasma renin activity increases in pregnancy, monitoring of mineralocorticoid action is limited to blood pressure and serum potassium. Particular attention needs to be given to factors that may interfere with medication adherence (eg, vomiting during pregnancy). From the standpoint of cortisol replacement, the peripartum period should be managed simi-larly to major surgery: stress doses (100–200 mg/24 h) followed by a rapid taper.

Outcomes of pregnancy are not as good in patients with AAD. In a population-based historical cohort study in Sweden consisting of 1188 women with AAD and 11,879 age-matched controls who delivered infants between 1973 and 2006, adjusted odds ratio (OR) for infants born to mothers with deliveries 3 years or less before the diagnosis of AAD were 2.40 (95% confidence interval [CI], 1.27–4.53) for preterm birth (≤37 wk), 3.50 (95% CI, 1.83–6.67) for low birth weight (<2500 g), and 1.74 (95% CI, 1.02–2.96) for cesarean section. Compared with controls, women who gave birth after their AAD diagnosis were at increased risk of both cesarean delivery (adjusted OR, 2.35; 95% CI, 1.68–3.27) and preterm delivery (adjusted OR, 2.61; 95% CI, 1.69–4.05). Stratifying by isolated AAD and concomitant type 1 diabetes and/or autoim-mune thyroid disease in the mother did not essentially influence these risks. There were no differences in risks of congenital malformations or infant death. Women with AAD had a reduced overall parity compared with controls (P<.001). Of note, in some women the diagnosis of AAD was made during pregnancy and delayed diagnosis could have accounted for some of the findings; women with deliveries 3 years or less before an AAD diagnosis may have undiagnosed AAD during pregnancy and these women had increased risks of preterm delivery and of having a low birth weight infant.[14]

Adrenal insufficiency manifesting during pregnancy presents its own set of problems.[14,18] Before the corticosteroid era, maternal mortality was as high as 35%. In most instances the diagnosis was proven at autopsy, therapeutic abortions were uniformly fatal, and one-third of the fetuses died at term delivery.[19] In the modern era, diagnosis of adrenal insufficiency during pregnancy may be difficult, especially in the first trimester because some of the symptoms are common in normal pregnancy (eg, nausea, vomiting, and fatigue.[20] A family history of autoimmune disorder should be sought. When accompanied by more specific findings, such as hyperkalemia, hypoglycemia, or skin hyperpigmentation (eg, of palmar creases), the diagnosis becomes more obvious. Hyperpigmentation of skin and mucosa can be present in normal pregnancy, but bluish-black spots on the lips, gums, and mucosal membranes of mouth, rectum, and vagina are more evident in adrenal insufficiency, as is darkening of the skin in unexposed regions of the body.[18] Pregnancy itself, especially labor and delivery, may precipitate an addisonian crisis (acute severe adrenal insufficiency).[21]

Pregnancy complicates the biochemical diagnosis of adrenal insufficiency. Such a patient may have total cortisol values that are within the normal laboratory range for nonpregnant women, reflecting cortisol bound to CBG (which makes a low cortisol level even more significant). Moreover, the relatively high corticotropin levels of pregnancy make this test somewhat less helpful in identifying adrenal insufficiency, though it is still useful in differentiating primary from secondary causes. Thus, when cortisol levels are low, the diagnosis is relatively straightforward. In primary adrenal insufficiency, corticotropin levels are elevated, whereas in secondary adrenal insufficiency they are not elevated. The 250-ug corticotropin stimulation test is the most widely available dynamic test of adrenocortical function in pregnancy and can be very helpful when baseline levels of cortisol are not inordinately low.[17]

CUSHING SYNDROME

Although Cushing syndrome occurs most commonly in women of childbearing age, pregnancy in Cushing syndrome is rare because of infertility associated with suppression of gonadotropin secretion by elevated cortisol levels and androgens. However, this rare co-occurrence has generated a large literature, perhaps because of the difficulties in diagnosis and management, as well as the unfavorable maternal and fetal outcomes.[22]

Clinical Features

Most of the reported cases of Cushing syndrome during pregnancy describe the typical signs and symptoms, including central obesity, thin skin, easy bruising, striae, and hypertension (**Table 1**). However, Cushing syndrome can present with much greater subtlety; it may go unrecognized and it may be underdiagnosed in pregnancy. Moreover, pregnancy itself often exhibits some of the clinical features seen in Cushing syndrome (eg, hypertension, hyperglycemia, and striae). Therefore, a high index of clinical suspicion must be maintained to prevent delay in diagnosis.[23,24]

The striae of Cushing syndrome are typically purplish, depressed and wide (often 0.5–2.0 cm) as compared with the pinkish-white striae seen in pregnant white women (**Fig. 2**). In addition to the abdominal wall, the striae in Cushing syndrome may also involve the axilla, thighs, and breasts. Signs and symptoms with the greatest discriminatory value are the catabolic features, such as bruising and proximal weakness,

Table 1
Major differences in Cushing syndrome between pregnant and nonpregnant states

	Pregnant State	Nonpregnant State
Prevalence	No incidence available; 120 cases in the literature	Incidence of endogenous Cushing syndrome estimated at 13 cases per million individuals
Presentation	Pregnant women without Cushing syndrome develop some features of Cushing syndrome, such as hypertension, hyperglycemia and striae A high index of clinical suspicion must be maintained to prevent delay in diagnosis	—
Cause	Adrenal adenomas 40%–50% Pituitary adenomas 30%	Adrenal adenomas 15% Pituitary adenomas 70%
Biochemical changes		
Corticotropin	Plasma corticotropin increases as pregnancy progresses Corticotropin levels not suppressed in half of those with primary adrenal disorders, possibly due to continued stimulation of the maternal HPA axis by placental CRH	—
Cortisol	Serum cortisol levels rise twofold to threefold in pregnancy, but diurnal variability is maintained Diurnal variation is lost	—
Salivary Cortisol	Salivary cortisol rises twofold during normal pregnancy	—
Urinary-free Cortisol	Concentrations increase during pregnancy to levels that may overlap with those observed the syndrome Not appropriately suppressed after dexamethasone	—
CBG	Plasma CBG levels increase in pregnancy due to increase in estrogen levels leading to elevated cortisol levels	—
Other factors	Placental degradation of cortisol seems to protect the fetus from glucocorticoid excess	—

From Abdelmannan D, Aron DC. Special aspects of Cushing's syndrome: pregnancy. In: Bronstein MD, editor. Contemporary endocrinology: Cushing's syndrome: pathophysiology, diagnosis and treatment. New York: Springer; 2010. p. 265. Chapter 21.

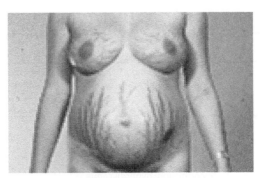

Fig. 2. Extensive striae affecting breasts and abdomen in a pregnant patient with Cushing syndrome.

especially if accompanied by hypertension and gestational diabetes.[23,25] Biochemical diagnosis presents its own set of challenges.

Establishing the Diagnosis of Cushing Syndrome in Pregnancy

The biochemical diagnosis of Cushing syndrome is challenging in the best of circumstances.[2,26] Pregnancy only complicates the diagnosis. Usual approaches to screening for and establishing the diagnosis of Cushing syndrome (eg, low dose dexamethasone suppression testing, assessment of 24-hour urinary-free cortisol, and midnight salivary cortisol) perform relatively poorly during pregnancy. Elevated CBG levels in pregnancy lead to high total cortisol levels. Starting from a higher baseline means that even a normally suppressible HPA axis will not show the levels of suppression achieved in normal circumstances (ie, those for which the standards have been developed). Thus, there are more false-positive tests. Though normal in the first trimester, 24-hour–free urinary free cortisol excretion increases to as high as three times the normal upper limit during the second and third trimesters, resulting in a high false-positive rate.

Salivary cortisol levels also rise twofold to threefold during pregnancy, a magnitude similar to the increase in total plasma cortisol. Scott and colleagues[27] found that the mean ($\pm$ 1 SD) hourly salivary cortisol level was 5.0 $\pm$ 1.4, 7.2 $\pm$ 1.2, and 13.6 $\pm$ 3.6 nmol/L in normal nonpregnant women, early pregnancy, and late pregnancy, respectively. These levels are still below those usually observed in Cushing syndrome.[28] Although diurnal rhythm for cortisol, both serum and salivary, is preserved, the diagnostic thresholds for evening serum or salivary cortisol in pregnant patients have not been clearly established. Data related to other tests (eg, corticotropin-releasing hormone or low-dose dexamethasone suppression) are quite limited.

Determining the Cause of Cushing Syndrome in Pregnancy

Once the diagnosis of Cushing syndrome is made, the next step is to determine the cause and differentiate between corticotropin-secreting pituitary tumors, ectopic corticotropin syndrome, adrenal tumors (benign and malignant), and other rarer causes. About half of the cases of Cushing syndrome in pregnancy are caused by adrenal adenomas and only about one-third are caused by pituitary tumors. This contrasts with the distribution of causes in the nonpregnant state in which adrenal adenomas account for only 15% of cases, whereas about 70% are caused by pituitary adenomas. Although diagnosis of autonomous cortisol secretion by adrenal tumors is usually straightforward, it is more difficult in pregnancy because, in contrast to the corticotropin suppression observed in nonpregnant women with cortisol-producing adrenal tumors, pregnant patients with such tumors may not have a suppressed corticotropin, probably a consequence of stimulation by placental CRH. If the pregnant patient does have a suppressed corticotropin, the diagnosis of corticotropin-independent disease is confirmed and imaging can be performed to localize the adrenal tumor (adenoma or carcinoma) or identify nodular adrenal hyperplasia. Ultrasound is preferred because of its record of safe use. Ultrasound has reasonably good sensitivity for the adrenal tumors associated with Cushing syndrome, but it is more operator-dependent than CT scan or MRI.[29] When ultrasound is nondiagnostic, non-contrast MRI can be performed.[30]

In addition to the usual diagnostic difficulties, further complicating the diagnosis is that several cases of corticotropin-independent pregnancy-dependent Cushing syndrome have been reported that either showed no radiologic evidence of adrenal tumors[31] or had spontaneous remission postpartum.[32–34] It has been suggested that the expression of "illicit" luteinizing hormone receptors and β-human chorionic gonadotropin receptors on the adrenal gland could account for adrenal Cushing syndrome that resolves after delivery because the placenta is removed and, therefore, β-human chorionic gonadotropin production ceases.[35] Finally, there is the issue of adrenal incidentalomas (see later discussion).

When the corticotropin is not suppressed, high-dose dexamethasone suppression testing can be tried. If there is suppression of cortisol, the likelihood of a cortisol-producing adrenal tumor is very low, but lack of suppression is less informative because of the effect of higher false-positive rates related to high bound-cortisol levels. Both pituitary Cushing and ectopic corticotropin syndrome may fail to suppress. The role of CRH testing in pregnancy is unclear. Few cases of ectopic corticotropin syndrome during pregnancy have been reported and whether the prevalence of this disorder is the same during pregnancy as the nonpregnant state is unknown. Moreover, many corticotropin-secreting tumors, both pituitary and ectopic, are small, which makes them difficult to localize by imaging studies. However, among patients with pituitary Cushing syndrome, the prevalence of pituitary macroadenomas is much higher in pregnancy. However, whether this is a function of publication bias or the effects of pregnancy on the pituitary is not clear.[4]

Lindsay and colleagues have suggested an approach recommending that pregnant women with CRH and dexamethasone test responses consistent with pituitary Cushing syndrome and pituitary lesions larger than at least 6 mm often require no additional testing.[4,5] Petrosal sinus sampling may be necessary in other cases, although the usual criteria to establish a pituitary or systemic gradient may not apply in the pregnant state.[4,5] There are several reports of this procedure being performed in which the pregnancies were uneventful. However, notwithstanding the special attention that can be paid to minimizing fetal exposure to ionizing radiation, the potential deleterious effects of ionizing radiation is a serious limitation.[4,36]

Outcomes of Cushing Syndrome in Pregnancy

Maternal morbidity occurs in about 70% of cases, although maternal mortality is mercifully infrequent, at least in the developed world. The frequency of hypertension and gestational diabetes are much greater than during normal pregnancy. In addition, preeclampsia and eclampsia seem to occur more commonly. Other reported problems include infection, osteoporotic fracture, and congestive heart failure.[22]

The risk to the fetus depends on the effects of glucocorticoids on both the fetus directly and the maternal-placental unit. The fetus itself is relatively protected from glucocorticoids.[37] Nevertheless, fetal mortality is as high as 25% to 40% owing to spontaneous abortion, stillbirth, and early neonatal death due to prematurity. There is little indication of increased risk of congenital anomalies.[38] The actual fetal loss rate may be higher because of underdiagnosis of Cushing syndrome. Preterm delivery rate may be as high as 50%. These complications are the likely result of the adverse effects on the placenta of the complications associated with hypercortisolemia (eg, hypertension and hyperglycemia). Adrenal insufficiency in the newborn resulting from suppression of fetal corticotropin by maternal cortisol levels is uncommon. Comparison of fetal outcomes suggests that treatment during pregnancy is beneficial. Lindsey and Nieman[4] reviewed 136 pregnancies in which treatment outcomes were available. When no active treatment was given, there were 59 live births (76%) compared with 50 live births (89%) in women in whom treatment was instituted at a mean gestational age of 20 plus or minus 1 week. Most patients reviewed had undergone adrenalectomy for adrenal adenomas. The live birth rate after unilateral or bilateral adrenalectomy was approximately 87%. Of the 40 women with pituitary Cushing syndrome, most were treated medically; 20% underwent transsphenoidal surgery.[4] This review suggests that treatment during pregnancy is associated with better fetal outcomes. However, there are important limitations of the data, especially in terms of the comparability of the groups who did and did not undergo surgery.

Management of Cushing Syndrome in Pregnancy

Decision-making process about therapy must take into account the stage of pregnancy at the time of diagnosis, cause and severity of hypercortisolism, and the potential benefits of therapy. Unfortunately, the literature on which to base decisions is very limited. Moreover, the choice of therapy and its timing must be individualized because prognostication is so difficult. Maternal and fetal outcomes of untreated Cushing syndrome are poor. The data that treatment during pregnancy has a positive impact on maternal outcomes is modest. However, the data provide stronger support for treatment for the purpose of improving fetal outcomes. However, the issue of timing of treatment of Cushing syndrome in the pregnant patient remains somewhat uncertain. The management of pituitary Cushing syndrome is described in the article by Motivala and colleagues elsewhere in this issue. For adrenal tumors, unilateral adrenalectomy for adrenal adenoma has been performed safely even into the early third trimester, although most surgery was performed between 6 and 28 weeks of gestation. Medical treatment in pregnancy is usually avoided to minimize the potential for teratogenesis and induction of fetal adrenal insufficiency. It will be most useful given either as preparation or as a substitute for surgery for those patients with persistent disease postoperatively and for those who are not good surgical candidates.[39] Generally, cesarean delivery should be avoided because of the problems of wound healing in hypercortisolism. If cesarean section is performed, stress dose steroids are not recommended. Further details on Cushing disease in pregnancy are discussed in the article by Motivala and colleagues elsewhere in this issue.

PRIMARY HYPERALDOSTERONISM

Primary hyperaldosteronism, or Conn syndrome, results from an adrenal adenoma, hyperplasia, or rarely, an adrenal carcinoma. A classic presentation includes hypertension, hypokalemia, and a mild metabolic alkalosis. The diagnosis during pregnancy is very uncommon with fewer than 50 cases reported in the literature. Diagnosis is complicated by the normal increase in aldosterone during pregnancy. Plasma renin activity also rises during pregnancy, but it should be suppressed in the presence of primary hyperaldosteronism so that the plasma aldosterone-to-renin ratio rises.

Reported cases have involved imaging with ultrasound or MRI. The main goal is control of the hypertension, whether by tumor resection or medical management, with deferral of surgery until the postpartum period. Both approaches have been effective. Medical management includes potassium repletion and standard antenatal antihypertensive treatment. Spironolactone (an aldosterone antagonist) should be avoided in pregnancy because of its antiandrogenic effects. Although there are no definitive data pointing to fetal risk of eplerenone, another aldosterone antagonist, there are relatively few data on its safety in pregnancy in humans.

Pregnancy in women with glucocorticoid-remediable aldosteronism (GRA), a hereditary form of primary hyperaldosteronism, seems to be associated with exacerbation of their hypertension, but no increase in the rate of preeclampsia.[40,41] In a review of 35 pregnancies in 16 women, 6% of pregnancies in women with GRA were complicated by preeclampsia as compared with published rates in general obstetric populations varying from 2.5% to 10%.[41] However, 39% had pregnancy-aggravated hypertension. Infants of GRA mothers with pregnancy-aggravated hypertension tended to have lower birth weights than those that did not (3019 g vs 3385 g, respectively; $P = .08$). The primary cesarean section rate was 32%, which is approximately double that seen in other general or hypertensive obstetric populations.[41]

PHEOCHROMOCYTOMA

Pheochromocytoma in pregnancy is rare with an incidence of 0.007%.[16] Despite being rare, it is crucial to recognize and treat pheochromocytoma in pregnancy as early as possible to avoid maternal and fetal complications of hypertensive crisis.[23] In undiagnosed cases, maternal and fetal mortality may be as high as 15% and 25%, respectively.[16] It has been suggested that the maximum estrogen levels in pregnancy may serve as a growth factor leading to adrenal tumor amplification and presentation during gestation.[42] Similar to the general population, most cases are sporadic and unilateral, with 10% being malignant, bilateral, or familial (multiple endocrine neoplasia II, von Hippel-Lindau syndrome, and neurofibromatosis).

Clinical Features

Clinical features of pheochromocytoma are similar to those of nonpregnant women, the chief presentation being labile or sustained hypertension, headache, excessive sweating, palpitations, and impaired glucose tolerance.[23] In pregnancy, it is more difficult to attribute these symptoms to pheochromocytoma because of the differential diagnosis of the more common condition, preeclampsia, especially if proteinuria is present.[43] Symptoms are usually more obvious as pregnancy progresses (possibly related to tumor growth from estrogen). Symptoms also are more likely to manifest when the mother assumes a supine position, which causes the gravid uterus to compress the tumor and results in paradoxic supine hypertension with normal blood pressure in the sitting or erect position.[16] In general, uncontrolled hypertension is the most common presenting feature and it can present at any time throughout pregnancy and less commonly in the postpartum period. Other presenting symptoms include palpitations, sweating, abdominal pain, and pulmonary edema.[16,44] Kamari and colleagues[44] reported a case of persistent uncontrolled hypertension during pregnancy and after delivery, as well as postpartum pulmonary edema. Work-up revealed a left adrenal mass and the pathology was consistent with pheochromocytoma. This case illustrates the possibility of presentation of pheochromocytoma even in the postpartum period. Rarely, the adrenal tumor may be a neuroblastoma and not a pheochromocytoma. The diagnosis is usually made postoperatively through tissue diagnosis.

Neuroblastomas are rare tumors that arise from the neural crest cells of the adrenal medulla. Although rare in adulthood, there have been case reports of presentation during pregnancy.[42] Catecholamine levels can be elevated; however, more commonly, the presentation is with abdominal pain from the mass effect. If catecholamines are elevated the presentation is similar to that of a pheochromocytoma with hypertension, palpitations, sweating, and so forth. Pathology is the gold standard test for diagnosis and it reveals primitive-appearing, round, blue cells with hyperchromatic nuclei and scant cytoplasm in a lobular pattern with sheets of neuroblasts surrounding eosinophilic neutrophils that are pathognomic.[42]

Diagnosis

Once suspected clinically, the diagnosis of pheochromocytoma (as in nonpregnant women) is usually based on the results of 24-hour urinary fractionated metanephrines and catecholamines and/or plasma fractionated metanephrines. The levels of urinary catecholamines (adrenaline, noradrenaline, and dopamine) are at least two times the upper limit of the normal range. Adrenal imaging with ultrasound or MRI is also done. MRI without gadolinium is the imaging test of choice in the pregnant woman with 98% of the tumors detected within the abdomen. Because of the possible effects on the fetal thyroid, meta-iodobenzylguanidine (iobenguane I 123) scintigraphy is not considered safe for pregnant women.[45]

Treatment

The optimal therapy for pheochromocytoma in pregnancy is not clearly defined because the published literature largely consists of case reports or case series.[46–55] Whether or not surgery is chosen, it is necessary to optimize medical therapy before surgical intervention. Medical therapy should be initiated with alpha-adrenergic blockade (usually phenoxybenzamine) followed by beta-adrenergic blockade (propranolol). Phenoxybenzamine has generally been safe for the fetus.[56] However, it does cross the placenta and can cause perinatal depression and transient hypotension in selected cases.[57] Patients should also receive intravenous fluids to maintain adequate volume and minimize the risk of hypotension.[16] The timing of surgical intervention, which may be performed laparoscopically, is still controversial. Some investigators recommend surgery if the pregnancy is early (<6–7 months) and medical management when the pregnancy is farther along (last trimester).[45,57] If medical management is chosen, a cesarean section can be planned when the fetus is near term.[56]

Adrenal tumors incidental and otherwise

Although adrenal tumors account for most of the patients with Cushing syndrome, primary hyperaldosteronism, and pheochromocytoma during pregnancy, they may also become evident as incidentalomas. The term adrenal incidentaloma is usually defined as an adrenal mass unexpectedly detected through an imaging procedure performed for reasons a priori unrelated to adrenal dysfunction or suspected dysfunction. Although the identification of an adrenal mass as an incidental finding is not uncommon in the general adult population,[58] such findings have been only rarely described during pregnancy. This probably relates to the limited amount of imaging conducted during pregnancy apart from ultrasound directed toward the fetus. Although the differential diagnosis of an incidentally discovered mass is quite extensive, most are nonsecreting cortical adenomas. The challenge is to recognize and treat the small percentage of adrenal incidentalomas that do pose a significant risk, either because of their hormonal activity or because of their malignant histology, while leaving the rest alone.[59] The preferred approach to their management in terms of diagnosis, follow-up, and treatment remain controversial despite a state-of-the-science conference sponsored by the National Institutes of Health.[60] Although most experts' recommendations tend to be relatively minor variations of the conference's approach, dissenting voices have been heard.[60–69] In general, the approach is to screen for the more "common" causes of hormonal hypersecretion (Cushing syndrome, pheochromocytoma, and hyperaldosteronism) and rely on imaging characteristics to differentiate benign and malignant lesions, noninvasively if possible.[70] Occasionally, adrenal lesions in the fetus are discovered.[71]

Most adenomas are small, but large ones have been seen. Findings suggestive of malignancy include large size (>4 cm), irregular shape, vague contour, heterogeneous enhancement or attenuation, poor margination, and, of course, invasion into surrounding structures. Adrenal cortical adenomas typically exhibit homogeneous signal intensity and enhancement with T2-weighted intensity similar to liver tissue with MRI. In contrast, malignant masses are typically hypointense on both T1- and T2-weighted images with strong enhancement after contrast injection and delayed washout. MRI characteristics of benign adrenal adenomas and adrenal metastases overlap significantly. Specialized techniques such as chemical-shift MRI may be useful; however, the lipid content of adenomas causes a loss in signal intensity on chemical-shift MRI.[72,73] High signal intensity on T2-weighted MRI is suggestive of pheochromocytoma; however, initial optimistic findings of nearly 100% sensitivity and specificity have not been confirmed. For adrenal lesions overall, ultrasonography has a sensitivity of 74% to 97%, a specificity of 61% to 96%, and an accuracy of 70% to 97%.[74] Until recently, there has been relatively little diagnostic utility of ultrasound in terms of differentiating benign from malignant incidentalomas other than by size, although it might have a larger role in follow-up because it does not involve radiation exposure.[64,75]

If hormonal hypersecretion or findings suggestive of adrenal carcinoma are found, appropriate specific management can be performed. Whether surgical removal of a hormonally active or malignant adrenal tumor should take place during the pregnancy or be deferred depends on the balance between risks and benefits. Fallo and colleagues[76] reported a case of a pregnant woman with an adrenal mass discovered serendipitously, who had follow-up during gestation and underwent adrenalectomy shortly after delivery. No evidence of adrenal change in morphology and function was found in the patient throughout pregnancy, as shown by adrenal ultrasound imaging and adrenal hormone measurements. Four months after delivery, the patient underwent laparoscopic right adrenalectomy and pathologic analysis revealed a 2.7 cm benign adrenocortical adenoma. The diameter of the adrenal mass at ultrasonography correlated highly with postpartum mass diameter measured by abdominal CT scan. Quantitative expression of both estrogen receptor alpha and estrogen receptor beta by real-time polymerase chain reaction analysis and Western blotting findings did not differ among adenoma, normal adjacent adrenal, and normal adrenal control tissues, which indicates that the receptors are likely not estrogen dependant. The investigators suggested that close observation with endocrine investigations and ultrasonography could be an appropriate approach, delaying the decision of surgical intervention after delivery.[76] A retrospective cohort study that included cases of adrenal carcinoma diagnosed in women between 1963 and 2007 (n = 110) was reported. Twelve of these women were pregnant or in the first 6 months after delivery. Adrenocortical tumors diagnosed during pregnancy or in the postpartum period tended to be cortisol-secreting tumors ($P = .06$) and to be discovered at a more advanced stage than those in nonpregnant women, although the differences were not significant. Fetal outcome was poor. Overall survival of the mother was worse than that of matched controls (hazard ratio of death: 3.98, CI = 1.34–11.85, $P = .013$).

Pregnancy in Women with Congenital Adrenal Hyperplasia

A practice guideline from pediatric endocrinology specialty societies states that pregnant women with congenital adrenal hyperplasia should be monitored and delivered in a tertiary center equipped and experienced to handle such pregnancies.[77] It recommended the use of hydrocortisone or prednisolone as replacement therapy and doses adjusted to maintain maternal serum testosterone concentrations near the upper range of normal for pregnancy. It was recommended that dexamethasone should be avoided except when used in prenatal therapy. When reconstructive surgery has been performed, elective cesarean section is recommended to avoid damage to the genital tract. When cesarean section is performed, doses of hydrocortisone have to be increased before and tapered after delivery. Finally, a pediatrician should be present during delivery to take care of the newborn and to initiate diagnostic procedures when an affected child is expected according to the results of prenatal testing.[77] Prenatal diagnosis and management for the fetus at risk is beyond the scope of this article and readers are referred to the practice guideline.[77]

SUMMARY

Adrenal disorders may manifest during pregnancy de novo, or before pregnancy undiagnosed or diagnosed and treated. Adrenal disorders may present as hormonal hypofunction or hyperfunction, or with mass effects or other nonendocrine effects. Pregnancy presents special problems in the evaluation of the hypothalamic-pituitary-adrenal axis in addition to the usual considerations. The renin-angiotensin-aldosterone axis undergoes major changes during pregnancy. Nevertheless, the common adrenal disorders are associated with morbidity during pregnancy and their management is more complicated. A high index of suspicion must be maintained for these disorders lest they go unrecognized and untreated.

REFERENCES

1. Aron DC. Diagnostic implications of adrenal physiology and clinical epidemiology for evaluation of glucocorticoid excess and deficiency. In: DeGroot LJ, Jameson JL, editors. Endocrinology. Philadelphia: Saunders; 2000.
2. Findling J, Raff H. Cushing's syndrome: important issues in diagnosis and management. J Clin Endocrinol Metab 2009;91(10):3746–53.
3. Chrousos GP, Torpy DJ, Gold PW. Interactions between the hypothalamic-pituitary-adrenal axis and the female reproductive systems: clinical implications. Ann Intern Med 1998;129:229–40.
4. Lindsay J, Jonklaas J, Oldfield E, et al. Cushing's syndrome during pregnancy: personal experience and review of the literature. J Clin Endocrinol Metab 2005; 90(5):3077–83.
5. Lindsay J, Nieman L. The hypothalamic-pituitary-adrenal axis in pregnancy: challenges in disease detection and treatment. Endocr Rev 2005;26(6):775–99.
6. Magiakou MA, Mastorakos H, Rabin D, et al. The maternal hypothalamic-pituitary-adrenal axis in third trimester human pregnancy. Clin Endocrinol (Oxf) 1996;44: 419–28.
7. Magiakou MA, Mastorakos G, Webster E, et al. The hypothalamic-pituitary-adrenal axis and the female reproductive system. Ann N Y Acad Sci 1997;816: 42–56.
8. Nolten WE, Lindheimer MD, Rveckert PA, et al. Diurnal patterns and regulation of cortisol secretion in pregnancy. J Clin Endocrinol Metab 1980;31:466–72.

9. Cousins L, Rigg L, Hollingsworth D, et al. Qualitative and quantitative assessment of the circadian rhythm of cortisol in pregnancy. Am J Obstet Gynecol 1983;145: 411–6.

10. Campbell EA, Linton EA, Wolfe CD, et al. Plasma corticotrophin-releasing hormone concentration during pregnancy and parturition. J Clin Endocrinol Metab 1987;64:1054–9.

11. Robinson BG, Emanuel RL, Frim DM, et al. Glucocorticoid stimulates expression of corticotropin-releasing hormone gene in human placenta. Proc Natl Acad Sci U S A 1988;85:5244–8.

12. Trainer PJ, Woods RJ, Korbonits M, et al. The pathophysiology of circulating corticotropin-releasing hormone-binding protein levels in the human. J Clin Endocrinol Metab 1998;83:1611–4.

13. Escher G. Hyperaldosteronism in pregnancy. Ther Adv Cardiovasc Dis 2009;3(2): 123–32.

14. Björnsdottir S, Cnattingius S, Brandt L, et al. Addison's disease in women is a risk factor for an adverse pregnancy outcome. J Clin Endocrinol Metab 2010;95(12): 5249–57.

15. Arlt W, Alliolo B. Adrenal insufficiency. Lancet 2003;361:1881–93.

16. Girling J, Martineau M. Thyroid and other endocrine disorders in pregnancy. Obstet Gynaecol Reprod Med 2010;20(9):265–71.

17. Suri D, Moran J, Hibbbard J, et al. Assessment of adrenal reserve in pregnancy: defining the normal response to the adrenocorticotropin stimulation test. J Clin Endocrinol Metab 2006;9(10):3866–72.

18. Otta C, de Mereshian P, Iraci G, et al. Pregnancies associated with primary adrenal insufficiency. Fertil Steril 2008;90(4):e17–20.

19. Cohen M. Addison's disease complicated by toxemia of pregnancy. Review of the literature. Arch Intern Med 1948;81(6):879–87.

20. Lewandowski K, Hincz P, Grzesiak M, et al. New onset Addison's disease presenting as prolonged hyperemesis in early pregnancy. Ginekol Pol 2010;81(7): 537–40.

21. Hahner S, Loeffier M, Bleicken B, et al. Epidemiology of adrenal crisis in chronic adrenal insufficiency: the need for new prevention strategies. Eur J Endocrinol 2010;162(3):597–602.

22. Abdelmannan D, Aron DC. Special aspects of Cushing's syndrome: pregnancy. In: Bronstein MD, editor. Contemporary endocriminology: Cushing's syndrome: pathophysiology, diagnosis and treatment. New York: Springer; 2010. p. 259–71.

23. Keely E. Endocrine causes of hypertension in pregnancy—when to start looking for zebras. Semin Perinatol 1998;22(6):471–84.

24. Kreisberg R. Clinical problem-solving. Half a loaf. N Engl J Med 1994;330(18): 1295–9.

25. Ross EJ, Linch DC. Cushing's syndrome–killing disease: discriminatory value of signs and symptoms aiding early diagnosis. Lancet 1982;2:646–9.

26. Nieman LK, Biller BM, Findling JW, et al. The diagnosis of Cushing's syndrome: an Endocrine Society Clinical Practice Guideline. J Clin Endocrinol Metab 2008;93(5):1526–40.

27. Scott EM, McGarrigle HH, Lachelin CL. The increase in plasma and saliva cortisol levels in pregnancy is not due to the increase in corticosteroid-binding globulin levels. J Clin Endocrinol Metab 1990;71:639–44.

28. Billaud L, Sanson ML, Guilhaume B, et al. Cushing syndrome during pregnancy. New diagnostic methods used in 3 cases of adrenal cortex carcinoma. Presse Med 1992;21(42):2041–5.

29. Resnek RM, Armstrong P. The adrenal gland. Clin Endocrinol 1994;40:561–76.
30. Wieseler KM, Bhargava P, Kanal KM, et al. Imaging in pregnant patients: examination appropriateness. Radiographics 2010;30(5):1215–29.
31. Close CF, Mann MC, Watts JF, et al. ACTH-independent Cushing's syndrome in pregnancy with spontaneous resolution after delivery: control of the hypercortisolism with metyrapone. Clin Endocrinol (Oxf) 1993;39(3):375–9.
32. Margulies PL, Imperato-McGinley J, Arthur A, et al. Remission of Cushing's syndrome during pregnancy. Int J Gynaecol Obstet 1983;21(1):77–83.
33. Parra A, Cruz-Krohn J. Intercurrent Cushing's syndrome and pregnancy. Am J Med 1966;40(6):961–6.
34. Verdugo C, Donoso J, Meza H, et al. Cushing's syndrome and pregnancy with spontaneous remission after delivery. Rev Med Chil 1982;110(6):564–9.
35. Polli N, Giraldi F, Cavagnini F. Cushing's disease and pregnancy. Pituitary 2004;7: 237–41.
36. Pinette MG, Pan YQ, Oppenheim D, et al. Bilateral inferior petrosal sinus corticotropin sampling with corticotropin-releasing hormone stimulation in a pregnant patient with Cushing's syndrome. Am J Obstet Gynecol 1994;171(2):563–4.
37. Hillman DA, Giroud CJ. Plasma cortisone and cortisol levels at birth and during the neonatal period. J Clin Endocrinol Metab 1995;25:243–8.
38. Fitzsimons R, Greenberger PA, Patterson MD. Outcome of pregnancy in women requiring corticosteroids for severe asthma. J Allergy Clin Immunol 2009;78: 349–53.
39. Sonino N, Boscaro M. Medical therapy for Cushing's disease. Endocrinol Metab Clin North Am 1999;28:211–22.
40. Hamilton E, o'Callaghan C, O'Brien R, et al. Familial hyperaldosteronism type 1 in pregnancy. Intern Med J 2009;39(2):135–6.
41. Wyckoff JA, Seely EW, Hurwitz S, et al. Glucocorticoid-remediable aldosteronism and pregnancy. Hypertension 2000;35:668–72.
42. Refaat M, Idriss S, Blaszkowsky L. Case report: an unusual case of adrenal neuroblastoma in pregnancy. Oncologist 2008;13(2):152–6.
43. Wolf A, Goretzki P, Röhrborn A, et al. Pheochromocytoma during pregnancy: laparoscopic and conventional surgical treatment of two cases. Exp Clin Endocrinol Diabetes 2004;112:98–101.
44. Kamari Y, Sharabi Y, Leiba A, et al. Peripartum hypertension from pheochromocytoma: a rare and challenging entity. Am J Hypertens 2005;18:1306–12.
45. Finkenstedt G, Gasser RW, Hofle G. Pheochromocytoma and sub-clinical Cushing's syndrome during pregnancy: diagnosis, medical pre-treatment and cure by laparoscopic unilateral adrenalectomy. J Endocrinol Invest 1999;22(7):551.
46. Schenker J, Chowers I. Pheochromocytoma and pregnancy: review of 89 cases. Obstet Gynecol 1971;26:739–47.
47. Kariya N, Nishi S, Hosono Y, et al. Cesarean section at 28 weeks' gestation with resection of pheochromocytoma: perioperative antihypertensive management. J Clin Anesth 2005;17:296–9.
48. Junglee N, Harries S, Davies N, et al. Pheochromocytoma in pregnancy: when is operative intervention indicated? J Womens Health (Larchmt) 2007;16: 1362–5.
49. Griffin J, Norman P, Douvas P, et al. Pheochromocytoma in pregnancy: diagnosis and collaborative management. South Med J 1984;77:1325–7.
50. Asensio MM, Pavon B, Barrena S, et al. Anesthesia for surgical removal of a pheochromocytoma during the first trimester of pregnancy. Rev Esp Anestesiol Reanim 2009;56:129–31 [in Spanish].

51. Kennelly M, Ball S, Robson V, et al. Difficult alpha-adrenergic blockade of a phaeochromocytoma in a twin pregnancy. J Obstet Gynaecol 2007;27: 729–30.
52. Kondziella D, Lycke J, Szentgyorgy E. A diagnosis not to miss: pheochromocytoma during pregnancy. J Neurol 2007;254:1612–3.
53. Ahlawat S, Jain S, Kumari S, et al. Pheochromocytoma associated with pregnancy: case report and review of the literature. Obstet Gynecol Surv 1999;54: 728–37.
54. Dugas G, Fuller J, Singh S, et al. Pheochromocytoma and pregnancy: a case report and review of anesthetic management. Can J Anaesth 2004;51:134–8.
55. Oliva R, Angelos P, Kaplan E, et al. Pheochromocytoma in pregnancy: a case series and review. Hypertension 2010;2010(600):606.
56. Stenstrom G, Sjostrom L, Smith U. Diabetes mellitus in phaeochromocytoma: fasting blood glucose levels before and after surgery in 60 patients with phaeochromocytoma. Acta Endocrinol 1984;106:511–5.
57. Santeiro ML, Stromquist C, Wyble L. Phenoxybenzamine placental transfer during the third trimester. Ann Pharmacother 1996;30(11):1249–51.
58. Lau J, Balk E, Rothberg M, et al. Management of clinically inapparent adrenal mass. Evidence Report/Technology Assessment, Number 56 [pamphlet]. Rockville (MD): Agency for Healthcare Research and Quality; 2002.
59. Aron DC. Endocrine incidentalomas. Endocrinol Metab Clin North Am 2002;29: 1–238.
60. Grumbach M, Biller B, Braunstein G, et al. Management of the clinically inapparent adrenal mass ("incidentaloma"). Ann Intern Med 2003;138(5):424–9.
61. Anagnostis P, Karagiannis A, Tziomalos K, et al. Adrenal incidentaloma: a diagnostic challenge. Hormones (Athens) 2009;8(3):163–84.
62. Aron D, Kievit J. Adrenal Incidentalomas. In: Schwartz AE, Pertsemlidis D, Gagner M, editors. Endocrine Surgery. New York: Marcel Dekker; 2004. p. 411–27.
63. Bertherat J, Mosnier-Pudar H, Bertagna X. Adrenal incidentalomas. Curr Opin Oncol 2002;14:58–63.
64. Mansmann G, Lau J, Balk E, et al. The clinically inapparent adrenal mass: update in diagnosis and management. Endocr Rev 2004;25:309–40.
65. Mantero F, Albiger N. A comprehensive approach to adrenal incidentalomas. Arq Bras Endocrinol Metabol 2004;48:583–91.
66. Nawar R, Aron D. Adrenal incidentalomas—a continuing management dilemma. Endocr Relat Cancer 2005;12:585–98.
67. Terzolo M, Bovio S, Pia A, et al. Management of adrenal incidentaloma. Best Pract Res Clin Endocrinol Metab 2009;23:233–43.
68. Young WF Jr. Management approaches to adrenal incidentalomas. A view from Rochester, Minnesota. Endocrinol Metab Clin North Am 2000;29:159–85.
69. Nieman L. Approach to the patient with an adrenal incidentaloma. J Clin Endocrinol Metab 2010;95(9):4106–13.
70. Berland L, Silverman S, Gore R, et al. Managing Incidental Findings on Abdominal CT: White Paper of the ACR Incidental Findings Committee. Am Coll Radiol 2010;7:754–73.
71. Holgersen LO, Subramanian S, Kirpekar M, et al. Spontaneous resolution of antenatally diagnosed adrenal masses. J Pediatr Surg 1996;31(1):153–5.
72. Outwater EK, Siegelman ES, Radecki PD, et al. Distinction between benign and malignant adrenal masses: value of T1-weighted chemical-shift MR imaging. AJR Am J Roentgenol 1995;165(3):579–83.

73. Outwater EK, Siegelman ES, Huang AB, et al. Adrenal masses: correlation between CT attenuation value and chemical shift ratio at MR imaging with in-phase and opposed-phase sequences. Radiology 1996;200(3):749–52.

74. Wan YL. Ultrasonography of the adrenal gland. J Med Ultrasound 2007;15(4): 213–27.

75. Fontana D, Porpiglia F, Destefanis P, et al. What is the role of ultrasonography in the follow-up of adrenal incidentalomas? The Gruppo Piemontese Incidentalomi Surrenalici. Urology 1999;54(4):612–6.

76. Fallo F, Pezzi V, Sonino N, et al. Adrenal incidentaloma in pregnancy: clinical, molecular and immunohistochemical findings. J Endocrinol Invest 2005;28(5): 459–63.

77. Joint LWPES/ESPE CAH Working Group. Consensus statement on 21-hydroxy-lase deficiency from the Lawson Wilkins Pediatric Endocrine Society and the European Society for Paediatric Endocrinology. J Clin Endocrinol Metab 2002; 87(9):4048–53.

Calcium and Bone Metabolism Disorders During Pregnancy and Lactation

Christopher S. Kovacs, MD, FRCPC

KEYWORDS
- Pregnancy • Lactation • Fetus • Neonate
- Parathyroid hormone-related protein
- Primary hyperparathyroidism • Hypoparathyroidism
- Pseudohypoparathyroidism • Vitamin D deficiency

Pregnancy and lactation require women to mobilize calcium to provide to the offspring. A common assumption is that higher intakes of calcium and vitamin D are required during these periods or else maternal and child health is impaired. However, several physiologic adaptations are invoked during pregnancy and lactation to supply the required calcium, such that the maternal requirements for calcium and vitamin D are unchanged. Intestinal calcium absorption is upregulated during pregnancy, and bone resorption provides much of the calcium in breast milk (**Fig. 1**). These adaptations may cause short-term fragility and depletion of skeletal mineral content but seem to have no adverse long-term consequences.

This article begins by reviewing the adaptations in mineral metabolism that occur during pregnancy and lactation, and then addresses how the presentation, diagnosis, and management of disorders of calcium and bone metabolism can be significantly altered by pregnancy and lactation. Other articles provide detailed references about the physiologic adaptations.[1–3]

Financial Disclosure: Nothing to disclose.
Grant Support: Supported in part by grant support from the Canadian Institutes of Health Research.
Faculty of Medicine–Endocrinology, Health Sciences Centre, Memorial University of Newfoundland, 300 Prince Philip Drive, St John's, Newfoundland, A1B 3V6, Canada
E-mail address: ckovacs@mun.ca

Endocrinol Metab Clin N Am 40 (2011) 795–826
doi:10.1016/j.ecl.2011.08.002
0889-8529/11/$ – see front matter © 2011 Elsevier Inc. All rights reserved.

endo.theclinics.com

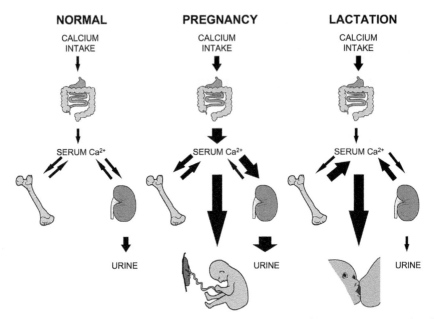

Fig. 1. Contrast of calcium homeostasis in human pregnancy and lactation, compared with normal. The thickness of arrows indicates a relative increase or decrease with respect to the normal and nonpregnant state. (*Adapted from* Kovacs CS, Kronenberg HM. Maternal-fetal calcium and bone metabolism during pregnancy, puerperium and lactation. Endocr Rev 1997;18:859; with permission.)

ADAPTATIONS DURING PREGNANCY

The human fetus accretes about 30 g of calcium by term, with 80% of it obtained during the third trimester.[4–6] Intestinal calcium absorption more than doubles during pregnancy to meet this increased demand for calcium; this upregulation is mediated by 1,25-dihydroxyvitamin D_3 (calcitriol), prolactin/placental lactogen, and possibly by other factors.

Mineral Ions and Calciotropic Hormones

Normal pregnancy alters serum calcium and calciotropic hormones as depicted in **Fig. 2.**[1] Most laboratories do not state pregnancy-specific ranges and so this schematic should serve as a guide. The total serum calcium (sum of the ionized, complexed, and albumin-bound fractions) decreases because of a decline in serum albumin but this has no physiologic significance. The ionized calcium is the physiologically important fraction and it remains unchanged throughout normal pregnancy. The ionized calcium or albumin-corrected serum calcium should be measured to know the correct value during the pregnant as well as nonpregnant states. Serum magnesium and phosphorus levels also remain normal.

First-generation parathyroid hormone (PTH) assays in the 1970s and 1980s detected multiple biologically inactive fragments of PTH, and some studies reported high levels of PTH during pregnancy, leading (together with the artifactual decrease in serum calcium) to the erroneous concept of physiologic hyperparathyroidism of pregnancy. With modern intact and biointact assays, PTH is normal or suppressed during pregnancy in North American women who consume diets adequate in calcium.[7–11] PTH

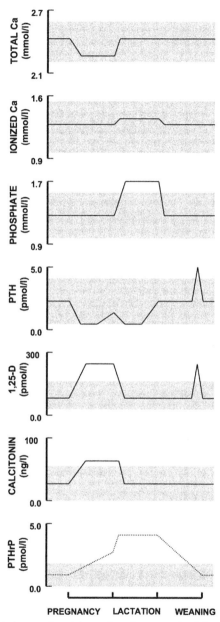

Fig. 2. The longitudinal changes in calcium, phosphorus, and calcitropic hormone levels that occur during pregnancy and lactation. Normal adult ranges are indicated by the shaded areas. The progression in parathyroid hormone-related protein (PTHrP) levels has been depicted by a dashed line to reflect that the data are less complete; the implied comparison of PTHrP levels in late pregnancy and lactation are uncertain extrapolations because no reports followed patients serially. In both situations PTHrP levels are increased. (*Adapted from* Kovacs CS, Kronenberg HM. Maternal-fetal calcium and bone metabolism during pregnancy, puerperium and lactation. Endocr Rev 1997;18:832–72; with permission.)

reaches a trough level in the low to normal range (becoming undetectable in some women) during the first trimester, and then increases steadily to the midnormal range by term.[7–11] Conversely in women consuming very low calcium intakes, such as in Asia and Africa, the serum PTH may exceed the normal range.[12]

Total calcitriol levels more than double during the first trimester and maintain this increase until term; however, free calcitriol levels do not increase until the third trimester.[1,13] PTH is suppressed and therefore is not the source driving the increase in calcitriol. Evidence from animal models suggests that prolactin or placental lactogen may stimulate renal 1α-hydroxylase.[1] Although the placenta expresses 1α-hydroxylase, it seems that the maternal kidneys account for most of the circulating calcitriol during pregnancy, as illustrated by an anephric woman on hemodialysis who had low calcitriol before and during her pregnancy.[1,14]

Serum calcitonin increases during pregnancy and may derive from thyroidal C cells, breast, and placenta. Although high calcitonin levels theoretically protect the maternal skeleton from excessive resorption during pregnancy, available animal data indicate that absence of calcitonin does not perturb the maternal skeleton during pregnancy.[15]

Parathyroid hormone-related protein (PTHrP), the mediator of humoral hypercalcemia of malignancy, is normally undetectable in the adult circulation but increases during late pregnancy. It may derive from diverse tissues including placenta, amnion, decidua, umbilical cord, fetal parathyroid glands, and breast. Whether PTHrP has functional significance for the pregnant mother is uncertain. Because of its late-pregnancy increase it is probably not responsible for the high calcitriol and suppressed PTH that occurs earlier in pregnancy. Moreover, PTHrP is less potent than PTH in stimulating renal 1α-hydroxylase.[16,17] Hypercalcemia caused by increased PTHrP secretion has been reported in late pregnancy and the puerperium.[18] PTHrP does regulate placental calcium transport at least from the fetal side,[19,20] and because its carboxyl-terminal end inhibits osteoclast-mediated bone resorption, it may protect the maternal skeleton against excessive bone resorption during pregnancy.[21–23]

Other hormones are significantly altered during pregnancy, including the sex steroids, prolactin, placental lactogen, and insulin-like growth factor 1. The effects that these alterations may have on maternal calcium and bone metabolism have been largely unexplored.

Intestinal Absorption of Calcium

Intestinal calcium absorption doubles from as early as the 12th week of pregnancy, the earliest time point studied.[1] This early increase in absorption leads to a positive calcium balance,[24] and may allow the maternal skeleton to store calcium before the peak fetal demands during the third trimester. Whether the increase in total calcitriol levels explains the increase in intestinal calcium absorption is uncertain. Animal studies have shown that intestinal calcium absorption upregulates during pregnancy despite severe vitamin D deficiency or absence of the vitamin D receptor.[25–27] Other animal studies indicate that prolactin and placental lactogen may stimulate intestinal calcium absorption during pregnancy.[28,29]

Renal Handling of Calcium

Enhanced intestinal calcium absorption leads to increased 24-hour urine calcium excretion, also beginning from at least the 12th week of gestation.[1] For many women the 24-hour value exceeds the normal range although the fasting urine calcium is low, confirming that this is absorptive hypercalciuria. High calcitonin levels may also promote renal calcium excretion.

Skeletal Calcium Metabolism

Although the doubling of intestinal calcium absorption may completely meet the calcium requirements of the fetus, there is inconsistent evidence that the maternal skeleton undergoes resorption during pregnancy. In 1 study, 15 women who electively terminated a pregnancy in the first trimester (8–10 weeks) had bone biopsy evidence of increased bone resorption, which was not present in biopsies obtained from nonpregnant controls.[30] No other studies have examined bone histomorphometry during human pregnancy, and instead alterations in steady-state levels of biomarkers of bone metabolism have been used to infer whether bone resorption and formation are altered during pregnancy. Use of these markers during pregnancy invokes several confounding variables that have been discussed in detail elsewhere.[13] Despite these limitations, many studies have consistently found that bone resorption is increased from early pregnancy to midpregnancy (based on 24-hour urine excretion of deoxypyridinoline, pyridinoline, and hydroxyproline). Conversely bone formation is suppressed from prepregnancy values before increasing to normal or higher by the late third trimester (based on osteocalcin, procollagen I carboxypeptides, and bone specific alkaline phosphatase). Total alkaline phosphatase increases early because of the placental fraction, and is not a useful marker of bone formation in pregnancy.

Alterations in bone turnover may also be implied by net changes in skeletal calcium content, but few studies have examined sequential bone density measurements during pregnancy. Using the now outdated technology of single-photon absorptiometry (SPA) or dual-photon absorptiometry (DPA), several prospective studies did not find a significant change in cortical or trabecular bone density during pregnancy.[1] The modern technique of dual radiograph absorptiometry (DXA) has been used 1 to 8 months before pregnancy and 1 to 6 weeks post partum in order to avoid fetal radiation exposure.[31–37] These studies were small (16 or fewer subjects) and found either no change or up to a 5% decrease in lumbar spine bone density at the postpartum measurement. Peripheral ultrasonographic bone mineral density (BMD) measurements at the heel also decreased in a prospective study of pregnant women.[38] Thus, although the longitudinal studies with SPA/DPA during pregnancy suggested no change in trabecular or cortical bone density, the subsequent evidence from preconception and postdelivery DXA, and peripheral ultrasonography, suggest that a small net loss of maternal bone mineral content (BMC) may occur.

These alterations in skeletal turnover during pregnancy do not normally cause long-term changes in skeletal calcium content or strength. Numerous studies of osteoporotic or osteopenic women have failed to find a significant association of parity with bone density or fracture risk.[1,39] A study of twins indicated that there may be a protective effect of parity and lactation on maintaining BMC.[40]

ADAPTATIONS DURING LACTATION

Women typically lose 210 mg of calcium through breast milk daily, and more if nursing twins. The main adaptation to provide this calcium seems to be skeletal resorption, stimulated in part by the effects of mammary-derived PTHrP and low estradiol.

Mineral Ions and Calciotropic Hormones

The normal lactational changes in maternal serum chemistries and calciotropic hormones are depicted in **Fig. 2**.[1] Laboratories do not provide lactation-specific ranges and so this schematic should serve as a guide. The mean ionized calcium and albumin-corrected serum calcium are modestly higher than prepregnant values but remain normal. Serum phosphorus increases and exceeds the normal range in some women. This mild hyperphosphatemia is likely caused by increased bone resorption and active reabsorption of phosphorus by the kidneys.

PTH, measured by intact or biointact assays, remains low during the first several months of exclusive lactation and is undetectable in many women. It increases to normal at weaning or slightly higher at weaning. Conversely, during the puerperium, calcitriol decreases to normal from the high values of pregnancy and remains normal throughout lactation.

PTHrP increases markedly in the blood of lactating women and seems to derive from the breast. It is released into milk at 10,000 times the concentration observed in the blood of patients with hypercalcemia of malignancy or normal human controls. Suckling may force PTHrP into the maternal bloodstream as shown by a small increase in PTHrP that has been observed after suckling in humans.[41] In addition, suckling-induced increases in urinary cAMP (a downstream mediator of the action of PTHrP on the kidney) have been observed in rodents.[42] Mammary tissue is likely the source of PTHrP in the maternal circulation, as confirmed by ablating the PTHrP gene only from mammary tissue in mice, resulting in a significant reduction in circulating PTHrP.[43] Moreover, a woman with massive mammary hyperplasia had increased PTHrP and hypercalcemia, which was corrected by reduction mammoplasty.[44]

PTHrP plays a central role during lactation by stimulating resorption of calcium from the maternal skeleton, renal tubular reabsorption of calcium, and (indirectly) suppression of PTH (**Fig. 3**). The breast becomes an accessory parathyroid during lactation, but the hyperparathyroidism of lactation is caused by increased secretion of PTHrP and not PTH. This role for PTHrP was confirmed when the PTHrP gene was ablated from mammary tissue at the onset of lactation and the mice lost significantly less BMC during lactation.[43] Clinical confirmation of the role of PTHrP in lactation includes that PTHrP correlates negatively with PTH and positively with the ionized calcium levels of lactating women,[41,45] and that higher plasma PTHrP correlates with greater loss of BMD during lactation.[46] Perhaps the most convincing confirmation of the role of PTHrP role during lactation is the normalization of mineral homeostasis that occurs in hypothyroid and aparathyroid women, as discussed later.

Calcitonin levels are increased in the first 6 weeks of lactation. Calcitonin may protect the maternal skeleton against excessive resorption during lactation, as suggested by calcitonin-depleted mice that lost twice the normal amount of BMC during lactation but restored their skeletons fully after weaning.[15] Available clinical data are conflicting on whether thyroidectomy-induced calcitonin deficiency leads to bone loss or an increase in fracture risk,[47–51] but no study has examined the bone mass of thyroidectomized women during pregnancy and lactation. Extrathyroidal production of calcitonin in placenta, pituitary, and lactating mammary tissues suggests that thyroidectomized women are not fully calcitonin-deficient.[52–54]

Intestinal Absorption of Calcium

Intestinal calcium absorption decreases to the nonpregnant rate from the high rate of pregnancy. This decrease coincides with the decrease in calcitriol levels to normal.

Renal Handling of Calcium

In humans, the glomerular filtration rate decreases during lactation, and renal excretion of calcium decreases to low levels. Renal tubular reabsorption of calcium must be increased to account for reduced calcium excretion in the setting of increased serum calcium.

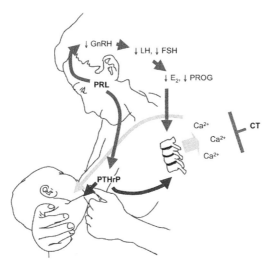

Fig. 3. The breast is a central regulator of skeletal demineralization during lactation. Suckling and prolactin both inhibit the hypothalamic gonadotropin-releasing hormone pulse center, which in turn suppresses the gonadotropins (luteinizing hormone [LH], follicle-stimulating hormone [FSH]), leading to low levels of the ovarian sex steroids (estradiol and progesterone). PTHrP production and release from the breast are controlled by several factors, including suckling, prolactin, and the calcium receptor. PTHrP enters the bloodstream and combines with systemically low estradiol levels to markedly upregulate bone resorption. Increased bone resorption releases calcium and phosphate into the blood stream, which then reaches the breast ducts and is actively pumped into the breast milk. PTHrP also passes into the milk at high concentrations, but whether swallowed PTHrP plays a role in regulating calcium physiology of the neonate is unknown. (*Reproduced from* Kovacs CS. Calcium and bone metabolism during pregnancy and lactation. J Mammary Gland Biol Neoplasia 2005;10(2):113; with permission.)

Skeletal Calcium Metabolism

Women lose 3% to 10% of trabecular BMC and smaller amounts from cortical sites during 2 to 6 months of lactation.[1,39,55] This skeletal resorption is not suppressed by increasing the dietary intake of calcium in women,[56–59] and the magnitude of decline in BMD correlates with the breast milk output.[60] The use of bone formation and resorption markers is fraught with confounding factors because of changes in blood volume and other factors, but resorption markers are consistently increased several-fold during lactation, and bone formation markers are also increased.

The bone loss seems to be regulated only in part by the hypoestrogenemia that occurs during lactation (estradiol values in the postmenopausal range of less than 150 pmol/L may occur). Bone density losses from lactation (5%–10% over 2–6 months) are more rapid than what occurs early after menopause, or in women of reproductive age who have acute estrogen deficiency induced by gonadotropin-releasing hormone (GnRH) agonist therapy.[1] PTHrP synergizes with low estradiol to enhance bone resorption and stimulates renal calcium reabsorption (**Fig. 4**). Studies in lactating mice have helped confirm the relative roles of estrogen deficiency and PTHrP in regulating lactational bone resorption.[43,61] It is likely that other factors play a role as well.

After weaning, the bone density is fully restored over the subsequent 6 to 12 months.[1,39,58] The mechanism for this recovery is uncertain and largely unexplored, but evidence from lactating rodents suggests that PTH, PTHrP, calcitriol, calcitonin,

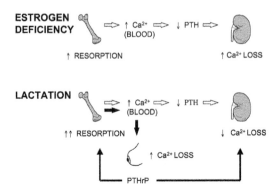

Fig. 4. Acute estrogen deficiency (eg, GnRH analogue therapy) increases skeletal resorption and increases the blood calcium; in turn, PTH is suppressed and renal calcium losses are increased. During lactation, the combined effects of PTHrP (secreted by the breast) and estrogen deficiency increase skeletal resorption, reduce renal calcium losses, and raise the blood calcium, but calcium is directed into the breast milk. (*Adapted from* Kovacs CS, Kronenberg HM. Maternal-fetal calcium and bone metabolism during pregnancy, puerperium and lactation. Endocr Rev 1997;18:854; with permission.)

and estrogen may not be required.[1,15,27] Lactation-induced depletion of bone mineral is clinically unimportant over the long-term, because most epidemiologic studies of premenopausal and postmenopausal women have found no adverse effect of a history of lactation on peak bone mass, bone density, or hip fracture risk.[1,39]

DISORDERS OF BONE AND MINERAL METABOLISM DURING PREGNANCY AND LACTATION

Pregnancy is characterized by increased intestinal calcium absorption, normal ionized or albumin-corrected calcium, high calcitriol, low PTH, gradually increasing PTHrP, and hypercalciuria (see **Fig. 2**). During lactation ionized calcium is slightly increased, PTHrP increases further, calcitriol and intestinal calcium resorption are normal, and bone resorption occurs (see **Figs. 2** and **3**). These differing hormonal changes can lead to nonclassic presentations of disorders of bone and mineral metabolism.

Primary Hyperparathyroidism

Incidence and epidemiology
Fewer than 200 cases of primary hyperparathyroidism during pregnancy have been reported in the English literature,[62,63] compared with the overall incidence of primary hyperparathyroidism in the general population of 4/100,000, with most cases older than 45 years.[64] An older series from an interval of automated screening of the serum calcium found the incidence of primary hyperparathyroidism in women of child-bearing age to be approximately 8/100,000 per year compared with 188/100,000 per year in women older than 60 years.[65] In 2 large retrospective case series parathyroidectomies performed during pregnancy accounted for 0.8% to 1.4% of the total.[62,66] In addition to being rare, the diagnosis may be confounded by the normal pregnancy-related decrease in serum albumin and suppressed PTH. If the ionized calcium or albumin-corrected serum calcium is increased with a detectable PTH level, this reliably indicates primary hyperparathyroidism even during pregnancy.

Maternal hypercalcemia can result in significant maternal and fetal morbidity and mortality. Complications have been found in up to 67% of mothers and 80% of their babies.[67] The relative distribution of adenomas versus hyperplasia is no different than in nonpregnant cases.[68] Among 100 cases of pregnancy-associated primary hyperparathyroidism, the histology was adenomas in 89%, hyperplasia in 9%, and carcinoma in 2%.[62]

Clinical features of the pregnant woman

Normal pregnancy is associated with many nonspecific symptoms that overlap with symptoms of hypercalcemia, such as nausea, hyperemesis, constipation, fatigue, weakness, and mental symptoms. The overlap of symptoms may delay the diagnosis of hyperparathyroidism. In a series of 45 pregnant women with hyperparathyroidism, 38% had nausea, vomiting or abdominal pain, 24% had renal colic, 22% had muscular weakness, 22% had mental symptoms, 11% had skeletal pain or fatigue and only 20% were asymptomatic.[69] Other symptoms may include hyperemesis gravidarum, weight loss, seizures, and features suggesting preeclampsia.[62,66] Clinical signs may include renal disease (nephrocalcinosis, nephrolithiasis, urinary tract infections), pancreatitis, and skeletal resorption on radiographs.[69,70] The absorptive hypercalciuria of pregnancy normally predisposes to nephrolithiasis and it is likely that this is aggravated by primary hyperparathyroidism. Pancreatitis may be the presenting manifestation in up to 15% of cases of primary hyperparathyroidism in pregnancy,[69,71–74] and usually occurs during the second or third trimester.[75] Severe hypercalcemia or parathyroid crisis can occur during the third trimester or especially post partum.[73,76–78] Rapid transfer of calcium across the placenta during the third trimester may protect against maternal hypercalcemia but this effect is abruptly lost after delivery of the placenta, thereby precipitating a postpartum hypercalcemic crisis.[76–78] Fractures are unlikely but have been reported in association with both marked hyperparathyroidism and parathyroid carcinoma.[79,80]

Fetal complications

Stillbirth, miscarriage, and neonatal tetany remain among the serious and common complications of primary hyperparathyroidism during pregnancy. The available data from case series suggest that the outcomes have improved over the past several decades as stillbirth declined from 13% to 2%, neonatal death from 8% to 2%, and neonatal tetany from 38% to 15% of cases.[70] The neonate is at high risk of hypocalcemia and tetany in the perinatal period as a result of suppression of the parathyroid glands in utero, and which remain suppressed for weeks afterward. In several case series, perinatal death occurred in 25% to 30%, whereas 50% of neonates had some complication, with the most common cause being tetany.[62,81–83] Hypocalcemia usually occurs in the perinatal period but presentations as late as 2.5 months post partum have been reported.[84] Although the neonatal hypoparathyroidism normally resolved within 3 to 5 months after birth,[70] some children have been left with permanent hypoparathyroidism, presumably because the development of the parathyroids was too suppressed in utero.[70,82,85] Hypocalcemia seems more likely in bottle-fed than breastfed infants because the higher phosphate/calcium ratio in formula and cow's milk binds calcium more tightly compared with breast milk.[70]

Management

There have been 3 international workshops to determine consensus guidelines for the management of asymptomatic primary hyperparathyroidism, but none has addressed pregnancy.[86] The preferred management of primary hyperparathyroidism during pregnancy is a parathyroidectomy, which should prevent fetal and neonatal morbidities, as well as a postpartum parathyroid crisis. However, the evidence is based on case series (which are subject to reporting biases) and not any randomized trials. A review of 39 surgically and 70 medically treated cases of hyperparathyroidism during pregnancy found 53% neonatal complications and 16% neonatal deaths in the medical group, compared with 12.5% neonatal complications and 2.5% neonatal deaths in those who underwent parathyroidectomy.[62] Parathyroidectomy is generally considered to be safest in the second trimester to avoid the complications of anesthesia, surgery, and precipitated delivery during the third trimester.[69,70,74,83] One case series reinforced this notion by observing that 4 of 7 third-trimester surgeries resulted in premature labor with neonatal death.[74] However, parathyroidectomy can be performed in the third trimester and should be done when the risks of surgery are considered lower than the risks of continued observation. Several case reports documented that third-trimester surgery was performed without adverse consequences.[63,78,87] A review of 3000 surgical cases determined that pregnancy significantly predicted a bilateral surgical approach to identifying all 4 glands, but the necessary absence of preoperative imaging likely played a role in the surgeon's decision.[88] On the other hand, minimally invasive surgery has been performed during pregnancy and may reduce the risks for mother and fetus.[89] Medical management is still appropriate for some women considered to have relatively benign hypercalcemia as long as careful attention in the postpartum interval avoids a parathyroid crisis.[90] A multidisciplinary approach to management is clearly needed with both maternal and fetal/neonatal outcomes considered in the decision-making process.

Localizing the adenoma preoperatively is difficult because the radioisotopes needed for parathyroid and thyroid scans must be avoided, ultrasonography has limited sensitivity, 10% of cases may involve hyperplasia of all 4 glands, and ectopic parathyroid glands occur. However, in 1 case ultrasound-guided needle aspiration of a suspected nodule enabled confirmation that it contained a high concentration of PTH, thereby enabling the surgeon to perform minimally invasive surgery.[89]

Medical treatment includes adequate hydration and correction of electrolyte abnormalities,[67] but pharmacologic agents approved to treat hypercalcemia have not been adequately studied in pregnancy. Calcitonin is a pregnancy category B medication of the US Food and Drug Administration that does not cross the placenta and has been used safely in pregnancy to suppress bone resorption and promote urine calcium excretion.[67] Oral phosphate is a pregnancy category C medication and has been used in pregnancy with modest efficacy to bind calcium. The most common side effects of phosphate are diarrhea and hypokalemia. It should be avoided in patients with renal failure and high serum phosphorus levels because of the risk of soft tissue calcifications.[67] Mithramycin is contradicted because of adverse effects on fetal development. Bisphosphonates cross the placenta and if received in sufficient doses may interfere with endochondral bone development,[91] but this effect has not yet been seen in any cases in which the mother received a bisphosphonate during pregnancy.[92–94] Cinacalcet is also a category C medication but has been used in pregnancy in at least 1 case.[90] This drug acts on the calcium receptor to suppress PTH synthesis and release and to stimulate calcitonin, thereby lowering the blood calcium, but its use is limited by the side effect of nausea. However, the calcium receptor is also expressed in placenta, fetal parathyroids, and C cells,[95–97] and so cinacalcet may also suppress the fetal parathyroid glands, stimulate fetal calcitonin, and alter the rate of placental calcium transfer. High-dose magnesium also acts on the calcium receptor to decrease PTH and calcium, and it is effective in delaying premature labor.[98,99] The clinical experience with any of these pharmacologic therapies is at the level of individual case reports and so the relative benefits and risks of each option are unknown. Moreover, the reported follow-up on the children is generally brief.

If medical management is undertaken there should be appropriate surveillance of maternal serum calcium and PTH, and regular biophysical profiles of the fetus by ultrasonography. In the postpartum interval the serum calcium should be expected to increase after the placenta is discharged and as the hemodilution of pregnancy resolves. Postpartum parathyroidectomy should be considered in cases that were medically managed during pregnancy.

Lactation adds a significant component of bone resorption because of the combined effects of PTHrP and low estradiol, and hypercalcemia can be expected to worsen in a woman who chooses to breastfeed. Potential maternal hypercalcemia is another consideration in deciding whether a postpartum parathyroidectomy is warranted versus ongoing surveillance.

Surveillance of the neonate is required for early detection and treatment of neonatal hypocalcemia. The blood calcium normally decreases about 20% over the first 12 hours with the onset of breathing, and rises to the adult normal range over the succeeding 24 to 48 hours.[100–102] Neonatal hypoparathyroidism caused by maternal hyperparathyroidism is usually transient and should be treated with calcium and calcitriol. If the infant is premature there may be no response to calcitriol because the intestine does not yet express the vitamin D receptor at high levels. Neonates should also be fed milk formulas high in calcium and low in phosphate to minimize the risk of hypocalcemia. Ongoing surveillance determines whether the hypoparathyroidism is permanent.

Neonatal hypocalcemia and other complications are not inevitable after marked maternal hypercalcemia during pregnancy. Conversely, some cases of neonatal hypocalcemia and tetany have occurred after mild, asymptomatic maternal hypocalcemia.[103] The variability of fetal and neonatal responses is best exemplified by a twin pregnancy in which 1 neonate developed hypocalcemia and tetanic seizures, whereas the other twin was completely normal.[104]

Poorly controlled maternal diabetes predisposes the infant to develop hypocalcemia, seizures, and tetany during the first 24 to 72 hours after birth. Hyperphosphatemia is often present, which, together with hypocalcemia, is consistent with transient hypoparathyroidism or failure of neonatal parathyroid function to increase normally after birth. A case series found that the ionized and total serum calcium were higher in cord blood of infants of diabetic mothers compared with control infants, and that the neonatal parathyroids remained suppressed longer after birth in infants of diabetic mothers.[105] A higher serum calcium in utero would suppress the parathyroids, but why the fetal calcium should be higher in the setting of maternal diabetes is unknown. Maternal magnesium wasting from glucosuria during pregnancy has been postulated to cause fetal and neonatal hypoparathyroidism, but a small clinical trial found no effect of postnatal magnesium supplementation on the incidence of neonatal hypocalcemia in infants of diabetic mothers.[106] Other factors such as prematurity, lung immaturity, and asphyxia increase the risk of hypocalcemia in these infants.

Familial Benign Hypocalciuric Hypercalcemia

Inactivating mutations in the calcium-sensing receptor cause autosomal-dominant hypercalcemia and hypocalciuria.[107] Because the condition develops in utero, maternal hypercalcemia is fully adapted to, asymptomatic, and free of the complications associated with hypercalcemia caused by primary hyperparathyroidism (eg, bone resorption, nephrolithiasis, nephrocalcinosis). Pregnancy seems to be uneventful in women with this condition.[108] However, the maternal hypercalcemia can cause suppression of the fetal parathyroids, followed by neonatal hypocalcemia and tetany.[108,109] The neonate of a woman known to have familial benign hypocalciuric hypercalcemia (FBHH) should undergo surveillance for hypocalcemia. Conversely, when a neonate presents with hypocalcemia the mother may be mistaken as having primary hyperparathyroidism. Treatment of the neonate is similar to that of children born to mothers with hyperparathyroidism (see earlier discussion).

The calcium-sensing receptor is expressed in the epithelial ducts of breast tissue, and has been shown to modulate the production of PTHrP and the transport of calcium into milk in mice.[110,111] Inactivating mutations of the receptor, analogous to the human mutation in FBHH, increase mammary gland PTHrP production but decrease milk calcium content.[111] Conversely, a calcimimetic drug similar to cinacalcet causes increased milk calcium content.[111] These data suggest that women with FBHH have more marked skeletal resorption during lactation and lower calcium content of milk, but no clinical studies have examined this observation.

Hypoparathyroidism

Most patients are known to have hypoparathyroidism or aparathyroidism before pregnancy, and the therapeutic challenge becomes how best to manage the blood calcium. The physiologic adaptations in pregnancy include upregulation of intestinal calcium absorption at a time when PTH becomes suppressed, and increasing levels of calcitriol, PTHrP, and other factors in the circulation. It is possible that women with hypoparathyroidism increase calcium delivery and attain a higher serum calcium level during pregnancy. Conversely, the fetal demand for calcium may overwhelm the mother's ability to maintain her own blood calcium, and hypocalcemic symptoms may worsen during pregnancy. The available case reports are consistent with both possibilities in that some women had lessening of symptoms and a lower requirement for calcium and calcitriol replacement during pregnancy, whereas others required higher doses of calcium and calcitriol.[1,112,113] It is also clear in a few reports that the normal decline in serum calcium caused by hemodilution was mistaken for worsening of hypocalcemia, and treatment was instituted based on that artifact and not hypocalcemic symptoms.[1]

The target for pregnancy should be to maintain the ionized calcium or albumin-corrected serum calcium in the low- to mid-normal range. An initial approach is to consider that because calcitriol levels normally double in the first trimester, therefore hypoparathyroid women should initially receive an increased dose of calcitriol or equivalent. Then, as pregnancy progresses, the calcitriol dose can be adjusted based on the ionized calcium level. Maternal hypocalcemia must be avoided because it increases the risk of premature labor and of fetal and neonatal secondary hyperparathyroidism, which in turn causes skeletal demineralization, subperiosteal bone resorption, and osteitis fibrosa cystica.[114] Conversely, overtreatment with calcitriol causes maternal hypercalcemia and suppression of the fetal and neonatal parathyroids, and there is the additional concern of teratogenicity that has been shown using older vitamin D preparations.[115,116] High-dose vitamin D (cholecalciferol) is still used to manage some cases of hypoparathyroidism but this requires high levels of 25-hydroxyvitamin D (>250 nmol/L or 100 ng/mL), for which fetal adverse effects remain uncertain. Calcitriol and 1α-calcidiol have shorter half-lives and lower risk of toxicity compared with the older preparations. In a recent case series of 10 women treated with calcitriol at doses of 0.25 to 3.25 μg/d, healthy babies were delivered to 10 women.[113] However, in 2 cases, serious adverse events occurred, including premature closure of the frontal fontanelle and stillbirth, but the causative role of calcitriol could not be established.[113] In 9 additional cases (summarized in the same report) of pregnancy in women with hypoparathyroidism or vitamin D–resistant rickets, no toxicity or teratogenicity was observed from use of high-dose cholecalciferol, calcitriol, or 1α-calcidiol, but only 2 women were treated with high-dose cholecalciferol.[113]

Calcium and calcitriol requirements decrease in hypoparathyroid patients during lactation, such that women become hypercalcemic unless the supplements are reduced substantially or discontinued.[117,118] The decreased requirement for calcium and calcitriol occurs when circulating PTHrP levels are high in the maternal circulation.[119–121] Mammary-derived PTHrP may stimulate endogenous calcitriol formation; in 1 patient the calcitriol level initially decreased less than normal when exogenous calcitriol was discontinued but thereafter the calcitriol level increased and remained in the lower half of the normal range as lactation proceeded.[119] These observations in hypoparathyroid women illustrate the impact of normal physiologic adaptations that invoke PTHrP and low estradiol-stimulated bone resorption during lactation and that may normalize mineral homeostasis for the duration of exclusive lactation.

The variability of responses during pregnancy and the subsequent alteration in calcium homeostasis during lactation make the management of hypoparathyroidism during pregnancy and lactation a challenge. During pregnancy, calcium supplementation should be maintained with an increased dose of calcitriol, but monitoring for hypocalcemic symptoms and use of the ionized calcium or albumin-corrected serum calcium to adjust the calcitriol dose as pregnancy progresses. The requirements for exogenous calcitriol vary during the second half of pregnancy but are expected to decrease substantially (if not completely) during lactation.

Pseudohypoparathyroidism

Pseudohypoparathyroidism or genetic resistance to PTH results in hypocalcemia, hyperphosphatemia, and high PTH. A few case reports have shown that this condition improved during pregnancy such that women became normocalcemic and did not require therapeutic doses of calcium or vitamin D analogues.[122] In contrast, other case reports have suggested that increased doses of calcium and calcitriol are needed to maintain the serum calcium in the normal range.[123,124] In 1 case a drop in the total serum calcium and not a change in symptoms prompted the dose increase,[123] whereas in the other case the woman recalled worsening of hypocalcemic symptoms during the second half of 2 pregnancies but did not receive treatment.[124]

The mechanism by which pseudohypoparathyroidism might be improved in pregnancy is unclear but may include effects of estradiol and other pregnancy-related hormones on the 1α-hydroxylase, because calcitriol levels more than doubled (similar to normal pregnancy) during the second and third trimester for 2 pseudohypoparathyroid women.[122] Placental production of calcitriol was identical to that of normal placentas in 4 pregnancies of pseudohypoparathyroid women,[125] but the significance of this observation is uncertain. As noted earlier, a case report from a pregnant anephric women suggests that most of the circulating calcitriol during pregnancy derives from the maternal kidneys with little or no contribution from the placenta.[14] The fetuses and neonates of women with pseudohypoparathyroidism are prone to secondary hyperparathyroidism and neonatal hypocalcemia unless maternal normocalcemia is maintained during pregnancy.[126]

The impact of lactation on calcium metabolism in pseudohypoparathyroidism is less well documented. These patients do not have skeletal resistance to PTH, and thus calcium and vitamin D requirements may decrease secondary to enhanced skeletal resorption because of the combined effects of endogenous high PTH levels, increasing PTHrP release from the breast, and lactation-induced estrogen deficiency. Women with pseudohypoparathyroidism might be anticipated to lose more bone density than normal during lactation.

Osteoporosis Associated with Pregnancy and Lactation

Epidemiology and pathogenesis
Osteoporosis usually presents as a fracture during late pregnancy or the first several months of lactation in women who have never had a baseline measure of bone density

or previous concern about skeletal strength.[127–130] Consequently, in most cases it remains unclear whether these osteoporotic fractures occurred in a previously abnormal skeleton, or whether skeletal resorption during pregnancy and lactation caused bone strength to become compromised.

Skeletal resorption normally occurs during lactation under the actions of mammary gland-derived PTHrP and low estradiol levels; therefore, lactation-induced osteoporotic fractures may occur when skeletal resorption is excessive or when the baseline bone mass is low and unable to tolerate the normal lactational losses of mineral. PTHrP levels were high in 1 case of lactational osteoporosis and remained increased for months after weaning.[131] A case series of 13 women with pregnancy-associated osteoporosis observed that BMD at the spine and hip increased significantly over time, suggesting that most of the apparent bone loss had been related to the pregnancy.[128] In another series, there were more fractures among the mothers of the women with pregnancy-associated osteoporosis than among the mothers of controls, indicating a possible genetic cause for fracture associated with pregnancy.[132] However, in that study too most of the women increased their BMD significantly during follow-up.[132] Because loss of endogenous calcitonin in mice more than doubles the lactation-induced losses of BMD,[15] it is possible that some women with lactation-induced osteoporosis might have a genetic deficiency in calcitonin or its receptor. Because the baseline BMD has been unknown in all reported cases, the relative contribution of baseline abnormalities in the skeleton versus pregnancy or lactation-associated changes in skeletal architecture remains unknown.

Clinical features

Osteoporosis during pregnancy usually presents in a first pregnancy or lactation at a mean of 27 to 28 years and increasing parity does not increase the risk of occurrence.[128–130] The most common presentation is a clinical or symptomatic vertebral compression fracture with significant pain in the lower thoracic or lumbar area.[128–130] Occasionally multiple fractures occur, as in 1 woman who had 8 at presentation.[133] Pain normally improves spontaneously over several weeks, as with most osteoporotic fractures, but may persist for years.[129] Most cases do not recur.

A distinct presentation, which may represent a different disorder, is hip pain and limp caused by transient osteoporosis of the hip.[128–130,134] Of the more than 200 cases of transient osteoporosis of the hip that have been reported in patients of both sexes, one-third occurred in women in the third trimester or early post partum.[134–136] The differential diagnosis includes inflammatory joint disorders, avascular necrosis of the hip, bone marrow edema, and reflex sympathetic dystrophy. There is usually no history of trauma, and no evidence of muscle spasm or the skin changes associated with reflex sympathetic dystrophy.[135] This condition does recur in about 40% of cases from both sexes, but how often the syndrome recurs in pregnant women is unknown.[134]

Pathogenesis and diagnostic studies

In most cases of pregnancy-associated or lactation-associated osteoporosis presenting with vertebral compression fractures there is no evident cause, but secondary causes of bone loss should be sought. In some cases, anorexia nervosa, hyperparathyroidism, osteogenesis imperfecta, corticosteroid or heparin therapy, and other secondary causes were identified.[129,130,132] In 1 case a woman with premature ovarian failure conceived after oocyte transfer and developed vertebral fractures; it seems probable that her bone mass had been low as a result of the preceding ovarian failure.[137] Pregnancy does not necessarily mean that bone mass decreases, as shown by a woman with very low bone density (−4.7 standard deviations [SD]) caused by chemotherapy-induced ovarian failure who gained 12% in the lumbar spine and 15% in the hip during pregnancy.[138]

Serum calcium, phosphorus, and calciotropic hormone levels have generally been normal in reported cases of osteoporosis associated with pregnancy or lactation.[129,130] The few available bone biopsies have shown evidence of osteoporosis but no osteomalacia.[129,130] Bone density is usually lower than expected but typically no prepregnancy baseline readings are available.[128,130] One series of 24 patients found low bone mass with mean Z-score −1.98 (±1.5, N = 15) at the lumbar spine and −1.48 (±1.5, N = 15) at the total hip.[130]

In transient osteoporosis of the hip, radiographs or magnetic resonance imaging show reduced bone density and increased water content of the marrow cavity.[134] A fracture may also be present. Serum chemistries and calciotropic hormone levels are normal.

Management

Any secondary causes of osteoporosis should be treated. For most patients none is identified and conservative treatment remains appropriate. The natural history of pregnancy and lactation-associated osteoporosis is for the BMD to increase substantially afterward, for pain to decrease, and for the condition not to recur in subsequent pregnancies. Most cases improve symptomatically within a few weeks with conservative measures.[129,134] Numerous pharmacologic agents have been used, including calcium, vitamin D, testosterone, estrogen, calcitonin, teriparatide,[139] and bisphosphonates,[129,133,140] although kyphoplasty[141] and vertebroplasty[142] have also been used to reduce pain. In most reports the investigators concluded that their treatment was effective and beneficial but do not acknowledge that the natural history is for the pain to subside and the BMD to increase substantially.[128,132] Because all of these cases lacked controls, the efficacy of such interventions remains unproved and they are therefore not warranted unless the clinical situation is considered desperate.

In severe cases of osteoporosis, it may be prudent to discourage breastfeeding, the rationale being that the skeleton may not be able to tolerate the normal resorption and demineralization that lactation induces. We advised so in the case of a 33-year-old woman with severe osteoporosis (BMD −4.7 SD and previous fracture), caused by chemotherapy-induced ovarian failure, who unexpectedly conceived a baby.[143] Patients should be cautioned against carrying heavy weights to avoid additional stress on the spine, and the use of a supportive corset may be helpful. They should also be reassured that the BMD should increase over the coming months,[128,132] and that the condition will most likely not recur.

Transient osteoporosis of the hip is usually self-limiting, and conservative measures including bed-rest are all that is required. Radiograph abnormalities resolve within a few months but the condition may recur.[134]

Magnesium Sulfate Administration During Pregnancy

Intravenous magnesium sulfate is typically used for 24 to 72 hours to treat preterm labor, preeclampsia, and eclampsia. Magnesium activates the calcium-sensing receptor to suppress PTH and thus disturbances in calcium metabolism may occur with long-term tocolytic therapy.[107]

Maternal complications

Hypocalcemia can occur with tocolytic therapy to suppress premature labor.[144–146] A typical pattern is for the serum PTH to decrease within the first hour and for the total and ionized serum calcium levels to remain below normal several hours later.[145,146]

Most cases seem asymptomatic but symptomatic hypocalcemia with positive Chvostek and Trousseau signs, or tetany, has been observed.[147]

When magnesium treatment continues beyond the initial 24 to 72 hours and into 2 to 3 weeks, the serum PTH may become stimulated above normal. The high PTH may be secondary hyperparathyroidism in response to prolonged hypocalcemia and urinary loss of calcium.[148] In a series of 20 women given intravenous magnesium sulfate for premature labor, serum magnesium and phosphorus increased, serum calcium decreased, serum PTH increased, and urinary excretion of magnesium and calcium increased 2-fold 3-fold.[148] Such secondary hyperparathyroidism can be expected to decrease bone mineralization and strength; prolonged magnesium administration for several weeks has also been associated with postpartum loss of BMD and calcaneal stress fractures.[148–150]

Neonatal complications

Magnesium is actively transported across the placenta; intravenous administration of magnesium to pregnant women causes fetal and neonatal hypermagnesemia, lower PTH levels, and variable effects on the total and ionized calcium of neonates.[144,146] Whether this hypermagnesemia has an adverse, neutral, or beneficial effect is unclear based on the aggregate results of several studies.[144,151–153] Two studies found that neonates were more likely to have respiratory depression and hypotonia if their mothers had received several days of intravenous magnesium sulfate.[152,153] Another study found that cord blood and neonatal serum magnesium levels were of no clinical value unless severe hypermagnesemia was present.[153,154] In contrast, the neonatal death rate was lower in infants whose mothers had received 10 to 95 g of intramuscular magnesium compared with those who had received no therapy; however, respiratory depression and hypotonia were not assessed in that report.[151] Several reports indicate that prolonged magnesium exposure in utero may cause bone abnormalities in the neonates, including defective ossification of bone and enamel in the teeth,[155] and abnormal mineralization of osteoid within the metaphyses.[156–158]

Within these reports there were variable dosing, duration, and routes of magnesium treatment, variable achieved cord blood magnesium levels, and variable gestational ages of the neonates. These factors may contribute to the apparently conflicting results of a beneficial, neutral, or adverse effect of neonatal hypermagnesemia.

Management

Maternal and cord blood magnesium are not routinely monitored. However, because severe hypermagnesemia (>7 mg/dL) can cause hypotonia, respiratory depression, and bone abnormalities,[144,153,154,158] it seems prudent to monitor maternal serum calcium and magnesium levels, and fetal movement, when tocolytic therapy is given for 2 days or more. Symptomatic neonates may need ventilation for 24 to 48 hours and intravenous fluids for electrolyte balance, with intravenous calcium used to antagonize the central nervous system depression and peripheral neuromuscular blockade.[153]

Low Calcium Intake

The doubling of intestinal calcium absorption implies that for most women there is no need for increased dietary intake of calcium during pregnancy. The 24-hour urine calcium excretion exceeds the normal range for many women and this suggests that calcium intake during pregnancy normally exceeds maternal requirements. Among women with documented low dietary calcium intake there was no consistent effect of calcium supplementation during pregnancy to improve maternal or neonatal bone density.[159] A double-blind study in 256 pregnant women found no effect of 2 g of calcium supplementation versus placebo on the BMC of the infants; however, a post-hoc subgroup analysis suggested that infants whose supplemented mothers were in the lowest quintile of calcium intake (<600 mg/d) did have a beneficial effect on BMC,[160] suggesting that calcium supplementation may benefit only those women (and their babies) with low dietary intakes of calcium.

Low calcium intake has been associated with increased risk of preeclampsia. Individual trials and meta-analyses have shown calcium supplementation reduces the risk of preeclampsia but only when the dietary calcium intake is low; there may be no effect when dietary calcium intake is adequate.[161–164]

During lactation the calcium that ends up in milk seems to derive largely from skeletal resorption; consistent with this finding, low calcium intake does not reduce breast milk calcium content nor does it accentuate maternal bone loss.[165] Even in women with very low calcium intakes, the breast milk calcium content was unchanged, and amount of mineral lost from the skeleton did not differ from those with the highest calcium or vitamin D intakes.[166–168] Conversely, high-calcium intakes do not reduce the magnitude of bone loss that occurs during lactation.[56–59]

In general, the physiologic changes in calcium and bone metabolism during pregnancy and lactation ensure fetal bone growth and breast-milk production in women with reasonable intakes of dietary calcium.[165] This finding is reflected in the 2011 Reference Dietary Intakes from the Institute of Medicine, which advise that calcium intakes during pregnancy and lactation should be no higher than in nonpregnant women of the same age.[169]

There has been lingering concern that adolescent pregnancy and lactation might impair achievement of expected peak bone mass, but the evidence suggests otherwise.[170] NHANES III (the National Health and Nutrition Examination Survey II) obtained BMD in 819 women aged 20 to 25 years and found that women who had been pregnant as adolescents had the same BMD as nulliparous women and women who had been pregnant as adults.[171] Also, women who had breastfed as adolescents had higher BMD than women who had not breastfed and nulliparous women, even after controlling for obstetric variables.[171] These findings reassure that the normal loss of BMD during lactation and full recovery afterward occurs in adolescent women too without any long-term deficit.

Vitamin D Deficiency and Genetic Vitamin D Resistance Syndromes

Maternal 25-hydroxyvitamin D levels do not change significantly during pregnancy,[172–175] even in women starting with the extremely low level of 20 nmol/L (8 ng/mL),[175] and thus it does not seem that pregnant women require higher intakes of vitamin D to maintain a set 25-hydroxyvitamin D level. Severe vitamin D deficiency causes hypocalcemia, hypophosphatemia, secondary hyperparathyroidism, muscle weakness/myopathy, and rickets or osteomalacia. Pregnancy in a woman with severe vitamin D deficiency can lead to worsening of hypocalcemia and also significant obstetric problems during labor. If vitamin D deficiency is recognized during pregnancy, the mother should be treated with calcium as well as a loading and maintenance dose of cholecalciferol to increase the maternal 25-hydroxyvitamin D level to at least 50 nmol/L (20 ng/mL). High-dose vitamin D has been proposed to have nonskeletal benefits such as reduced preterm delivery, preeclampsia, and vaginal infections. Two trials of high-dose vitamin D in pregnancy have been completed (4000 IU vs 2000 IU or 400 IU daily), 30% to 40% of participants dropped out, and neither trial showed any skeletal or nonskeletal benefit to mother or child apart from higher 25-hydroxyvitamin D levels.[176,177]

The genetic forms of vitamin D resistance can also lead to worsening during pregnancy but if normocalcemia is maintained the pregnancy should be uneventful.[178,179]

In women with absent 1α-hydroxylase (vitamin D-dependent rickets type 1, VDDR-I) treatment with calcium and physiologic doses of calcitriol or 1α-cholecalciferol should be adjusted as needed (similar to the management of hypoparathyroidism) to maintain a normal ionized or albumin-corrected serum calcium. In women with absent vitamin D receptor (VDDR-II) there may no responsiveness to even extremely high doses of calcitriol or cholecalciferol, but a high-calcium diet should be sufficient to maintain a normal ionized or albumin-corrected serum calcium.

Because of relatively free passage of 25-hydroxyvitamin D across the placenta, cord blood values are 75% to 100% of the maternal level at term.[180–184] Animal models have clearly shown that severe vitamin D deficiency, absent 1α-hydroxylase, or absent vitamin D receptor do not affect the fetus, which is born with a normally formed and fully mineralized skeleton, and normal blood calcium, phosphorus, and PTH.[185–191] It is not until the time of weaning, when intestinal calcium absorption becomes an active, calcitriol-dependent process,[192–194] that the untreated neonate begins to develop hypocalcemia and rickets. Even then, a high-calcium diet prevents the skeletal and biochemical abnormalities.[190,195–199] Available data from human babies suggest that those with severe vitamin D deficiency (including mean fetal 25-hydroxyvitamin D of 10 nmol/L [4 ng/mL]), VDDR-I, or VDDR-II, all have normal cord blood calcium, phosphorus, PTH, ash weight, and mineral content of the skeleton, and no radiological signs of rickets.[175,200–203] Even when 126 pregnant mothers were treated in a randomized controlled trial with an apparent dose of 10,000 IU of cholecalciferol per day versus placebo, and the achieved cord blood 25-hydroxyvitamin D levels were 138 nmol/L (55 ng/mL) versus 10 nmol/L (4 ng/mL), there was no change in cord blood calcium or phosphorus, and no radiological signs of rickets.[175] In regions where vitamin D deficiency is endemic and there is increased vigilance for early signs of rickets, none is evident until days to weeks after birth.[201–205]

The untreated (especially breastfed[206]) vitamin-D–deficient neonate eventually develops progressive problems of hypocalcemia, secondary hyperparathyroidism, and rickets, with the peak incidence of rickets occurring at 18 months of age in most surveys.[201–204,206] Neonatal hypocalcemia after 48 hours is the earliest manifestation at which time the skeleton is likely to be radiographically normal; hypocalcemia attributable to vitamin D deficiency does not occur with 25-hydroxyvitamin D levels greater than 30 nmol/L (12 ng/mL).[175,207,208] Rickets caused by vitamin D deficiency also does not develop if the 25-hydroxyvitamin D level is maintained greater than 30 nmol/L (12 ng/mL)[209]; conversely, if dietary calcium intake is low or blocked by high dietary phytate, rickets develops even if the 25-hydroxyvitamin D level is near 100 nmol/L (40 ng/mL) because the problem is one of calcium deficiency.[210–213] Children with VDDR-I usually present later in the first year of life, whereas those with VDDR-II present in the second year[214–219]; in both conditions the rickets can be prevented or healed with high dietary calcium intake or intermittent intravenous infusions of calcium.[217,220,221] Collectively these data indicate that the main role of calcitriol with respect to the skeleton is an indirect one to ensure adequate calcium delivery, and it is a role that can be bypassed by adjusting calcium intake.

Recent associational studies that have gathered much attention have suggested, for example, that a maternal 25-hydroxyvitamin D level less than 27.5 nmol/L (11 ng/mL) is associated with a lower skeletal BMC of the child at 9 years of age, although no skeletal abnormality was detected at birth or 9 months of age.[222] This has been interpreted to indicate that fetal exposure to 25-hydroxyvitamin D programs the peak bone mass achieved later in life.[223] Other studies have assessed the fetal skeleton in utero or at birth and found contradictory results, such that fetuses whose mothers had the lowest 25-hydroxyvitamin D levels had either shorter tibial lengths[173] and smaller tibial cross-sectional areas[184] versus the longest femoral lengths and highest cross-sectional areas.[224] These studies are confounded by the maternal factors that led to the lower 25-hydroxyvitamin D level (eg, maternal obesity, nutrition, and socioeconomic status) and may not indicate a causal relationship between maternal 25-hydroxyvitamin D and skeletal parameters in the fetus or child. Consequently, low levels of 25-hydroxyvitamin D in utero may imply continued low levels in childhood because of maternally shared characteristics of higher body weight, poorer nutrition, lower socioeconomic status, and so forth.

During lactation maternal 25-hydroxyvitamin D levels are unchanged[225,226] because little vitamin D or 25-hydroxyvitamin D passes into breast milk. Typical maternal cholecalciferol doses of 400 to 2000 IU per day do not alter breast milk content of vitamin D, 25-hydroxyvitamin D, or calcium.[227–232] Animal studies have shown that, despite severe vitamin D deficiency or absent vitamin D receptor, lactation proceeds normally, with skeletal resorption providing the milk calcium content followed by increases in skeletal mineral content after weaning.[27,233,234] Clinical trials of high-dose (4000–6400 IU daily) cholecalciferol supplementation showed no effect on milk calcium content[227,235,236]; the mean maternal 25-hydroxyvitamin D level was 160 nmol/L (64 ng/mL) in women taking 6400 IU daily.[236] In that small study of 19 women (10 on vitamin D and 9 on placebo), all babies achieved a 25-hydroxyvitamin D level greater than 75 nmol/L (30 ng/mL) regardless of whether the babies received 300 IU daily directly versus indirectly in breast milk from mothers consuming 6400 IU per day.[236] It had been suggested that high-dose vitamin D supplementation of lactating women would improve vitamin D nutrition in the mother and breastfeeding infant[237] but no benefits have been clearly shown in these small trials.

These findings explain why the 2011 Reference Dietary Intakes from the Institute of Medicine advise that vitamin D intakes during pregnancy and lactation should be no higher than in nonpregnant women of the same age but enough to maintain the 25-hydroxyvitamin D level greater than 50 nmol/L (20 ng/mL).[169] Breastfed infants should receive 400 IU of vitamin D supplementation directly to prevent nutritional rickets until solid, vitamin-D–fortified foods are initiated. The approach of giving 6400 IU directly to the mother requires additional study to know if it is safe and whether it provides benefits over giving vitamin D directly to the baby.

Hypercalcemia of Malignancy

Hypercalcemia of malignancy during pregnancy is rare, with fewer than 10 reported cases,[238–244] although the author is aware of other unpublished cases. The outcome of the baby was not mentioned in several reports. The available data indicate that the neonate may be hypercalcemic at birth,[238,239,243] after which the serum calcium normalizes or hypocalcemia and respiratory distress may occur,[240,241] and the baby died in 1 of 4 cases in which the outcome was reported.[240] In 2 cases intravenous pamidronate was used to control maternal hypercalcemia during pregnancy and no adverse effect was noted in the neonate.[239,243] In another case chemotherapy (etoposide and cisplatin) was used to treat small cell carcinoma of the ovary when the mother declined to terminate the pregnancy and the outcome of the baby was not reported.[244] In several cases the mother died within a few months post partum.[238,239,244]

Treatment of hypercalcemia of malignancy during pregnancy should include debulking surgery where possible, adequate aggressive hydration with close monitoring, furosemide, and possibly calcitonin. Bisphosphonates cross the placenta and high doses could lead to fetal hypocalcemia and impaired endochondral bone development. Conversely, maternal hypercalcemia causes fetal hypoparathyroidism, neonatal hypocalcemia and tetany, and possibly permanent hypoparathyroidism.

Consequently, use of bisphosphonates should be considered but only after carefully considering relative benefits and risks.

IMPLICATIONS

The studies of pregnant women indicate that the fetal calcium demand is met in large part by a doubling of intestinal calcium absorption from early in pregnancy and possibly by a small contribution of mineral from the maternal skeleton. During lactation skeletal calcium resorption provides much of the calcium to breast milk, although renal calcium conservation is also apparent. Lactation programs an obligatory skeletal calcium loss irrespective of maternal calcium intake and vitamin D sufficiency, and after weaning the calcium is completely restored to the skeleton through mechanisms that remain to be elucidated. The adaptations during pregnancy and lactation lead to novel presentations and management issues for known disorders of calcium and bone metabolism, such as primary hyperparathyroidism, hypoparathyroidism and vitamin D deficiency. Although a few women experience fragility fractures during pregnancy or lactation, most women can be reassured that these changes in calcium and bone metabolism are normal, healthy, and without adverse consequences in the long-term.

REFERENCES

1. Kovacs CS, Kronenberg HM. Maternal-fetal calcium and bone metabolism during pregnancy, puerperium and lactation. Endocr Rev 1997;18:832–72.
2. Kovacs CS. Vitamin D in pregnancy and lactation: maternal, fetal, and neonatal outcomes from human and animal studies. Am J Clin Nutr 2008;88(2):520S–8S.
3. Kovacs CS. Fetus, neonate and infant. In: Feldman D, Pike WJ, Adams JS, editors. Vitamin D. 3rd edition. New York: Academic Press. p. 625–46.
4. Givens MH, Macy IC. The chemical composition of the human fetus. J Biol Chem 1933;102:7–17.
5. Trotter M, Hixon BB. Sequential changes in weight, density, and percentage ash weight of human skeletons from an early fetal period through old age. Anat Rec 1974;179:1–18.
6. Widdowson EM, Dickerson JW. Chemical composition of the body. In: Comar CL, Bronner F, editors. Mineral metabolism: an advanced treatise, Volume II, The Elements, Part A. New York: Academic Press; 1964. p. 1–247.
7. Dahlman T, Sjoberg HE, Bucht E. Calcium homeostasis in normal pregnancy and puerperium. A longitudinal study. Acta Obstet Gynecol Scand 1994;73: 393–8.
8. Gallacher SJ, Fraser WD, Owens OJ, et al. Changes in calciotrophic hormones and biochemical markers of bone turnover in normal human pregnancy. Eur J Endocrinol 1994;131:369–74.
9. Cross NA, Hillman LS, Allen SH, et al. Calcium homeostasis and bone metabolism during pregnancy, lactation, and postweaning: a longitudinal study. Am J Clin Nutr 1995;61:514–23.
10. Rasmussen N, Frolich A, Hornnes PJ, et al. Serum ionized calcium and intact parathyroid hormone levels during pregnancy and postpartum. Br J Obstet Gynaecol 1990;97:857–9.
11. Seki K, Makimura N, Mitsui C, et al. Calcium-regulating hormones and osteocalcin levels during pregnancy: a longitudinal study. Am J Obstet Gynecol 1991; 164:1248–52.
12. Singh HJ, Mohammad NH, Nila A. Serum calcium and parathormone during normal pregnancy in Malay women. J Matern Fetal Med 1999;8(3):95–100.

13. Kovacs CS. Calcium and bone metabolism in pregnancy and lactation. J Clin Endocrinol Metab 2001;86(6):2344–8.

14. Turner M, Barre PE, Benjamin A, et al. Does the maternal kidney contribute to the increased circulating 1,25-dihydroxyvitamin D concentrations during pregnancy? Miner Electrolyte Metab 1988;14:246–52.

15. Woodrow JP, Sharpe CJ, Fudge NJ, et al. Calcitonin plays a critical role in regulating skeletal mineral metabolism during lactation. Endocrinology 2006;147: 4010–21.

16. Horwitz MJ, Tedesco MB, Sereika SM, et al. Direct comparison of sustained infusion of human parathyroid hormone-related protein-(1-36). J Clin Endocrinol Metab 2003;88(4):1603–9.

17. Horwitz MJ, Tedesco MB, Sereika SM, et al. Continuous PTH and PTHrP infusion causes suppression of bone formation and discordant effects on 1,25(OH)2 vitamin D. J Bone Miner Res 2005;20(10):1792–803.

18. Sato K. Hypercalcemia during pregnancy, puerperium, and lactation: review and a case report of hypercalcemic crisis after delivery due to excessive production of PTH-related protein (PTHrP) without malignancy (humoral hypercalcemia of pregnancy). Endocr J 2008;55(6):959–66.

19. Kovacs CS, Lanske B, Hunzelman JL, et al. Parathyroid hormone-related peptide (PTHrP) regulates fetal-placental calcium transport through a receptor distinct from the PTH/PTHrP receptor. Proc Natl Acad Sci U S A 1996;93: 15233–8.

20. Care AD, Abbas SK, Pickard DW, et al. Stimulation of ovine placental transport of calcium and magnesium by mid-molecule fragments of human parathyroid hormone-related protein. Exp Physiol 1990;75:605–8.

21. Cornish J, Callon KE, Nicholson GC, et al. Parathyroid hormone-related protein-(107-139) inhibits bone resorption in vivo. Endocrinology 1997;138:1299–304.

22. Fenton AJ, Kemp BE, Hammonds RG Jr, et al. A potent inhibitor of osteoclastic bone resorption within a highly conserved pentapeptide region of parathyroid hormone-related protein; PTHrP[107-111]. Endocrinology 1991;129:3424–6.

23. Fenton AJ, Kemp BE, Kent GN, et al. A carboxyl-terminal peptide from the parathyroid hormone-related protein inhibits bone resorption by osteoclasts. Endocrinology 1991;129:1762–8.

24. Heaney RP, Skillman TG. Calcium metabolism in normal human pregnancy. J Clin Endocrinol Metab 1971;33:661–70.

25. Halloran BP, DeLuca HF. Calcium transport in small intestine during pregnancy and lactation. Am J Physiol 1980;239:E64–8.

26. Brommage R, Baxter DC, Gierke LW. Vitamin D-independent intestinal calcium and phosphorus absorption during reproduction. Am J Physiol 1990;259: G631–8.

27. Fudge NJ, Kovacs CS. Pregnancy up-regulates intestinal calcium absorption and skeletal mineralization independently of the vitamin D receptor. Endocrinology 2010;151(3):886–95.

28. Pahuja DN, DeLuca HF. Stimulation of intestinal calcium transport and bone calcium mobilization by prolactin in vitamin D-deficient rats. Science 1981; 214:1038–9.

29. Mainoya JR. Effects of bovine growth hormone, human placental lactogen and ovine prolactin on intestinal fluid and ion transport in the rat. Endocrinology 1975;96:1165–70.

30. Purdie DW, Aaron JE, Selby PL. Bone histology and mineral homeostasis in human pregnancy. Br J Obstet Gynaecol 1988;95(9):849–54.

31. Naylor KE, Iqbal P, Fledelius C, et al. The effect of pregnancy on bone density and bone turnover. J Bone Miner Res 2000;15(1):129–37.

32. Black AJ, Topping J, Durham B, et al. A detailed assessment of alterations in bone turnover, calcium homeostasis, and bone density in normal pregnancy. J Bone Miner Res 2000;15(3):557–63.

33. Ritchie LD, Fung EB, Halloran BP, et al. A longitudinal study of calcium homeostasis during human pregnancy and lactation and after resumption of menses. Am J Clin Nutr 1998;67(4):693–701.

34. Ulrich U, Miller PB, Eyre DR, et al. Bone remodeling and bone mineral density during pregnancy. Arch Gynecol Obstet 2003;268(4):309–16.

35. Kaur M, Pearson D, Godber I, et al. Longitudinal changes in bone mineral density during normal pregnancy. Bone 2003;32(4):449–54.

36. Gambacciani M, Spinetti A, Gallo R, et al. Ultrasonographic bone characteristics during normal pregnancy: longitudinal and cross-sectional evaluation. Am J Obstet Gynecol 1995;173:890–3.

37. Pearson D, Kaur M, San P, et al. Recovery of pregnancy mediated bone loss during lactation. Bone 2004;34(3):570–8.

38. To WW, Wong MW, Leung TW. Relationship between bone mineral density changes in pregnancy and maternal and pregnancy characteristics: a longitudinal study. Acta Obstet Gynecol Scand 2003;82(9):820–7.

39. Sowers M. Pregnancy and lactation as risk factors for subsequent bone loss and osteoporosis. J Bone Miner Res 1996;11:1052–60.

40. Paton LM, Alexander JL, Nowson CA, et al. Pregnancy and lactation have no long-term deleterious effect on measures of bone mineral in healthy women: a twin study. Am J Clin Nutr 2003;77(3):707–14.

41. Dobnig H, Kainer F, Stepan V, et al. Elevated parathyroid hormone-related peptide levels after human gestation: relationship to changes in bone and mineral metabolism. J Clin Endocrinol Metab 1995;80:3699–707.

42. Yamamoto M, Duong LT, Fisher JE, et al. Suckling-mediated increases in urinary phosphate and 3′,5′-cyclic adenosine monophosphate excretion in lactating rats: possible systemic effects of parathyroid hormone-related protein. Endocrinology 1991;129:2614–22.

43. VanHouten JN, Dann P, Stewart AF, et al. Mammary-specific deletion of parathyroid hormone-related protein preserves bone mass during lactation. J Clin Invest 2003;112(9):1429–36.

44. Khosla S, van Heerden JA, Gharib H, et al. Parathyroid hormone-related protein and hypercalcemia secondary to massive mammary hyperplasia [letter]. N Engl J Med 1990;322:1157.

45. Kovacs CS, Chik CL. Hyperprolactinemia caused by lactation and pituitary adenomas is associated with altered serum calcium, phosphate, parathyroid hormone (PTH), and PTH-related peptide levels. J Clin Endocrinol Metab 1995;80:3036–42.

46. Sowers MF, Hollis BW, Shapiro B, et al. Elevated parathyroid hormone-related peptide associated with lactation and bone density loss. J Am Med Assoc 1996;276:549–54.

47. Hurley DL, Tiegs RD, Wahner HW, et al. Axial and appendicular bone mineral density in patients with long-term deficiency or excess of calcitonin. N Engl J Med 1987;317(9):537–41.

48. Gonzalez DC, Mautalen CA, Correa PH, et al. Bone mass in totally thyroidectomized patients. Role of calcitonin deficiency and exogenous thyroid treatment. Acta Endocrinol (Copenh) 1991;124(5):521–5.

49. Giannini S, Nobile M, Sartori L, et al. Bone density and mineral metabolism in thyroidectomized patients treated with long-term L-thyroxine. Clin Sci (Lond) 1994;87(5):593–7.
50. Nguyen TT, Heath H 3rd, Bryant SC, et al. Fractures after thyroidectomy in men: a population-based cohort study. J Bone Miner Res 1997;12(7):1092–9.
51. Mirzaei S, Krotla G, Knoll P, et al. Possible effect of calcitonin deficiency on bone mass after subtotal thyroidectomy. Acta Med Austriaca 1999;26(1):29–31.
52. Bucht E, Telenius-Berg M, Lundell G, et al. Immunoextracted calcitonin in milk and plasma from totally thyroidectomized women. Evidence of monomeric calcitonin in plasma during pregnancy and lactation. Acta Endocrinol (Copenh) 1986;113:529–35.
53. Balabanova S, Kruse B, Wolf AS. Calcitonin secretion by human placental tissue. Acta Obstet Gynecol Scand 1987;66(4):323–6.
54. Ren Y, Chien J, Sun YP, et al. Calcitonin is expressed in gonadotropes of the anterior pituitary gland: its possible role in paracrine regulation of lactotrope function. J Endocrinol 2001;171(2):217–28.
55. Laskey MA, Prentice A. Effect of pregnancy on recovery of lactational bone loss [letter]. Lancet 1997;349:1518–9.
56. Cross NA, Hillman LS, Allen SH, et al. Changes in bone mineral density and markers of bone remodeling during lactation and postweaning in women consuming high amounts of calcium. J Bone Miner Res 1995;10:1312–20.
57. Kalkwarf HJ, Specker BL, Bianchi DC, et al. The effect of calcium supplementation on bone density during lactation and after weaning. N Engl J Med 1997; 337(8):523–8.
58. Polatti F, Capuzzo E, Viazzo F, et al. Bone mineral changes during and after lactation. Obstet Gynecol 1999;94(1):52–6.
59. Kolthoff N, Eiken P, Kristensen B, et al. Bone mineral changes during pregnancy and lactation: a longitudinal cohort study. Clin Sci (Lond) 1998;94(4):405–12.
60. Laskey MA, Prentice A, Hanratty LA, et al. Bone changes after 3 mo of lactation: influence of calcium intake, breast-milk output, and vitamin D-receptor genotype. Am J Clin Nutr 1998;67(4):685–92.
61. VanHouten JN, Wysolmerski JJ. Low estrogen and high parathyroid hormone-related peptide levels contribute to accelerated bone resorption and bone loss in lactating mice. Endocrinology 2003;144(12):5521–9.
62. Kelly TR. Primary hyperparathyroidism during pregnancy. Surgery 1991;110(6): 1028–33 [discussion: 1033–4].
63. Haenel LC, Mayfield RK. Primary hyperparathyroidism in a twin pregnancy and review of fetal/maternal calcium homeostasis. Am J Med Sci 2000;319(3): 191–4.
64. Wermers RA, Khosla S, Atkinson EJ, et al. The rise and fall of primary hyperparathyroidism: a population-based study in Rochester, Minnesota, 1965-1992. Ann Intern Med 1997;126(6):433–40.
65. Heath H, Hodgson SF, Kennedy MA. Primary hyperparathyroidism. Incidence, morbidity, and potential economic impact in a community. N Engl J Med 1980;302(4):189–93.
66. Kort KC, Schiller HJ, Numann PJ. Hyperparathyroidism and pregnancy. Am J Surg 1999;177(1):66–8.
67. Schnatz PF, Curry SL. Primary hyperparathyroidism in pregnancy: evidence-based management. Obstet Gynecol Surv 2002;57(6):365–76.
68. El-Hajj Fuleihan G. Pathogenesis and etiology of primary hyperparathyroidism. In: Rose BD, editor. UpToDate 13.1. Wellesley (MA): UpToDate; 2005.

69. Kristoffersson A, Dahlgren S, Lithner F, et al. Primary hyperparathyroidism in pregnancy. Surgery 1985;97(3):326–30.
70. Shangold MM, Dor N, Welt SI, et al. Hyperparathyroidism and pregnancy: a review. Obstet Gynecol Surv 1982;37:217–28.
71. Croom RD, Thomas CG. Primary hyperparathyroidism during pregnancy. Surgery 1984;96(6):1109–18.
72. Krysiak R, Wilk M, Okopien B. Recurrent pancreatitis induced by hyperparathyroidism in pregnancy. Arch Gynecol Obstet 2011;284(3):531–4.
73. Clark D, Seeds JW, Cefalo RC. Hyperparathyroid crisis and pregnancy. Am J Obstet Gynecol 1981;140(7):840–2.
74. Carella MJ, Gossain VV. Hyperparathyroidism and pregnancy: case report and review. J Gen Intern Med 1992;7:448–53.
75. Inabnet WB, Baldwin D, Daniel RO, et al. Hyperparathyroidism and pancreatitis during pregnancy. Surgery 1996;119(6):710–3.
76. Matthias GS, Helliwell TR, Williams A. Postpartum hyperparathyroid crisis. Case report. Br J Obstet Gynaecol 1987;94(8):807–10.
77. Salem R, Taylor S. Hyperparathyroidism in pregnancy. Br J Surg 1979;66(9): 648–50.
78. Nilsson IL, Adner N, Reihner E, et al. Primary hyperparathyroidism in pregnancy: a diagnostic and therapeutic challenge. J Womens Health (Larchmt) 2010; 19(6):1117–21.
79. Negishi H, Kobayashi M, Nishida R, et al. Primary hyperparathyroidism and simultaneous bilateral fracture of the femoral neck during pregnancy. J Trauma 2002;52(2):367–9.
80. Hess HM, Dickson J, Fox HE. Hyperfunctioning parathyroid carcinoma presenting as acute pancreatitis in pregnancy. J Reprod Med 1980;25(2):83–7.
81. Wagner G, Transhol L, Melchior JC. Hyperparathyroidism and pregnancy. Acta Endocrinol (Copenh) 1964;47:549–64.
82. Ludwig GD. Hyperparathyroidism in relation to pregnancy. N Engl J Med 1962; 267:637–42.
83. Delmonico FL, Neer RM, Cosimi AB, et al. Hyperparathyroidism during pregnancy. Am J Surg 1976;131:328–37.
84. Ip P. Neonatal convulsion revealing maternal hyperparathyroidism: an unusual case of late neonatal hypoparathyroidism. Arch Gynecol Obstet 2003;268(3): 227–9.
85. Bruce J, Strong JA. Maternal hyperparathyroidism and parathyroid deficiency in the child, with account of effect of parathyroidectomy on renal function, and of attempt to transplant part of tumor. Q J Med 1955;24:307–19.
86. Bilezikian JP, Khan AA, Potts JT Jr. Guidelines for the management of asymptomatic primary hyperparathyroidism: summary statement from the third international workshop. J Clin Endocrinol Metab 2009;94(2):335–9.
87. Schnatz PF. Surgical treatment of primary hyperparathyroidism during the third trimester. Obstet Gynecol 2002;99(5 Pt 2):961–3.
88. Norman J, Politz D. Prospective study in 3,000 consecutive parathyroid operations demonstrates 18 objective factors that influence the decision for unilateral versus bilateral surgical approach. J Am Coll Surg 2010;211(2):244–9.
89. Pothiwala P, Levine SN. Parathyroid surgery in pregnancy: review of the literature and localization by aspiration for parathyroid hormone levels. J Perinatol 2009;29(12):779–84.
90. Horjus C, Groot I, Telting D, et al. Cinacalcet for hyperparathyroidism in pregnancy and puerperium. J Pediatr Endocrinol Metab 2009;22(8):741–9.

91. Patlas N, Golomb G, Yaffe P, et al. Transplacental effects of bisphosphonates on fetal skeletal ossification and mineralization in rats. Teratology 1999;60(2):68–73.

92. Mastaglia SR, Watman NP, Oliveri B. Intravenous bisphosphonate treatment and pregnancy: its effects on mother and infant bone health. Osteoporos Int 2010; 21(11):1959–62.

93. Djokanovic N, Klieger-Grossmann C, Koren G. Does treatment with bisphosph-onates endanger the human pregnancy? J Obstet Gynaecol Can 2008;30(12): 1146–8.

94. Levy S, Fayez I, Taguchi N, et al. Pregnancy outcome following in utero expo-sure to bisphosphonates. Bone 2009;44(3):428–30.

95. Kovacs CS, Chafe LL, Woodland ML, et al. Calcitropic gene expression suggests a role for intraplacental yolk sac in maternal-fetal calcium exchange. Am J Physiol Endocrinol Metab 2002;282(3):E721–32.

96. Kovacs CS, Ho-Pao CL, Hunzelman JL, et al. Regulation of murine fetal-placental calcium metabolism by the calcium-sensing receptor. J Clin Invest 1998;101:2812–20.

97. Fudge NJ, Kovacs CS. Physiological studies in heterozygous calcium sensing receptor (CaSR) gene-ablated mice confirm that the CaSR regulates calcitonin release in vivo. BMC Physiol 2004;4:5.

98. Rajala B, Abbasi RA, Hutchinson HT, et al. Acute pancreatitis and primary hyperparathyroidism in pregnancy: treatment of hypercalcemia with magnesium sulfate. Obstet Gynecol 1987;70(3 Pt 2):460–2.

99. Dahan M, Chang RJ. Pancreatitis secondary to hyperparathyroidism during pregnancy. Obstet Gynecol 2001;98(5 Pt 2):923–5.

100. Loughead JL, Mimouni F, Tsang RC. Serum ionized calcium concentrations in normal neonates. Am J Dis Child 1988;142:516–8.

101. Schauberger CW, Pitkin RM. Maternal-perinatal calcium relationships. Obstet Gynecol 1979;53:74–6.

102. David L, Anast CS. Calcium metabolism in newborn infants. The interrelationship of parathyroid function and calcium, magnesium, and phosphorus metabolism in normal, sick, and hypocalcemic newborns. J Clin Invest 1974;54:287–96.

103. Pieringer H, Hatzl-Griesenhofer M, Shebl O, et al. Hypocalcemic tetany in the newborn as a manifestation of unrecognized maternal primary hyperparathy-roidism. Wien Klin Wochenschr 2007;119(3–4):129–31.

104. McDonnell CM, Zacharin MR. Maternal primary hyperparathyroidism: discor-dant outcomes in a twin pregnancy. J Paediatr Child Health 2006;42(1–2):70–1.

105. Tsang RC, Chen I, Friedman MA, et al. Parathyroid function in infants of diabetic mothers. J Pediatr 1975;86:399–404.

106. Mehta KC, Kalkwarf HJ, Mimouni F, et al. Randomized trial of magnesium admin-istration to prevent hypocalcemia in infants of diabetic mothers. J Perinatol 1998;18(5):352–6.

107. Brown EM. The calcium-sensing receptor: physiology, pathophysiology and CaR-based therapeutics. Subcell Biochem 2007;45:139–67.

108. Powell BR, Buist NR. Late presenting, prolonged hypocalcemia in an infant of a woman with hypocalciuric hypercalcemia. Clin Pediatr (Phila) 1990;29:241–3.

109. Thomas BR, Bennett JD. Symptomatic hypocalcemia and hypoparathyroidism in two infants of mothers with hyperparathyroidism and familial benign hypercal-cemia. J Perinatol 1995;15:23–6.

110. VanHouten J, Dann P, McGeoch G, et al. The calcium-sensing receptor regu-lates mammary gland parathyroid hormone-related protein production and calcium transport. J Clin Invest 2004;113(4):598–608.

111. Ardeshirpour L, Dann P, Pollak M, et al. The calcium-sensing receptor regulates PTHrP production and calcium transport in the lactating mammary gland. Bone 2006;38(6):787–93.

112. Sweeney LL, Malabanan AO, Rosen H. Decreased calcitriol requirement during pregnancy and lactation with a window of increased requirement immediately post partum. Endocr Pract 2010;16(3):459–62.

113. Callies F, Arlt W, Scholz HJ, et al. Management of hypoparathyroidism during pregnancy–report of twelve cases. Eur J Endocrinol 1998;139(3):284–9.

114. Landing BH, Kamoshita S. Congenital hyperparathyroidism secondary to maternal hypoparathyroidism. J Pediatr 1970;77:842–7.

115. Taussig HB. Possible injury to the cardiovascular system from vitamin D. Ann Intern Med 1966;65(6):1195–200.

116. Friedman WF, Mills LF. The relationship between vitamin D and the craniofacial and dental anomalies of the supravalvular aortic stenosis syndrome. Pediatrics 1969;43(1):12–8.

117. Salle BL, Berthezene F, Glorieux FH, et al. Hypoparathyroidism during pregnancy: treatment with calcitriol. J Clin Endocrinol Metab 1981;52:810–3.

118. Sadeghi-Nejad A, Wolfsdorf JI, Senior B. Hypoparathyroidism and pregnancy. Treatment with calcitriol. J Am Med Assoc 1980;243:254–5.

119. Mather KJ, Chik CL, Corenblum B. Maintenance of serum calcium by parathyroid hormone-related peptide during lactation in a hypoparathyroid patient. J Clin Endocrinol Metab 1999;84(2):424–7.

120. Caplan RH, Beguin EA. Hypercalcemia in a calcitriol-treated hypoparathyroid woman during lactation. Obstet Gynecol 1990;76:485–9.

121. Shomali ME, Ross DS. Hypercalcemia in a woman with hypoparathyroidism associated with increased parathyroid hormone-related protein during lactation. Endocr Pract 1999;5(4):198–200.

122. Breslau NA, Zerwekh JE. Relationship of estrogen and pregnancy to calcium homeostasis in pseudohypoparathyroidism. J Clin Endocrinol Metab 1986;62: 45–51.

123. O'Donnell D, Costa J, Meyers AM. Management of pseudohypoparathyroidism in pregnancy. Case report. Br J Obstet Gynaecol 1985;92(6):639–41.

124. Saito H, Saito M, Saito K, et al. Subclinical pseudohypoparathyroidism type II: evidence for failure of physiologic adjustment in calcium metabolism during pregnancy. Am J Med Sci 1989;297:247–50.

125. Zerwekh JE, Breslau NA. Human placental production of 1a,25-dihydroxyvitamin D_3: biochemical characterization and production in normal subjects and patients with pseudohypoparathyroidism. J Clin Endocrinol Metab 1986;62: 192–6.

126. Glass EJ, Barr DG. Transient neonatal hyperparathyroidism secondary to maternal pseudohypoparathyroidism. Arch Dis Child 1981;56:565–8.

127. Nordin BE, Roper A. Postpregnancy osteoporosis: a syndrome? Lancet 1955; 268(6861):431–4.

128. Phillips AJ, Ostlere SJ, Smith R. Pregnancy-associated osteoporosis: does the skeleton recover? Osteoporos Int 2000;11(5):449–54.

129. Khovidhunkit W, Epstein S. Osteoporosis in pregnancy. Osteoporos Int 1996; 6(5):345–54.

130. Smith R, Athanasou NA, Ostlere SJ, et al. Pregnancy-associated osteoporosis. QJM 1995;88:865–78.

131. Reid IR, Wattie DJ, Evans MC, et al. Post-pregnancy osteoporosis associated with hypercalcaemia. Clin Endocrinol (Oxf) 1992;37:298–303.

132. Dunne F, Walters B, Marshall T, et al. Pregnancy associated osteoporosis. Clin Endocrinol (Oxf) 1993;39:487–90.
133. Ofluoglu O, Ofluoglu D. A case report: pregnancy-induced severe osteoporosis with eight vertebral fractures. Rheumatol Int 2008;29(2):197–201.
134. Lakhanpal S, Ginsburg WW, Luthra HS, et al. Transient regional osteoporosis. A study of 56 cases and review of the literature. Ann Intern Med 1987;106(3): 444–50.
135. Arayssi TK, Tawbi HA, Usta IM, et al. Calcitonin in the treatment of transient osteoporosis of the hip. Semin Arthritis Rheum 2003;32(6):388–97.
136. Curtiss PH Jr, Kincaid WE. Transitory demineralization of the hip in pregnancy: a report of three cases. J Bone Joint Surg Am 1959;41:1327–33.
137. Khastgir G, Studd JW, King H, et al. Changes in bone density and biochemical markers of bone turnover in pregnancy-associated osteoporosis. Br J Obstet Gynaecol 1996;103(7):716–8.
138. Kovacs CS. Severe low bone mass partly rescued by normal pregnancy [abstract]. J Bone Miner Res 2006;21(Suppl 1):S310.
139. Hellmeyer L, Boekhoff J, Hadji P. Treatment with teriparatide in a patient with pregnancy-associated osteoporosis. Gynecol Endocrinol 2010;26(10):725–8.
140. Sarikaya S, Ozdolap S, Acikgoz G, et al. Pregnancy-associated osteoporosis with vertebral fractures and scoliosis. Joint Bone Spine 2004;71(1):84–5.
141. Bayram S, Ozturk C, Sivrioglu K, et al. Kyphoplasty for pregnancy-associated osteoporotic vertebral fractures. Joint Bone Spine 2006;73(5):564–6.
142. Kim HW, Song JW, Kwon A, et al. Percutaneous vertebroplasty for pregnancy-associated osteoporotic vertebral compression fractures. J Korean Neurosurg Soc 2010;47(5):399–402.
143. Kovacs CS, El-Hajj Fuleihan G. Calcium and bone disorders during pregnancy and lactation. Endocrinol Metab Clin North Am 2006;35(1):21–51.
144. Donovan EF, Tsang RC, Steichen JJ, et al. Neonatal hypermagnesemia: effect on parathyroid hormone and calcium homeostasis. J Pediatr 1980;96(2):305–10.
145. Cholst IN, Steinberg SF, Tropper PJ, et al. The influence of hypermagnesemia on serum calcium and parathyroid hormone levels in human subjects. N Engl J Med 1984;310(19):1221–5.
146. Cruikshank DP, Pitkin RM, Reynolds WA, et al. Effects of magnesium sulfate treatment on perinatal calcium metabolism. I. Maternal and fetal responses. Am J Obstet Gynecol 1979;134(3):243–9.
147. Koontz SL, Friedman SA, Schwartz ML. Symptomatic hypocalcemia after tocolytic therapy with magnesium sulfate and nifedipine. Am J Obstet Gynecol 2004; 190(6):1773–6.
148. Smith LG Jr, Burns PA, Schanler RJ. Calcium homeostasis in pregnant women receiving long-term magnesium sulfate therapy for preterm labor. Am J Obstet Gynecol 1992;167:45–51.
149. Hung JW, Tsai MY, Yang BY, et al. Maternal osteoporosis after prolonged magnesium sulfate tocolysis therapy: a case report. Arch Phys Med Rehabil 2005;86(1):146–9.
150. Levav AL, Chan L, Wapner RJ. Long-term magnesium sulfate tocolysis and maternal osteoporosis in a triplet pregnancy: a case report. Am J Perinatol 1998;15(1):43–6.
151. Stone SR, Pritchard JA. Effect of maternally administered magnesium sulfate on the neonate. Obstet Gynecol 1970;35(4):574–7.
152. Lipsitz PJ, English IC. Hypermagnesemia in the newborn infant. Pediatrics 1967; 40(5):856–62.

153. Lipsitz PJ. The clinical and biochemical effects of excess magnesium in the newborn. Pediatrics 1971;47(3):501–9.
154. Savory J, Monif GR. Serum calcium levels in cord sera of the progeny of mothers treated with magnesium sulfate for toxemia of pregnancy. Am J Obstet Gynecol 1971;110(4):556–9.
155. Lamm CI, Norton KI, Murphy RJ, et al. Congenital rickets associated with magnesium sulfate infusion for tocolysis. J Pediatr 1988;113(6):1078–82.
156. Santi MD, Henry GW, Douglas GL. Magnesium sulfate treatment of preterm labor as a cause of abnormal neonatal bone mineralization. J Pediatr Orthop 1994;14(2):249–53.
157. Cumming WA, Thomas VJ. Hypermagnesemia: a cause of abnormal metaphyses in the neonate. AJR Am J Roentgenol 1989;152(5):1071–2.
158. Malaeb SN, Rassi AI, Haddad MC, et al. Bone mineralization in newborns whose mothers received magnesium sulphate for tocolysis of premature labour. Pediatr Radiol 2004;34(5):384–6.
159. Prentice A. Pregnancy and lactation. In: Glorieux FH, Petifor JM, Jüppner H, editors. Pediatric bone: biology & diseases. New York: Academic Press; 2003. p. 249–69.
160. Koo WW, Walters JC, Esterlitz J, et al. Maternal calcium supplementation and fetal bone mineralization. Obstet Gynecol 1999;94(4):577–82.
161. Hofmeyr GJ, Atallah AN, Duley L. Calcium supplementation during pregnancy for preventing hypertensive disorders and related problems. Cochrane Database Syst Rev 2006;3:CD001059.
162. Kumar A, Devi SG, Batra S, et al. Calcium supplementation for the prevention of pre-eclampsia. Int J Gynaecol Obstet 2009;104(1):32–6.
163. Hiller JE, Crowther CA, Moore VA, et al. Calcium supplementation in pregnancy and its impact on blood pressure in children and women: follow up of a randomised controlled trial. Aust N Z J Obstet Gynaecol 2007;47(2):115–21.
164. Villar J, Abdel-Aleem H, Merialdi M, et al. World Health Organization randomized trial of calcium supplementation among low calcium intake pregnant women. Am J Obstet Gynecol 2006;194(3):639–49.
165. Prentice A. Calcium in pregnancy and lactation. Annu Rev Nutr 2000;20:249–72.
166. Prentice A, Jarjou LM, Cole TJ, et al. Calcium requirements of lactating Gambian mothers: effects of a calcium supplement on breast-milk calcium concentration, maternal bone mineral content, and urinary calcium excretion. Am J Clin Nutr 1995;62:58–67.
167. Prentice A, Jarjou LM, Stirling DM, et al. Biochemical markers of calcium and bone metabolism during 18 months of lactation in Gambian women accustomed to a low calcium intake and in those consuming a calcium supplement. J Clin Endocrinol Metab 1998;83(4):1059–66.
168. Prentice A, Yan L, Jarjou LM, et al. Vitamin D status does not influence the breast-milk calcium concentration of lactating mothers accustomed to a low calcium intake. Acta Paediatr 1997;86(9):1006–8.
169. IOM. Dietary reference intakes for calcium and vitamin D. Washington, DC: The National Academies Press; 2011.
170. Bezerra FF, Mendonca LM, Lobato EC, et al. Bone mass is recovered from lactation to postweaning in adolescent mothers with low calcium intakes. Am J Clin Nutr 2004;80(5):1322–6.
171. Chantry CJ, Auinger P, Byrd RS. Lactation among adolescent mothers and subsequent bone mineral density. Arch Pediatr Adolesc Med 2004;158(7):650–6.

172. Hillman LS, Slatopolsky E, Haddad JG. Perinatal vitamin D metabolism. IV. Maternal and cord serum 24,25-dihydroxyvitamin D concentrations. J Clin Endocrinol Metab 1978;47:1073–7.

173. Morley R, Carlin JB, Pasco JA, et al. Maternal 25-hydroxyvitamin D and parathyroid hormone concentrations and offspring birth size. J Clin Endocrinol Metab 2006;91(3):906–12.

174. Ardawi MS, Nasrat HA, BA'Aqueel HS. Calcium-regulating hormones and parathyroid hormone-related peptide in normal human pregnancy and postpartum: a longitudinal study. Eur J Endocrinol 1997;137(4):402–9.

175. Brooke OG, Brown IR, Bone CD, et al. Vitamin D supplements in pregnant Asian women: effects on calcium status and fetal growth. Br Med J 1980;280:751–4.

176. Hollis BW, Johnson D, Hulsey TC, et al. Vitamin D supplementation during pregnancy: double blind, randomized clinical trial of safety and effectiveness. J Bone Miner Res 2011. [Epub ahead of print].

177. Wagner CL. Vitamin D supplementation during pregnancy: impact on maternal outcomes. Presented at the Centers for Disease Control and Prevention Conference on Vitamin D Physiology in Pregnancy: Implications for Preterm Birth and Preeclampsia. Atlanta (GA), April 26-7, 2011.

178. Glorieux FH, St-Arnaud R. Vitamin D pseudodeficiency. In: Feldman D, Glorieux FH, Pike JW, editors. Vitamin D. San Diego (CA): Academic Press; 1997. p. 755–64.

179. Malloy PJ, Pike JW, Feldman D. Hereditary 1,25-dihydroxyvitamin D resistant rickets. In: Feldman D, Glorieux FH, Pike JW, editors. Vitamin D. San Diego (CA): Academic Press; 1997. p. 765–87.

180. Wieland P, Fischer JA, Trechsel U, et al. Perinatal parathyroid hormone, vitamin D metabolites, and calcitonin in man. Am J Physiol 1980;239:E385–90.

181. Fleischman AR, Rosen JF, Cole J, et al. Maternal and fetal serum 1,25-dihydroxyvitamin D levels at term. J Pediatr 1980;97:640–2.

182. Seki K, Furuya K, Makimura N, et al. Cord blood levels of calcium-regulating hormones and osteocalcin in premature infants. J Perinat Med 1994;22:189–94.

183. Hollis BW, Pittard WB. Evaluation of the total fetomaternal vitamin D relationships at term: evidence for racial differences. J Clin Endocrinol Metab 1984;59:652–7.

184. Viljakainen HT, Saarnio E, Hytinantti T, et al. Maternal vitamin D status determines bone variables in the newborn. J Clin Endocrinol Metab 2010;95(4): 1749–57.

185. Halloran BP, De Luca HF. Effect of vitamin D deficiency on skeletal development during early growth in the rat. Arch Biochem Biophys 1981;209:7–14.

186. Miller SC, Halloran BP, DeLuca HF, et al. Studies on the role of vitamin D in early skeletal development, mineralization, and growth in rats. Calcif Tissue Int 1983; 35:455–60.

187. Lachenmaier-Currle U, Harmeyer J. Placental transport of calcium and phosphorus in pigs. J Perinat Med 1989;17:127–36.

188. Panda DK, Miao D, Tremblay ML, et al. Targeted ablation of the 25-hydroxyvitamin D 1alpha-hydroxylase enzyme: evidence for skeletal, reproductive, and immune dysfunction. Proc Natl Acad Sci U S A 2001;98(13):7498–503.

189. Dardenne O, Prud'homme J, Arabian A, et al. Targeted inactivation of the 25-hydroxyvitamin D(3)-1(alpha)-hydroxylase gene (CYP27B1) creates an animal model of pseudovitamin D-deficiency rickets. Endocrinology 2001;142(7): 3135–41.

190. Li YC, Amling M, Pirro AE, et al. Normalization of mineral ion homeostasis by dietary means prevents hyperparathyroidism, rickets, and osteomalacia, but not

alopecia in vitamin D receptor-ablated mice. Endocrinology 1998;139(10): 4391–6.

191. Li YC, Pirro AE, Amling M, et al. Targeted ablation of the vitamin D receptor: an animal model of vitamin D dependent rickets type II with alopecia. Proc Natl Acad Sci U S A 1997;94:9831–5.

192. Halloran BP, DeLuca HF. Calcium transport in small intestine during early development: role of vitamin D. Am J Physiol 1980;239:G473–9.

193. Ghishan FK, Parker P, Nichols S, et al. Kinetics of intestinal calcium transport during maturation in rats. Pediatr Res 1984;18:235–9.

194. Ghishan FK, Jenkins JT, Younoszai MK. Maturation of calcium transport in the rat small and large intestine. J Nutr 1980;110:1622–8.

195. Amling M, Priemel M, Holzmann T, et al. Rescue of the skeletal phenotype of vitamin D receptor-ablated mice in the setting of normal mineral ion homeostasis: formal histomorphometric and biomechanical analyses. Endocrinology 1999;140(11):4982–7.

196. Van Cromphaut SJ, Dewerchin M, Hoenderop JG, et al. Duodenal calcium absorption in vitamin D receptor-knockout mice: functional and molecular aspects. Proc Natl Acad Sci U S A 2001;98(23):13324–9.

197. Dardenne O, Prudhomme J, Hacking SA, et al. Rescue of the pseudo-vitamin D deficiency rickets phenotype of CYP27B1-deficient mice by treatment with 1,25-dihydroxyvitamin D3: biochemical, histomorphometric, and biomechanical analyses. J Bone Miner Res 2003;18(4):637–43.

198. Rowling MJ, Gliniak C, Welsh J, et al. High dietary vitamin D prevents hypocalcemia and osteomalacia in CYP27B1 knockout mice. J Nutr 2007;137(12): 2608–15.

199. Hoenderop JG, Dardenne O, Van Abel M, et al. Modulation of renal Ca2+ transport protein genes by dietary Ca2+ and 1,25-dihydroxyvitamin D3 in 25-hydroxyvitamin D3-1alpha-hydroxylase knockout mice. FASEB J 2002;16(11): 1398–406.

200. Maxwell JP, Miles LM. Osteomalacia in China. J Obstet Gynaecol Br Empire 1925;32(3):433–73.

201. Campbell DE, Fleischman AR. Rickets of prematurity: controversies in causation and prevention. Clin Perinatol 1988;15:879–90.

202. Pereira GR, Zucker AH. Nutritional deficiencies in the neonate. Clin Perinatol 1986;13:175–89.

203. Specker BL. Do North American women need supplemental vitamin D during pregnancy or lactation? Am J Clin Nutr 1994;59:484S–90S.

204. Beck-Nielsen SS, Brock-Jacobsen B, Gram J, et al. Incidence and prevalence of nutritional and hereditary rickets in southern Denmark. Eur J Endocrinol 2009;160(3):491–7.

205. Teotia M, Teotia SP, Nath M. Metabolic studies in congenital vitamin D deficiency rickets. Indian J Pediatr 1995;62(1):55–61.

206. Ward LM, Gaboury I, Ladhani M, et al. Vitamin D-deficiency rickets among children in Canada. CMAJ 2007;177(2):161–6.

207. Ashraf A, Mick G, Atchison J, et al. Prevalence of hypovitaminosis D in early infantile hypocalcemia. J Pediatr Endocrinol Metab 2006;19(8):1025–31.

208. Teaema FH, Al Ansari K. Nineteen cases of symptomatic neonatal hypocalcemia secondary to vitamin D deficiency: a 2-year study. J Trop Pediatr 2010;56(2): 108–10.

209. Cranney A, Horsley T, O'Donnell S, et al. Effectiveness and Safety of Vitamin D in Relation to Bone Health. Evidence Report/Technology Assessment No. 158.

AHRQ Publication No. 07-E013. Rockville (MD): Agency for Healthcare Research and Quality; 2007.

210. Pettifor JM. Vitamin D &/or calcium deficiency rickets in infants & children: a global perspective. Indian J Med Res 2008;127(3):245–9.

211. Thacher TD, Fischer PR, Pettifor JM, et al. A comparison of calcium, vitamin D, or both for nutritional rickets in Nigerian children. N Engl J Med 1999;341(8): 563–8.

212. Fischer PR, Rahman A, Cimma JP, et al. Nutritional rickets without vitamin D deficiency in Bangladesh. J Trop Pediatr 1999;45(5):291–3.

213. Thacher TD, Obadofin MO, O'Brien KO, et al. The effect of vitamin D2 and vitamin D3 on intestinal calcium absorption in Nigerian children with rickets. J Clin Endocrinol Metab 2009;94(9):3314–21.

214. Rauch F. Etiology and treatment of hypocalcemic rickets in children. In: Rose BD, editor. UpToDate 17.3. Wellesley (MA): UpToDate; 2009.

215. Bouillon R, Verstuyf A, Mathieu C, et al. Vitamin D resistance. Best Pract Res Clin Endocrinol Metab 2006;20(4):627–45.

216. Takeda E, Yamamoto H, Taketani Y, et al. Vitamin D-dependent rickets type I and type II. Acta Paediatr Jpn 1997;39(4):508–13.

217. Kitanaka S, Takeyama K, Murayama A, et al. Inactivating mutations in the 25-hydroxyvitamin D3 1alpha-hydroxylase gene in patients with pseudovitamin D-deficiency rickets. N Engl J Med 1998;338(10):653–61.

218. Silver J, Landau H, Bab I, et al. Vitamin D-dependent rickets types I and II. Diagnosis and response to therapy. Isr J Med Sci 1985;21(1):53–6.

219. Teotia M, Teotia SP. Nutritional and metabolic rickets. Indian J Pediatr 1997; 64(2):153–7.

220. Balsan S, Garabedian M, Larchet M, et al. Long-term nocturnal calcium infusions can cure rickets and promote normal mineralization in hereditary resistance to 1,25-dihydroxyvitamin D. J Clin Invest 1986;77(5):1661–7.

221. Hochberg Z, Tiosano D, Even L. Calcium therapy for calcitriol-resistant rickets. J Pediatr 1992;121(5 Pt 1):803–8.

222. Javaid MK, Crozier SR, Harvey NC, et al. Maternal vitamin D status during pregnancy and childhood bone mass at age 9 years: a longitudinal study. Lancet 2006;367(9504):36–43.

223. Cooper C, Westlake S, Harvey N, et al. Review: developmental origins of osteoporotic fracture. Osteoporos Int 2006;17(3):337–47.

224. Mahon P, Harvey N, Crozier S, et al. Low maternal vitamin D status and fetal bone development: cohort study. J Bone Miner Res 2010;25(1):14–9.

225. Kent GN, Price RI, Gutteridge DH, et al. Human lactation: forearm trabecular bone loss, increased bone turnover, and renal conservation of calcium and inorganic phosphate with recovery of bone mass following weaning. J Bone Miner Res 1990;5:361–9.

226. Sowers M, Zhang D, Hollis BW, et al. Role of calciotrophic hormones in calcium mobilization of lactation. Am J Clin Nutr 1998;67(2):284–91.

227. Hollis BW, Wagner CL. Vitamin D requirements during lactation: high-dose maternal supplementation as therapy to prevent hypovitaminosis D for both the mother and the nursing infant. Am J Clin Nutr 2004;80(Suppl 6):1752S–8S.

228. Rothberg AD, Pettifor JM, Cohen DF, et al. Maternal-infant vitamin D relationships during breast-feeding. J Pediatr 1982;101(4):500–3.

229. Ala-Houhala M, Koskinen T, Parviainen MT, et al. 25-Hydroxyvitamin D and vitamin D in human milk: effects of supplementation and season. Am J Clin Nutr 1988;48(4):1057–60.

230. Ala-Houhala M. 25-Hydroxyvitamin D levels during breast-feeding with or without maternal or infantile supplementation of vitamin D. J Pediatr Gastroenterol Nutr 1985;4(2):220–6.

231. Greer FR, Searcy JE, Levin RS, et al. Bone mineral content and serum 25-hydroxyvitamin D concentrations in breastfed infants with and without supplemental vitamin D: one-year follow-up. J Pediatr 1982;100(6):919–22.

232. Greer FR, Marshall S. Bone mineral content, serum vitamin D metabolite concentrations, and ultraviolet B light exposure in infants fed human milk with and without vitamin D2 supplements. J Pediatr 1989;114(2):204–12.

233. Halloran BP, DeLuca HF. Skeletal changes during pregnancy and lactation: the role of vitamin D. Endocrinology 1980;107:1923–9.

234. Miller SC, Halloran BP, DeLuca HF, et al. Role of vitamin D in maternal skeletal changes during pregnancy and lactation: a histomorphometric study. Calcif Tissue Int 1982;34:245–52.

235. Basile LA, Taylor SN, Wagner CL, et al. The effect of high-dose vitamin D supplementation on serum vitamin D levels and milk calcium concentration in lactating women and their infants. Breastfeed Med 2006;1(1):27–35.

236. Wagner CL, Hulsey TC, Fanning D, et al. High-dose vitamin D3 supplementation in a cohort of breastfeeding mothers and their infants: a 6-month follow-up pilot study. Breastfeed Med 2006;1(2):59–70.

237. Hollis BW, Wagner CL. Assessment of dietary vitamin D requirements during pregnancy and lactation. Am J Clin Nutr 2004;79(5):717–26.

238. Usta IM, Chammas M, Khalil AM. Renal cell carcinoma with hypercalcemia complicating a pregnancy: case report and review of the literature. Eur J Gynaecol Oncol 1998;19(6):584–7.

239. Illidge TM, Hussey M, Godden CW. Malignant hypercalcaemia in pregnancy and antenatal administration of intravenous pamidronate. Clin Oncol (R Coll Radiol) 1996;8(4):257–8.

240. Montoro MN, Paler RJ, Goodwin TM, et al. Parathyroid carcinoma during pregnancy. Obstet Gynecol 2000;96(5 Pt 2):841.

241. Abraham P, Ralston SH, Hewison M, et al. Presentation of a PTHrP-secreting pancreatic neuroendocrine tumour, with hypercalcaemic crisis, pre-eclampsia, and renal failure. Postgrad Med J 2002;78(926):752–3.

242. Hwang CS, Park SY, Yu SH, et al. Hypercalcemia induced by ovarian clear cell carcinoma producing all transcriptional variants of parathyroid hormone-related peptide gene during pregnancy. Gynecol Oncol 2006;103(2):740–4.

243. Culbert EC, Schfirin BS. Malignant hypercalcemia in pregnancy: effect of pamidronate on uterine contractions. Obstet Gynecol 2006;108(3 Pt 2):789–91.

244. McCormick TC, Muffly T, Lu G, et al. Aggressive small cell carcinoma of the ovary, hypercalcemic type with hypercalcemia in pregnancy, treated with conservative surgery and chemotherapy. Int J Gynecol Cancer 2009;19(8):1339–41.

Pituitary Disorders During Pregnancy

Soriaya Motivala, MD, Yakov Gologorsky, MD,
Jane Kostandinov, NP, RN, Kalmon D. Post, MD*

KEYWORDS

- Pituitary • Apoplexy • Sheehan • Prolactinoma • Adenoma
- Pregnancy

There is a myriad of hormone changes associated with pregnancy, so it is no surprise that the pituitary gland undergoes much anatomic and physiologic variation at this time. It has been known for centuries that the pituitary gland enlarges during gestation. In vivo magnetic resonance imaging (MRI) studies by Gonzalez and colleagues[1] showed that pituitary hyperplasia led to an overall increase in size in all dimensions of 136% compared with the control group, attributable mainly to an increase in size and number of the lactotroph cells, which are responsible for prolactin secretion. The gland continues to grow significantly in the immediate postpartum period as well. While the height of the gland rarely increases beyond 10 mm during pregnancy, it has been found to exceed 10 mm in height in the early postpartum period.[2] It has been reported that the gland returns to its normal size at 6 months postpartum[3]; however, the authors have noted a persistent pituitary plumping in many patients for many more months after childbirth.

This growth can render diagnosis of pituitary disorders during pregnancy very difficult based on imaging studies alone.[4] Differentiating benign expansion of the gland from other more serious gland disorders such as pituitary adenoma, lymphocytic hypophysitis, Sheehan syndrome, or apoplexy must involve a thorough review of the patient's history, clinical presentation, endocrinologic workup, and MRI of the pituitary sella. Current guidelines do not recommend the routine use of gadolinium contrast for MRI in pregnancy, given the unknown risk to the fetus; however, it may be used on a case-by-case basis after carefully documented risk-benefit analysis.[5]

Pituitary disease may have a significant impact on a patient before conception as well as throughout her pregnancy. It is imperative to provide care to patients affected by pituitary disease with a multidisciplinary approach involving endocrinologists, obstetricians and, when appropriate, neurosurgical care, as this group of disorders can represent a substantial level of morbidity and mortality for both mother and fetus.

The authors have nothing to disclose.
Department of Neurosurgery, Mount Sinai Hospital, 1 Gustave Levy Place, New York, NY 10029, USA
* Corresponding author.
E-mail address: kalmon.post@mountsinai.org

Endocrinol Metab Clin N Am 40 (2011) 827–836
doi:10.1016/j.ecl.2011.08.007

PROLACTINOMAS

Prolactinomas are pituitary adenomas derived from the lactotroph cells. Prolactinomas remain the most frequent of pituitary tumors in both the pregnant and nonpregnant state, accounting for approximately 40% of adenomas. The tumors are diagnosed based on their hypersecretion of prolactin and associated MRI findings in the pituitary gland. Prolactin levels in the nonpregnant state are considered to be normal at less than 25 µg per liter.[6] Prolactinomas are predominantly benign tumors that are classified by size as either microprolactinomas (<10 mm) or macroprolactinomas (>10 mm), with the majority being the microprolactinoma variety that rarely increase in size over time. Ten percent of prolactinomas are macroprolactinomas, and are more frequent in men. This finding has been postulated to be due to a delay in diagnosis because of the propensity for premenopausal women to present with oligorrhea/amenorrhea, galactorrhea, and infertility, whereas men of a similar age bracket tend to present with much more subtle findings, except where the tumor growth causes local compression leading to visual field deficits and/or headache.[6] Overall, prolactinomas represent the most frequent cause of persistent pathologic hyperprolactinemia.

In pregnancy, placentally derived estrogens stimulate lactotroph function and lead to hypertrophy and rising prolactin levels during gestation, which drop sharply after delivery, thus rendering the measurement of prolactin levels during pregnancy of little value.

There are 3 confounding issues for physicians and patients surrounding prolactinomas and pregnancy: (1) their being a frequent cause of infertility in women; (2) the effects of dopamine agonists used in the treatment of prolactinomas on the fetus itself; and (3) the effect of a pregnancy on the prolactinoma and its possible growth in addition to the normal pituitary enlargement of pregnancy.

The increased prolactin levels seen with prolactinomas cause hormonal effects analogous to those seen in women in the postpartum period. There is suppression of gonadotropin-releasing hormone from the hypothalamus, leading to inhibition of secretion of luteinizing hormone and follicular stimulating hormone. This process leads to suppressed gonadal function and increased milk production, resulting in one of the most frequent causes of anovulation.[7] Often the diagnosis of a prolactinoma is made during the medical workup for infertility, resulting in most prolactinomas in pregnancy having been identified prior to conception.

For those patients with prolactinomas and hyperprolactinemia wishing to restore fertility, medical treatment with dopamine agonists to reduce tumor size and level of prolactin secretion should be considered as first-line therapy. Surgery is generally reserved for those patients with acute symptoms secondary to mass effect such as visual compromise, or for those resistant to pharmacotherapy. Fertility rates after initiating treatment with dopamine agonists have been found to be very high. A recent study of 85 women with microprolactinomas and macroprolactinomas treated with the dopamine agonist cabergoline had a 94% conception rate.[8]

Given the frequent usage of dopamine agonists in the treatment of prolactinomas to induce fertility, much has been written about their safety as regards the fetus, as it is likely that the fetus will be exposed at least for the initial few weeks of pregnancy. Dopamine, an endogenous ligand, binds to dopamine receptors on the lactotroph cells in the anterior pituitary lobe and downregulates adenylyl cyclase activity, thus resulting in inhibition of prolactin secretion. There are several agonists on the market available for treatment, all of which have been shown to cross the placental barrier.[9] In general, dopamine agonist therapy is usually discontinued once a pregnancy has been positively confirmed, particularly with microadenomas.[10]

Bromocriptine historically has been the longest used therapy in the treatment of prolactinomas. In general, it is considered safe for the fetus when terminated at the time of definitive diagnosis of pregnancy. In more than 6000 pregnancies whereby bromocriptine was being used at conception, it was not found to cause any increase in spontaneous abortion, ectopic pregnancies, trophoblastic disease, or frequency of multiple pregnancies, and led to congenital malformations in only 1.8% of births, which was comparable if not lower than the rate of congenital defects found in the general population.[11] There are limited data on the use of bromocriptine throughout pregnancy.

Cabergoline, an increasingly popular dopamine agonist, is currently considered the first-line treatment for hyperprolactinemia in the nonpregnant state. The data on cabergoline's effects on the fetus were relatively unknown until recently. Lebbe and colleagues[12] published their review of 100 cases of pregnancy in which women were being treated with cabergoline at the time of conception. The incidence of spontaneous abortion was found to be 10% and the rate of neonatal malformation was 3.4%, both concordant to rates in the general population in Belgium at the time of study. Another recent study in Japan showed that for 85 women treated with high-dose cabergoline who achieved pregnancy, there were 83 live births, 1 stillbirth, and 2 abortions. There were no significant congenital malformations seen at birth. The incidence of infants of low birth weight (10%) and stillbirths (1.2%) was similar to those of the general Japanese population.[8] Given the increasing amount of data regarding the safety of cabergoline in early fetal development, it is increasingly used as the first0line agent to promote fertility in women of childbearing age with prolactinoma.

Quinagolide is a nonergot-derived dopamine agonist that is infrequently used despite its preferred once-a-day dosing. Quinagolide is currently not approved for use in the United States and, due to the increased prevalence of adverse outcomes, is not currently recommended for women with prolactinomas who desire pregnancy.[10]

Of course the greatest concern physicians have when a woman with a prolactinoma becomes pregnant is whether the tumor will enlarge and produce symptoms requiring intervention secondary to (1) stimulatory effect of increased endogenous estrogen on lactotrophs and (2) the discontinuation of dopamine agonist treatment. A review of the literature by Molitch[13] pooled information from 514 women with either microadenoma or macroadenoma. Of the women with microadenomas, none of whom had received prior radiation or surgical intervention, only 5 (1.4%) had symptomatic enlargement defined as headache, visual field deficit, or both. In no case was surgical intervention necessary. However, regarding macroadenomas the story was quite different. In the 84 women with macroadenomas who did not have prior treatment with radiation or surgery, 26% had symptomatic tumor enlargement. Four of these women required surgery during pregnancy, and 15 patients required bromocriptine therapy. Of the 67 women with macroadenomas who were previously treated with surgery or radiation, only 2 had enlargement.[13]

In general, few microprolactinomas will show significant growth during pregnancy to become symptomatic from mass effect. Such patients can be followed clinically and should only undergo follow-up visual field testing or noncontrast MRI if they become symptomatic. Macroprolactinomas, however, have a greater propensity toward symptomatic growth, and such patients should be followed more closely.

Dopamine agonist therapy with cabergoline or bromocriptine should be reinitiated if there is symptomatic tumor growth, as it is generally considered to place the mother and fetus at less risk than operative intervention. If there is no response to the pharmacotherapy and there is a worsening of vision, transsphenoidal resection or delivery, if appropriate, should be undertaken.

Cesarean-section delivery is preferred for patients with macroprolactinoma, because of the potential increase in intracranial pressure during pushing. Although infant suckling causes an increase in prolactin secretion, there is little evidence to suggest that breastfeeding leads to tumor growth. In fact it has been noted that in some cases prolactinomas will shrink in the postpartum period,[14] and it has been suggested that this decrease in size may be due to hormonal effects on the pituitary vasculature resulting in infarction of the adenomatous tissue.

ACROMEGALY

Acromegaly is a disease caused by excessive growth hormone secretion from a generally benign pituitary adenoma. It results in a myriad of symptoms and complications caused by the systemic effects of the increase in growth hormone (GH) and the concomitant increase in insulin growth factor 1 (IGF-1). There have been fewer than 100 cases of active acromegaly during pregnancy. Infertility is common secondary to dysfunction of the hypothalamic-pituitary-gonadal axis. Hyperprolactinemia is often present from oversecretion due to mixed GH/prolactinoma tumor types, and/or from local stalk effect contributing to anovulation.[15]

Treatment of acromegaly includes transsphenoidal resection (generally considered to be first-line treatment), radiosurgery, or drugs (dopamine agonists, somatostatin analogues, or GH receptor analogues). Transsphenoidal resection and radiation therapy may worsen infertility by further disrupting the hypothalamic-pituitary-gonadal axis.[16] Furthermore, surgery in the early stages of pregnancy carries a high risk of spontaneous abortion.

The number of acromegalics who are able to conceive is likely to increase as treatment paradigms and in vitro fertilization techniques have improved. Given that 85% of tumors in acromegaly are macroadenomas, this has resulted in the theoretical concern of tumor enlargement during pregnancy leading to exacerbation of symptoms and local compressive phenomena such as loss of visual acuity. Kupersmith and colleagues,[17] in their 1994 study of 65 pregnant patients with adenomas (prolactinomas and acromegaly), found that only those with macroadenomas were likely to develop visual field deficits. In a recent retrospective review in which MRI was performed at approximately 4 months and after delivery, out of 27 cases only 3 showed an increase in adenoma size, whereas 2 decreased and 22 remained stable.[16] There have been a few other reported cases of increase in tumor size during pregnancy.

Also of concern are the possible maternal and fetal affects of acromegaly during pregnancy. Possible maternal effects that have been reported to occur are impaired glucose tolerance or overt gestational diabetes, hypertension that could result in preeclampsia, or coronary artery disease. Increased birth weight has been observed in neonates born to women with active acromegaly. A recent retrospective multicenter trial looked at 49 women diagnosed with acromegaly either before conception or during pregnancy, and a total of 59 pregnancies resulted in 64 healthy babies. Gestational diabetes was seen in 6.8% while gravid hypertension was noted in 13.6% of patients. Maternal effects were more frequent in those patients whose hypersecretion of GH and IGF-1 were not well controlled before pregnancy. Of interest, 4 women gave birth to a small-for-gestational-age child; all had received a somatostatin analogue alone or in combination with a dopamine agonist during their pregnancy.[16]

Pharmacotherapy remains a highly used treatment option for acromegaly. At present, medical therapy is discontinued once a viable pregnancy has been identified. Dopamine agonists have been well studied in pregnancy and have not been shown to increase the risk of abortion or fetal defects as was previously discussed; however, this class of drugs is in general less efficacious at treating acromegaly (unless there is a significant prolactin secreting portion of the tumor). Somatostatin analogues have been anecdotally reported as being safe both to mother and fetus when taken during pregnancy, though definitive data currently do not exist.[18] GH receptor antagonist (pegvisomant) usage during pregnancy has not been reported in the current literature. Long-term usage of any of these drugs during pregnancy has not been well delineated, therefore they are currently not recommended.

There are several case reports of IGF-1 levels normalizing or decreasing during pregnancy and/or in the postpartum period, suggesting that biochemical improvement in these patients can occur with pregnancy (similar to improvement seen in prolactinomas and pregnancy). This process is postulated to be caused by increased concentrations of estrogens or other pregnancy hormones, though an exact mechanism has not been elucidated.[16,19,20] This aspect may prove to be an investigational avenue of possible future therapy for this disease.

CUSHING DISEASE

Cushing syndrome results in hypercortisolemia, hyperandrogenemia, and/or hyperprolactinemia, and may be caused by a corticotroph-secreting pituitary adenoma (Cushing disease), adrenal adenoma, or ectopic corticotropin production. This syndrome results in significantly impaired fertility, resulting in very few documented successful pregnancies with active disease.[21] The majority of cases documented in the literature of active Cushing syndrome during pregnancy are due to an adrenal adenoma. Only about 40% are attributable to a pituitary adenoma, making Cushing disease in pregnancy exceedingly rare.[4]

Hormonal changes in normal pregnancy profoundly affect the hypothalamic-pituitary-adrenal axis. There is a significant estrogen-induced increase in cortisol-binding globulin, coupled with the placental production of corticotropin-releasing hormone, which leads to an increase in cortisol. There is a threefold increase in total cortisol by week 26; both free and bound cortisol is increased. Dexamethasone suppression testing becomes abnormal, and a twofold to threefold increase in urine free cortisol measurements may be seen. One important difference between normal pregnancy and Cushing disease is that the circadian rhythm is preserved, though it may be blunted. The fetus is protected from this increase in cortisol by a placental enzyme (β-hydroxysteroid dehydrogenase 2), which converts active glucocorticoids into inactive metabolites.[22] Furthermore, a corticotropin surge is seen during delivery, which renders the diagnosis of Cushing syndrome very difficult in the peripartum period. It has been reported that abnormal dexamethasone suppression testing is very common in the peripartum period, and has been seen in up to 82% of the normal population.[23] This abnormality has been found to persist up to the fifth postpartum week.[24]

Adding to the dilemma of diagnosis are the similarities in clinical symptoms seen during normal pregnancy and in Cushing disease. Central obesity, striae, facial plethora, fatigue, emotional lability, glucose intolerance, and hypertension are symptoms that can easily be subscribed to either process.

Midnight salivary cortisol testing may provide a clue for Cushing syndrome, as loss of circadian rhythm is seen in Cushing syndrome and not pregnancy; however, its role has yet to be standardized.[4]

If Cushing disease is suspected, MRI may be performed, however, Cushing disease is often caused by a microadenoma, which may not be visible on MRI. Inferior petrosal sinus sampling should not be a routine tool of investigation in pregnancy, due to the necessary radiation. There has been one case report in the literature in which the jugular instead of the femoral vein was used for access to limit the radiation directly to the fetal area. There were no ill effects on the fetus; however, long-term follow-up continues to be needed.[25]

Early diagnosis and treatment are imperative as Cushing syndrome/Cushing disease poses a significant threat to both mother and fetus. In 1994 Sheeler and colleagues[26] reported on 69 women with pregnancy and active Cushing syndrome, 60 of whom developed significant complications. This study found that 69% developed gravid hypertension, 27% developed gestational diabetes, 7% developed preeclampsia, and 7% underwent congestive heart failure. Of significance, 3 patients in the series died of complications. Fetal effects such as intrauterine growth restriction (IUGR) (26.2%) and prematurity (64.6%) have also been noted.[27]

Given the high risk of complications to both mother and fetus, treatment is highly advocated. Medical therapy has had limited success in this regard. There have been reports of ketoconazole and metyrapone use during pregnancy. Ketoconazole has in general been well tolerated; however, IUGR has been reported.[28] Metyrapone has also been reported to cause IUGR, as well as fetal hypoadrenalism and coarctation of the aorta.[29,30] Mitotane, which is also used in the treatment of Cushing disease, is teratogenic, and therapeutic abortion is necessary in the case of fetal exposure.[31] In general transsphenoidal resection is the preferred treatment of choice, and has been done successfully in the second trimester. If hypercortisolemia is profound in the first trimester, medical therapy is often the first line of treatment, with surgical resection to follow when appropriate. Delayed diagnosis in the third trimester can be treated with pharmacotherapy, delivery of the baby when possible, or surgical resection with increased risk. It is important that pregnant patients treated for Cushing disease by either medical or surgical means should be followed closely and treated for any possible adrenal insufficiency that should result.

CLINICALLY NONFUNCTIONING ADENOMAS AND THYROID-STIMULATING HORMONE–SECRETING ADENOMAS

Nonsecretory pituitary adenomas are not common in pregnancy, as most lead to some degree of impaired fertility. These tumors are managed in the same manner as prolactinomas, and may be treated with bromocriptine because the DR2 dopamine receptor has been found in these tumors. However, tumor shrinkage is rarely seen with nonsecreting adenomas. Treatment with bromocriptine has resulted in spontaneous pregnancy.[32]

Thyroid-stimulating hormone–secreting tumors are also exceedingly rare in pregnancy. A few cases reported have been successfully treated with octreotide at various times during pregnancy.[33]

LYMPHOCYTIC HYPOPHYSITIS

Lymphocytic hypophysitis is a rare inflammatory lesion of the pituitary gland, which usually presents in the peripartum period (though there have been cases reported in men and children). It is a mass lesion that is usually indistinguishable from, and often mistaken for, an adenoma. Lymphocytic hypophysitis may present with headache, visual field defects, or signs of anterior pituitary deficiency. Diabetes insipidus is seen in cases of infundibulo-hypophysitis. It is speculated to be of autoimmune etiology and is associated with other autoimmune disorders (especially Hashimoto thyroiditis) in approximately 30% of cases.[34] Since its recognition, approximately 400 biopsy-proven cases of lymphocytic hypophysitis have been recorded in the literature. It typically presents in the third trimester of pregnancy or within 1 year post-partum, with symptoms related to mass effect and hypopituitarism.

Definitive diagnosis requires biopsy; however, peripartum hypopituitarism in the absence of hypovolemia or shock (Sheehan syndrome), a homogeneously enhancing sellar mass on MRI, and pituitary hormone deficiency pattern with early loss of cortico-trophs and thyrotrophs in an enlarging pituitary with late loss of gonadotrophs and somatotrophs are highly suggestive of lymphocytic hypophysitis. Furthermore, rapid onset of hypopituitarism with the degree of failure out of proportion to the size of the mass is also commonly seen.

The natural course of this disease is difficult to assess, as it is unclear how many women are never diagnosed or are misdiagnosed (ie, often confused with Sheehan syndrome). There have been several reported cases in the literature of spontaneous regression of the mass and return of normal pituitary function.[35–37] Corticosteroid therapy has been advocated to combat inflammation; however, current data do not clearly elucidate its efficacy, and given the known complications and side effects of high-dose steroid therapy it should be used judiciously. The authors advocate rapid surgical intervention for medically refractory cases with progressive neurologic dete-rioration. At present, transsphenoidal resection is used in a decompressive fashion, as aggressive resection rarely results in normalization of endocrine function.

Patients with lymphocytic hypophysitis may require hormone replacement and long-term endocrine follow-up for hormone therapy management as the inflammation resolves.

SHEEHAN SYNDROME

Sheehan syndrome consists of postpartum pituitary necrosis typically associated with severe hemorrhage, shock, or hypotension at delivery. It is uncommon in North America secondary to improved obstetric practices. As previously discussed, the pituitary gland enlarges substantially with normal pregnancy, which can result in compression of the superior hypophyseal artery leading to mild ischemia of the anterior pituitary gland. It is postulated that sudden changes in arterial pressure during delivery (hemorrhage, shock, hypovolemia) can tip the balance, resulting in pituitary necrosis. There are both acute and chronic forms. In the acute period one might see hypotension, failure to lactate, anorexia, extreme fatigue, nausea, vomiting, headache, meningismus, and hypoglycemia. In some cases severe hyponatremia and postpartum seizures have been reported.[38,39] In the chronic form, which is much more common and can present months to years postpartum, symptoms are much more indolent and difficult to differ-entiate, and often go undetected. Patients often complain of fatigue, anorexia, persis-tent amenorrhea, loss of libido, dry skin, and cold intolerance. In one study of 28 patients the average time to diagnosis from the obstetric event was 13.92 years.[40] Diabetes insipidus is a much less common manifestation, as the posterior pituitary gland is less sensitive to ischemia.

It is important to differentiate Sheehan syndrome from pituitary apoplexy in the acute setting, as apoplexy often requires emergent surgical intervention whereas Sheehan syndrome does not. Both are characterized by an enlarging gland acutely; however, Sheehan syndrome shows nonhemorrhagic enlargement followed by atrophy and involution to an empty sella with time. Lymphocytic hypophysitis should also be ruled out. Treatment of Sheehan syndrome consists of steroids in the acute period of pituitary enlargement, followed by hormone replacement with careful moni-toring for hypodrenalism.[4]

Continued fertility is possible, and there have been reports of improved function of the pituitary gland with subsequent pregnancy.[41]

PITUITARY APOPLEXY

Pituitary-tumor apoplexy is an acute hemorrhagic infarction of a preexisting pituitary adenoma or within a physiologically enlarged gland. It occurs rarely in pregnancy and results in sudden, severe headache, visual disturbances, and impairment of pituitary function. MRI is used to confirm the clinical diagnosis in pregnancy as computed tomography is contraindicated, though sellar hemorrhage is not always seen.[42] Treatment consists of acute medical stabilization with intravenous fluids, and intravenous steroids in the setting of profound hypoadrenalism. In the past, immediate transsphenoidal decompression was advocated. Increasingly it is now reserved for those patients who remain medically and neurologically unstable after aggressive medical management.[43]

Changes in hormone levels and pituitary morphology during pregnancy render it somewhat difficult to differentiate normal variation from pathology in the gravid period. Given the significant effects pituitary disease can have in the peripartum and postpartum period, prompt and accurate diagnosis as well as appropriate treatment is imperative. A multidisciplinary team approach involving endocrinologists, obstetricians and, when appropriate, neurosurgical care can greatly reduce the morbidity and mortality that result from this spectrum of pituitary disorders.

REFERENCES

1. Gonzalez JG, Elizondo G, Salvidar D, et al. Pituitary gland growth during normal pregnancy: an in vivo study using magnetic resonance imaging. Am J Med 1988; 85(2):217–20.
2. Dinc H, Esen F, Demirci A, et al. Pituitary dimensions and volume measurements in pregnancy and post partum. MR assessment. Acta Radiol 1998;39(1):64–9.
3. Elster AD, Sanders TG, Vines FS, et al. Size and shape of the pituitary gland during pregnancy and post partum: measurement with MR imaging. Radiology 1991;181(2):531–5.
4. Karaca Z, Tanriverdi F, Unluhizarci K, et al. Pregnancy and pituitary disorders. Eur J Endocrinol 2010;162(3):453–75.
5. Kanal E, Barkovich AJ, Bell C, et al. ACR guidance document for safe MR practices: 2007. AJR Am J Roentgenol 2007;188(6):1447–74.
6. Schlechte JA. Long-term management of prolactinomas. J Clin Endocrinol Metab 2007;92(8):2861–5.
7. Crosignani PG. Current treatment issues in female hyperprolactinaemia. Eur J Obstet Gynecol Reprod Biol 2006;125(2):152–64.
8. Ono M, Miki N, Amano K, et al. Individualized high-dose cabergoline therapy for hyperprolactinemic infertility in women with micro- and macroprolactinomas. J Clin Endocrinol Metab 2010;95(6):2672–9.
9. Kars M, Dekkers OM, Pereira AM, et al. Update in prolactinomas. Neth J Med 2010;68(3):104–12.
10. Molitch ME. Prolactinomas and pregnancy. Clin Endocrinol (Oxf) 2010;73(2):147–8.
11. Krupp P, Monka C. Bromocriptine in pregnancy: safety aspects. Klin Wochenschr 1987;65(17):823–7.
12. Lebbe M, Hubinot C, Bernard P, et al. Outcome of 100 pregnancies initiated under treatment with cabergoline in hyperprolactinaemic women. Clin Endocrinol (Oxf) 2010;73(2):236–42.
13. Molitch ME. Pituitary tumors and pregnancy. Growth Horm IGF Res 2003; 13(Suppl A):S38–44.

14. Badawy SZ, Marziale JC, Rosenbaum AE, et al. The long-term effects of pregnancy and bromocriptine treatment on prolactinomas—the value of radiologic studies. Early Pregnancy 1997;3(4):306–11.
15. Kaltsas GA, Androulakis II, Tziveriotis K, et al. Polycystic ovaries and the polycystic ovary syndrome phenotype in women with active acromegaly. Clin Endocrinol (Oxf) 2007;67(6):917–22.
16. Caron P, Broussaud S, Betherat J, et al. Acromegaly and pregnancy: a retrospective multicenter study of 59 pregnancies in 46 women. J Clin Endocrinol Metab 2010;95(10):4680–7.
17. Kupersmith MJ, Rosenberg C, Kleinberg D. Visual loss in pregnant women with pituitary adenomas. Ann Intern Med 1994;121(7):473–7.
18. Bornschein J, Drozdov I, Malfertheiner P. Octreotide LAR: safety and tolerability issues. Expert Opin Drug Saf 2009;8(6):755–68.
19. Lau SL, McGrath S, Evain-Brion D, et al. Clinical and biochemical improvement in acromegaly during pregnancy. J Endocrinol Invest 2008;31(3):255–61.
20. Ben Salem Hachmi L, Kammoun I, Bouzid C, et al. Management of acromegaly in pregnant woman. Ann Endocrinol (Paris) 2010;71(1):60–3 [in French].
21. Lado-Abeal J, Rodriguez-Arnao J, Newell-Price JD, et al. Menstrual abnormalities in women with Cushing's disease are correlated with hypercortisolemia rather than raised circulating androgen levels. J Clin Endocrinol Metab 1998;83(9): 3083–8.
22. Vilar L, Freitas Mda C, Lima LH, et al. Cushing's syndrome in pregnancy: an overview. Arq Bras Endocrinol Metabol 2007;51(8):1293–302.
23. Greenwood J, Parker G. The dexamethasone suppression test in the puerperium. Aust N Z J Psychiatry 1984;18(3):282–4.
24. Owens PC, Smith R, Brinsmead MW, et al. Postnatal disappearance of the pregnancy-associated reduced sensitivity of plasma cortisol to feedback inhibition. Life Sci 1987;41(14):1745–50.
25. Pinette MG, Pan YQ, Oppenheim D, et al. Bilateral inferior petrosal sinus corticotropin sampling with corticotropin-releasing hormone stimulation in a pregnant patient with Cushing's syndrome. Am J Obstet Gynecol 1994;171(2):563–4.
26. Sheeler LR. Cushing's syndrome and pregnancy. Endocrinol Metab Clin North Am 1994;23(3):619–27.
27. Buescher MA, McClamrock HD, Adashi EY. Cushing syndrome in pregnancy. Obstet Gynecol 1992;79(1):130–7.
28. Bronstein MD, Salgado LR, de Castro Musolino NR. Medical management of pituitary adenomas: the special case of management of the pregnant woman. Pituitary 2002;5(2):99–107.
29. Connell JM, Cordiner J, Davies DL, et al. Pregnancy complicated by Cushing's syndrome: potential hazard of metyrapone therapy. Case report. Br J Obstet Gynaecol 1985;92(11):1192–5.
30. Close CF, Mann MC, Watts JF, et al. ACTH-independent Cushing's syndrome in pregnancy with spontaneous resolution after delivery: control of the hypercortisolism with metyrapone. Clin Endocrinol (Oxf) 1993;39(3):375–9.
31. Leiba S, Weinstein R, Shindel B, et al. The protracted effect of o, p'-DDD in Cushing's disease and its impact on adrenal morphogenesis of young human embryo. Ann Endocrinol (Paris) 1989;50(1):49–53.
32. Murata Y, Ando H, Nagasaka T, et al. Successful pregnancy after bromocriptine therapy in an anovulatory woman complicated with ovarian hyperstimulation caused by follicle-stimulating hormone-producing plurihormonal pituitary microadenoma. J Clin Endocrinol Metab 2003;88(5):1988–93.

33. Caron P, Gerbeau C, Pradayrol L, et al. Successful pregnancy in an infertile woman with a thyrotropin-secreting macroadenoma treated with somatostatin analog (octreotide). J Clin Endocrinol Metab 1996;81(3):1164–8.

34. Nishiki M, Muarakami Y, Ozawa Y, et al. Serum antibodies to human pituitary membrane antigens in patients with autoimmune lymphocytic hypophysitis and infundibuloneurohypophysitis. Clin Endocrinol (Oxf) 2001;54(3):327–33.

35. Leiba S, Schindel B, Weinstein R, et al. Spontaneous postpartum regression of pituitary mass with return of function. JAMA 1986;255(2):230–2.

36. Castle D, de Villiers JC, Melvill R. Lymphocytic adenohypophysitis. Report of a case with demonstration of spontaneous tumour regression and a review of the literature. Br J Neurosurg 1988;2(3):401–5.

37. Ishihara T, Hino M, Kurahachi H, et al. Long-term clinical course of two cases of lymphocytic adenohypophysitis. Endocr J 1996;43(4):433–40.

38. Anfuso S, Patrelli TS, Soncini E, et al. A case report of Sheehan's syndrome with acute onset, hyponatremia and severe anemia. Acta Biomed 2009;80(1):73–6.

39. Jain G, Singh D, Kumar S. Sheehan's syndrome presenting as postpartum seizures. Anaesth Intensive Care 2010;38(3):571–3.

40. Sert M, Tetiker T, Krim S, et al. Clinical report of 28 patients with Sheehan's syndrome. Endocr J 2003;50(3):297–301.

41. See TT, Lee SP, Chen HF. Spontaneous pregnancy and partial recovery of pituitary function in a patient with Sheehan's syndrome. J Chin Med Assoc 2005;68(4):187–90.

42. Zak IT, Dulai HS, Kish KK. Imaging of neurologic disorders associated with pregnancy and the postpartum period. Radiographics 2007;27(1):95–108.

43. Murad-Kejbou S, Eggenberger E. Pituitary apoplexy: evaluation, management, and prognosis. Curr Opin Ophthalmol 2009;20(6):456–61.

Hyperprolactinemia and Infertility

Amal Shibli-Rahhal, MD, Janet Schlechte, MD*

KEYWORDS

- Prolactin • Infertility • Bromocriptine • Cabergoline
- Pituitary tumor

HYPERPROLACTINEMIA

Prolactin-secreting pituitary tumors are a common cause of gonadal dysfunction and infertility. This overview of the management of hyperprolactinemia in the infertile woman reviews the effect of pregnancy on tumor size, the choice of a dopamine agonist, and the potential effects of dopamine agonist therapy on fetal development. The article concludes with recommendations for treatment when fertility is not an issue and issues related to long-term follow-up of prolactinomas.

Clinical Presentation

When pregnancy, medications, thyroid, renal, and hepatic disease are excluded, the most likely cause of hyperprolactinemia is a prolactin-secreting pituitary tumor. Ninety percent of prolactinomas in women are microadenomas (<10 mm) (**Fig. 1**A) and present with menstrual dysfunction and infertility.[1] In general prolactin levels correlate with tumor size and hypopituitarism and neurologic deficits are uncommon in small tumors. Macroadenomas (>10 mm) (see **Fig. 1**B) are less common, are associated with higher prolactin levels, and usually present with neurologic dysfunction in addition to hypogonadism. Women with prolactinomas also present with low bone mass as a result of the inhibitory effect of prolactin on estrogen.[2,3]

Hyperprolactinemia is present in 15% to 20% of women undergoing evaluation for infertility.[4] In some studies the severity of hyperprolactinemia roughly correlates with the degree of menstrual dysfunction. In an infertility clinic in Brazil, Bahamondes and colleagues[5] reported hyperprolactinemia in 55% of women with amenorrhea, in 37% with oligomenorrhea, and in 9% with normal menses. Galactorrhea occurs in 50% to 80% of women with hyperprolactinemia and may occur with or without menstrual dysfunction.[1,4]

The authors have nothing to disclose.

Division of Endocrinology and Metabolism, Department of Internal Medicine, University of Iowa, 200 Hawkins Drive, Iowa City, IA 52242, USA

* Corresponding author.

E-mail address: janet-schlechte@uiowa.edu

Endocrinol Metab Clin N Am 40 (2011) 837–846

doi:10.1016/j.ecl.2011.08.008

endo.theclinics.com

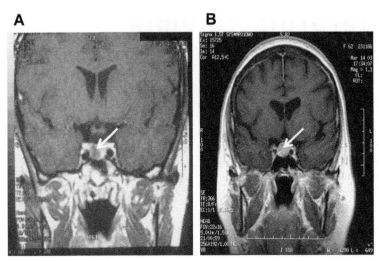

Fig. 1. (*A*) Pituitary microadenoma. (*B*) Pituitary macroadenoma.

Pathophysiology

The regulation of prolactin secretion is mediated through the inhibitory effects of hypothalamic dopamine. In animals and humans hypersecretion of prolactin leads to inhibition of gonadotropin-releasing hormone (GnRH) secretion. In hypogonadal rats hypothalamic GnRH secretion increases the number of pituitary GnRH receptors. In contrast, hypogonadal rats with hyperprolactinemia have fewer pituitary GnRH receptors, a diminished GnRH receptor response to GnRH, and a decline in luteinizing hormone (LH) pulse frequency and pulse amplitude, all of which reverse after correction of hyperprolactinemia.[6,7] Hyperprolactinemic women have diminished LH pulse frequency that normalizes after correction of hyperprolactinemia.[8,9] Except in women who have large tumors, treatment with physiologic doses of GnRH leads to normal or supranormal LH secretion in most patients with hyperprolactinemia.[9–11]

Although the primary abnormality in hyperprolactinemia is a decrease in hypothalamic GnRH secretion, prolactin also has a direct inhibitory effect on the ovaries, leading to decreased estrogen synthesis. Prolactin receptors are present in animal and human ovaries[12,13] and synthesis of estrogen and progesterone decreases when human ovarian cells are exposed to supraphysiologic concentrations of prolactin.[14,15]

Luteal phase insufficiency accounts for 3% to 10% of cases of infertility, and hyperprolactinemia has been reported in up to two-thirds of patients with luteal phase defects.[16,17] A luteal phase defect leads to poorly developed endometrium and failure of embryo implantation and is often the cause of infertility in hyperprolactinemic women who have normal menstrual cycles.[5,16] A small percentage of women with hirsutism have hyperprolactinemia but it is not clear how (or whether) the prolactin increase may contribute to increased hair growth. The underlying problem in many of these women is likely the polycystic ovarian syndrome.[18]

Principles of Treatment

The goals of therapy are to normalize prolactin, reduce tumor size, and restore gonadal function and fertility, and the treatment of choice is a dopamine agonist. Before the elucidation of the role of dopamine in the regulation of prolactin secretion, transsphenoidal surgery was the mainstay of therapy for prolactinomas. The success of the procedure is highly dependent on the experience of the neurosurgeon, and success rates range from 73% to 90% for microadenomas and 30% to 50% for macroadenomas.[19,20] Recurrence of hyperprolactinemia after surgery is common but is not usually associated with radiographic evidence of tumor regrowth.[21,22] Radiation has no role as primary therapy for prolactinomas but may be necessary in patients with large tumors who fail to respond to medical or surgical treatment.

Elucidating the inhibitory role of dopamine in prolactin secretion and the subsequent development of dopamine agonists revolutionized the treatment of prolactinomas so that now, with rare exception, the preferred therapy for hyperprolactinemia is a dopamine agonist.

DOPAMINE AGONISTS

Binding to D_2 receptors in the anterior pituitary, dopamine agonists decrease prolactin synthesis, limit cell multiplication, and reduce tumor size.[23,24] The decrease in prolactin occurs within days, and tumor shrinkage is usually apparent 3 to 6 months after initiation of therapy. Interruption or withdrawal of therapy leads to rapid recurrence of hyperprolactinemia and tumor regrowth.

In the United States the dopamine agonists approved for treatment of hyperprolactinemia are bromocriptine and cabergoline. Both are available in generic formulation and the major characteristics of the drugs are compared in **Table 1**. Bromocriptine is a semisynthetic ergot derivative that normalizes prolactin, restores regular menses, and reduces tumor size in 80% to 90% of patients with microadenomas.[25,26] Cabergoline is a selective D_2 agonist with high affinity for lactotroph dopamine receptors that normalizes prolactin in ∼95% of women with hyperprolactinemia.[27] When compared directly cabergoline is more effective than bromocriptine in normalizing prolactin (83% vs 59%), restoring ovulatory cycles, inducing pregnancy, and reducing tumor size. Patients are less likely to be resistant to the effects of cabergoline, and cabergoline is effective in 70% of patients who are unresponsive to bromocriptine.[28]

Side Effects

Administration of bromocriptine may cause nasal stuffiness, nausea, headache, drowsiness, and orthostatic hypotension. Cabergoline is associated with the same side effects but the symptoms are usually less severe and of shorter duration. In addition, fewer patients taking cabergoline discontinue therapy because of drug

Table 1 Comparison of approved dopamine agonists		
	Bromocriptine	**Cabergoline**
Half-life (h)	6–20	63–69
Duration of action	24 h	7–14 d
Dosing	Twice daily	Once or twice weekly
Recommended dose (mg)	5–7.5 daily	1–2 weekly
Normalization of prolactin (%)	48–59[25]	83–93[25]
Restoration of fertility (%)	48–52[25,27]	72[25,27]
Cost/y ($)	1156[a]	3600[b]

[a] 5 mg/d generic.
[b] 1 mg/wk generic.

intolerance. When the 2 drugs were compared directly, 53% to 68% of patients taking cabergoline developed gastrointestinal and other side effects compared with 65% to 78% with bromocriptine.[27,29] Side effects of both drugs can be limited by starting with a low dose and increasing the dose slowly.

Depression, digital vasospasm, pleural thickening, and retroperitoneal fibrosis are rare side effects of bromocriptine in patients receiving high doses.[30,31] An increase in cardiac valve regurgitation has been reported in patients with Parkinson disease treated with high doses of cabergoline (3 mg/d) but not with other dopamine agonists.[32,33] Although the doses of cabergoline used in treatment of prolactinomas are substantially lower (1 mg/wk) than those used in patients with Parkinson disease (3 mg/d) patients with large or invasive prolactinomas may require lifelong therapy, and sustained therapy (even at low doses) could potentially lead to valvular dysfunction. There has been no long-term prospective analysis of valve dysfunction in patients with prolactinomas taking cabergoline but the available data suggest no association between the use of cabergoline and cardiac valve regurgitation.[34,35] It is important that patients treated with cabergoline be apprised of the cardiac valve findings in Parkinson disease without causing undue alarm. There are no guidelines and no consensus on whether patients with prolactinomas treated with cabergoline should have echocardiographic monitoring. Large, prospective controlled studies are needed to answer this question.

Other Dopamine Agonists

Quinagolide is a nonergot dopamine agonist with specific D_2 receptor activity that reduces prolactin, decreases tumor size, and restores gonadal function in 70% to 95% of patients with hyperprolactinemia. It is also effective in 35% of patients resistant to or intolerant of bromocriptine.[36] The drug is not available in the United States, but is used in Europe and Canada. Quinagolide is associated with an increase in congenital malformations and should not be used if pregnancy is desired.[37]

MANAGEMENT OF HYPERPROLACTINEMIA IN THE INFERTILE WOMAN

In treatment of prolactin-induced infertility it is important to consider the potential effects of a dopamine agonist on fetal development, the effect of pregnancy on tumor size, and treatment options in the event of symptomatic tumor growth during pregnancy.

Effect of Dopamine Agonists on Fetal Development

Because a dopamine agonist is usually necessary to treat anovulation and infertility, a fetus is exposed to the drug during early gestation. Cabergoline and bromocriptine both cross the placenta. Neither drug is approved for use during pregnancy and the aim is to limit fetal exposure to the drug to the shortest possible period. Cabergoline has largely superseded bromocriptine in treatment of hyperprolactinemia because of the ease of administration, potency, and efficacy, except when fertility is the goal.

In more than 6000 pregnancies reported in the literature, babies born to mothers who took bromocriptine during early gestation did not differ in birth weight, incidence of congenital malformations, or perinatal disorders compared with the general population. In addition, bromocriptine administered during the first few weeks of gestation has not been associated with an increase in spontaneous abortions, ectopic or multiple pregnancies, or abnormal postnatal development.[38] In a review of 988 children exposed to bromocriptine in utero Krupp and Monka[38] reported normal physical development in 100% over a 4-month to 9-year follow-up. Bronstein and colleagues[39] noted normal psychomotor development in 68 of 70 children with intrauterine exposure to bromocriptine who were followed for 5.5 years (1–20 years).

In contrast, data on fetal exposure to cabergoline during early pregnancy are available from about 800 pregnancies. In a retrospective analysis of 763 cabergoline-induced pregnancies Stalldecker and colleagues[40] reported rates of miscarriage, preterm delivery, low birth weight, and congenital malformations comparable with those in the general population. With respect to postnatal development in children exposed to cabergoline, Ono and colleagues[41] and Lebbe and colleagues[42] reported normal development in 171 children followed for periods ranging between 2 months and 12 years. In contrast Stalldecker and colleagues[40] reported 2 cases of epilepsy and 2 cases of pervasive developmental disorder in 61 children exposed to cabergoline followed for up to 16 years.

Treatment Regimens

When fertility is the goal, 0.625 mg of bromocriptine should be initiated at bedtime with a snack. After 1 week, twice-daily dosing can be begun with the addition of a morning dose of 1.25 mg. The dose should be slowly increased (1.25 mg/wk) until a daily dose of 5 mg is reached. After the patient has taken 5 mg daily for 6 to 8 weeks a prolactin level should be repeated. The dose should be increased until normalization of prolactin or restoration of menses occurs. Most patients require 5 mg of bromocriptine daily. During therapy women should use a mechanical form of contraception and continue it until at least 2 regular menstrual cycles have occurred. Bromocriptine should be discontinued as soon as a pregnancy is confirmed.

In a woman who is resistant to or intolerant of bromocriptine it may be necessary to use cabergoline instead of bromocriptine to induce fertility. In these cases cabergoline should be initiated at a dose of 0.25 mg weekly. After 7 days, twice-weekly dosing should be initiated by adding 0.25 mg. At weekly intervals the dose should be increased to 0.5 mg twice weekly. A prolactin level should be obtained after 6 to 8 weeks and the dose should be adjusted until the prolactin normalizes or menses are restored. Most patients require 1 mg weekly. As is true for bromocriptine, gonadal function may be restored before the prolactin normalizes and it is not necessary to increase the dose of dopamine agonist merely to normalize prolactin. The lowest dose of either drug should always be used, and for cabergoline the dose should not exceed 2 mg weekly. As is true for bromocriptine, cabergoline should be discontinued as soon as pregnancy is confirmed.

Although not first-line therapy, transsphenoidal surgery is also an option in women who are resistant to or intolerant of both dopamine agonists. Although the overall success rate of transsphenoidal surgery is around 70%, higher rates have been achieved by experienced surgeons in selected young patients with prolactin levels less than 200 µg/L, small tumors, and short duration of amenorrhea.[19,20] When transsphenoidal surgery is performed by an experienced neurosurgeon, the complication and mortality rates are low.[43]

EFFECT OF PREGNANCY ON TUMOR GROWTH
Microadenomas

During pregnancy there is a progressive increase in prolactin, leading to a 10-fold increase at term. In lactating women prolactin levels remain increased until about 6 weeks after delivery. Because increasing levels of prolactin do not reliably correlate with tumor enlargement it is not necessary to serially measure prolactin levels during pregnancy.

The high levels of estrogen in pregnancy lead to lactotroph hyperplasia and a gradual increase in the size of the pituitary.[44] Whether the lactotroph hyperplasia becomes clinically significant depends on the size of the tumor and whether the patient has been treated with surgery or radiation before pregnancy. For women with microadenomas the risk of symptomatic tumor enlargement during pregnancy is 2.6%, and the risk of asymptomatic tumor enlargement documented by computed tomography or magnetic resonance imaging (MRI) is about 4.5%.[45] The risk of tumor enlargement with an intrasellar macroadenoma is the same as for microadenomas. Based on the low incidence of tumor expansion it is not necessary to perform serial MRI scans or visual field testing during pregnancy in women with microadenomas or intrasellar macroadenomas.[45]

Macroadenomas

For women with macroadenomas who achieved pregnancy using bromocriptine the risk of clinically significant tumor enlargement during pregnancy is 15% to 35% and the risk of asymptomatic growth ranges from 8.9% to 17%.[39,45] The risk of clinically significant tumor enlargement of a macroadenoma decreases to about 5% if a woman is treated with radiation or surgery before dopamine agonist therapy and pregnancy. In patients with large tumors formal visual field testing should be performed each trimester and more frequently if neurologic or visual symptoms develop. If visual field abnormalities develop an MRI without contrast should be used to assess the pituitary.

Most patients with macroadenomas who achieve fertility with bromocriptine have an uncomplicated pregnancy. However, in some cases significant neurologic or visual symptoms develop, and there is no consensus on how to treat symptomatic tumor growth during pregnancy. One option is to reinstitute bromocriptine and to continue it throughout pregnancy. Although no major complications or fetal abnormalities have been identified, information on the safety of bromocriptine used during pregnancy is limited to approximately 100 cases.[46,47] There is minimal information related to the use of cabergoline administered during pregnancy but no complications have been noted in ~200 cases.[41,42] Transsphenoidal surgery is another option in the case of symptomatic tumor growth but any surgery during pregnancy is associated with a 1.5-fold increase in fetal loss in the first trimester and a 5-fold increase in fetal loss in the second trimester, which limits its usefulness.[48]

Therapy for an invasive macroadenoma in a woman who wishes to achieve a pregnancy is complicated and must be individualized. In some cases cabergoline may be necessary to induce pregnancy because large tumors may be resistant to bromocriptine. Using 0.25 to 9 mg of cabergoline weekly and a rapid dose escalation Ono and colleagues[41] reported that pregnancy was achieved in 94% of patients including 57 with macroadenomas with no adverse outcomes. In other cases it may be necessary to surgically debulk the tumor before pregnancy followed by therapy with bromocriptine or cabergoline. A less desirable option is radiotherapy followed by treatment with bromocriptine. Although this protocol reduces the risk of tumor enlargement, the risk of hypopituitarism makes surgery and bromocriptine a more acceptable option.

The complex issues associated with management of a prolactin-secreting macroadenoma emphasize the importance of careful monitoring and the need for a multidisciplinary team (endocrinologist, obstetrician, neuro-ophthalmologist, and neurosurgeon) for the patient.

After Pregnancy

Breast-feeding stimulates prolactin release but is not associated with tumor growth and there is no contraindication to breast-feeding.[49] Pregnancy may have a favorable effect on the natural history of a prolactinoma. Prolactin levels are lower after delivery and remission of hyperprolactinemia has been reported in 17% to 37% of women after pregnancy.[50] After pregnancy a woman with a macroadenoma should resume therapy with a dopamine agonist, preferably cabergoline, unless there is a plan to breast-feed. Dopamine agonists cannot be used during lactation because the resulting decrease in serum prolactin levels hinders lactation. The postpartum management of amenorrheic women with microadenomas is discussed later.

WHEN FERTILITY IS NOT AN ISSUE
Microadenomas

After pregnancy some patients with hyperprolactinemia have regular menses and minimal galactorrhea and do not require therapy, but most remain amenorrheic. Because 95% of microadenomas do not progressively increase in size it is not necessary to treat to prevent tumor growth.[51] However, it is important to treat hypogonadism and to prevent bone loss. When fertility is not an issue the treatment options include cabergoline or an oral contraceptive. Treatment with cabergoline restores menses and improves bone density but negative aspects of dopamine agonist therapy include expense, side effects, and the possibility of pregnancy. An oral contraceptive is less expensive, has fewer side effects, effectively treats the hypogonadism, and prevents bone loss.

The observation that high doses of estrogen induce tumor growth in animals raised concerns that therapy with estrogen might accelerate tumor growth. Premenopausal women treated with conjugated estrogen or oral contraceptives for 2 to 6 years showed no evidence of tumor growth.[51–53] The low incidence of tumor growth during pregnancy is additional information supporting the safety of oral contraceptive therapy.[45] Treatment with estrogen may be associated with a mild increase in prolactin and may worsen galactorrhea, and estrogen should be used with caution in women with macroadenomas.

Long-term Follow-up

There is no consensus on how frequently to image the pituitary in patients with prolactinomas. For women with microadenomas we measure prolactin yearly and do not regularly repeat MRI scans. Because tumor growth usually parallels an increase in prolactin, an increase in prolactin (>250 ng/mL) or clinical signs of tumor expansion warrant an MRI or visual field examination.

Macroadenomas

All macroadenomas require long-term therapy irrespective of gonadal status, and cabergoline is the treatment of choice. A pituitary MRI scan should be obtained 3 months after initiation of therapy to confirm tumor shrinkage, and the dose of cabergoline should be increased until maximum tumor reduction has occurred. Because macroadenomas have a greater growth potential we repeat MRI 2 to 3 years after achieving a normal prolactin and reduction in tumor size to confirm tumor suppression and to ensure that serum prolactin remains a reliable indicator of tumor size.

A major drawback of dopamine agonist therapy is the need for continuous therapy. Recent analyses suggest that withdrawal of cabergoline may lead to remission of hyperprolactinemia without tumor regrowth in approximately 20% of patients treated for 2 years.[54] The optimal length of therapy with a dopamine agonist and the safety of drug withdrawal remain to be defined.

SUMMARY

Prolactin-secreting pituitary tumors are a common cause of amenorrhea and infertility in premenopausal women. Dopamine agonist therapy lowers prolactin, decreases tumor size, and restores menstrual function in more than 90% of cases. Withdrawal or interruption of therapy leads to recurrence of hyperprolactinemia and tumor regrowth. Based on an extensive safety record bromocriptine is the preferred dopamine agonist when fertility is desired, but accumulating data related to cabergoline-induced pregnancies suggest that it is not associated with an increase in congenital malformations or pregnancy complications. The high levels of estrogen achieved during pregnancy lead to pituitary enlargement and the risk of clinically significant tumor expansion during pregnancy depends on the size of the tumor and prepregnancy treatment. When fertility is not an issue an amenorrheic woman with hyperprolactinemia can be treated with cabergoline or an oral contraceptive. Macroadenomas require sustained therapy with cabergoline to prevent tumor enlargement.

REFERENCES

1. Klibanski A. Prolactinomas. N Engl J Med 2010;362:1219–26.
2. Klibanski A, Biller BM, Rosenthal DI, et al. Effects of prolactin and estrogen deficiency in amenorrheic bone loss. J Clin Endocrinol Metab 1988;67:124–30.
3. Schlechte J, Walker L, Kathol M. A longitudinal analysis of premenopausal bone loss in healthy women and women with hyperprolactinemia. J Clin Endocrinol Metab 1992;75:698–703.
4. Kredentser JV, Hoskins CF, Scott JZ. Hyperprolactinemia–a significant factor in female infertility. Am J Obstet Gynecol 1981;139:264–7.
5. Bahamondes L, Faundes A, Tambascia M, et al. Menstrual pattern and ovarian function in women with hyperprolactinemia. Int J Gynaecol Obstet 1985;23:31–6.
6. Fox SR, Hoefer MT, Bartke A, et al. Suppression of pulsatile LH secretion, pituitary GnRH receptor content and pituitary responsiveness to GnRH by hyperprolactinemia in the male rat. Neuroendocrinology 1987;46:350–9.
7. Garcia A, Herbon L, Barkan A, et al. Hyperprolactinemia inhibits gonadotropin-releasing hormone (GnRH) stimulation of the number of pituitary GnRH receptors. Endocrinology 1985;117:954–9.
8. Sartorio A, Pizzocaro A, Liberati D, et al. Abnormal LH pulsatility in women with hyperprolactinemic amenorrhea normalizes after bromocriptine treatment: deconvolution-based assessment. Clin Endocrinol (Oxf) 2000;52:703–12.
9. Sauder SE, Frager M, Case GD, et al. Abnormal patterns of pulsatile luteinizing hormone secretion in women with hyperprolactinemia and amenorrhea: response to bromocriptine. J Clin Endocrinol Metab 1984;59:941–8.
10. Asfour M, L'Hermite M, Hedouin-Quincampoix M, et al. Hypogonadism, galactorrhea and hyperprolactinemia: evaluation of pituitary gonadotrophins reserve before and under bromocriptine. Acta Endocrinol (Copenh) 1977;84:738–49.
11. Mortimer CH, Besser GM, McNeilly AS, et al. Luteinizing hormone and follicle stimulating hormone-releasing hormone test in patients with hypothalamic-pituitary-gonadal dysfunction. Br Med J 1973;4:73–7.
12. Saito T, Saxena BB. Specific receptors for prolactin in the ovary. Acta Endocrinol (Copenh) 1975;80:126–37.
13. Rolland R, Hammond JM. Demonstration of a specific receptor for prolactin in porcine granulosa cells. Endocr Res Commun 1975;2:281–98.
14. Dorrington J, Gore-Langton RE. Prolactin inhibits oestrogen synthesis in the ovary. Nature 1981;290:600–2.

15. Demura R, Ono M, Demura H, et al. Prolactin directly inhibits basal as well as gonadotropin-stimulated secretion of progesterone and 17β estradiol in the human ovary. J Clin Endocrinol Metab 1982;54:1246–50.

16. Dizerega GS, Ross GT. Luteal phase dysfunction. Clin Obstet Gynaecol 1981;8: 733–51.

17. Muhlenstedt D, Bohnet HG, Hanker JP, et al. Short luteal phase and prolactin. Int J Fertil 1978;23:213–8.

18. Franks S. Polycystic ovary syndrome. N Engl J Med 1995;333:853–61.

19. Jane JA Jr, Laws ER Jr. The surgical management of pituitary adenomas in a series of 3,093 patients. J Am Coll Surg 2001;193:651–9.

20. Nomikos P, Buchfelder M, Fahlbusch R. Current management of prolactinomas. J Neurooncol 2001;54:139–50.

21. Schlechte JA, Sherman BM, Chapler FK, et al. Long-term follow-up of women with surgically treated prolactin-secreting pituitary tumors. J Clin Endocrinol Metab 1986;62:1296–301.

22. Thompson JA, Gray CE, Teasdale GM. Relapse of hyperprolactinemia after trans-sphenoidal surgery for microprolactinoma: lesions from long-term follow-up. Neurosurgery 2002;50:36–40.

23. MacLeod RM, Lehmeyer JE. Suppression of pituitary tumor growth and function by ergot alkaloids. Cancer Res 1973;33:849–55.

24. Asa SL, Ezzat S. Medical management of pituitary adenomas: structural and ultrastructural changes. Pituitary 2002;5:133–9.

25. Molitch ME, Elton RL, Blackwell RE, et al. Bromocriptine as primary therapy for prolactin-secreting macroadenomas: results of a prospective multicenter study. J Clin Endocrinol Metab 1985;60:698–705.

26. Bevan JS, Webster J, Burke CW, et al. Dopamine agonists and pituitary tumor shrinkage. Endocr Rev 1992;13:220–40.

27. Webster J, Piscitelli G, Polli A, et al. A comparison of cabergoline and bromocriptine in the treatment of hyperprolactinemic amenorrhea. N Engl J Med 1994;331: 904–9.

28. Colao A, Di Sarno A, Sarnacchiaro S, et al. Prolactinomas resistant to standard dopamine agonists respond to chronic cabergoline treatment. J Clin Endocrinol Metab 1997;82:876–83.

29. Pascal-Vigneron V, Weryha G, Bosc M, et al. Cabergoline versus bromocriptine for hyperprolactinaemic amenorrhea. Results of a multicentric, randomized, double-blind trial in France. Presse Med 1995;24:753–7.

30. Demont JF, Rostin M, Dueymes JM, et al. Retroperitoneal fibrosis and treatment of Parkinson's disease with high doses of bromocriptine. Clin Neuropharmacol 1986;9:200–1.

31. McElvaney NG, Wilcox PG, Churg A, et al. Pleuropulmonary disease during bromocriptine treatment of Parkinson's disease. Arch Intern Med 1988;148: 2231–6.

32. Zanettini R, Antonini A, Gatto G, et al. Valvular heart disease and the use of dopamine agonists for Parkinson's disease. N Engl J Med 2007;356:39–46.

33. Schade R, Andersohn F, Suissa S, et al. Dopamine agonists and the risk of cardiac-valve regurgitation. N Engl J Med 2007;356:29–38.

34. Bogazzi F, Manetti L, Raffaelli V, et al. Cabergoline therapy and the risk of cardiac valve regurgitation in patients with hyperprolactinemia: a meta-analysis from clinical studies. J Endocrinol Invest 2008;31:1119–23.

35. Valassi E, Klibanski A, Biller BM. Potential cardiac valve effects of dopamine agonists in hyperprolactinemia. J Clin Endocrinol Metab 2010;95:1025–33.

36. Barlier A, Jaquet P. Quinagolide–a valuable treatment option for hyperprolactinaemia. Eur J Endocrinol 2006;154:187–95.

37. Webster J. A comparative review of the tolerability profiles of dopamine agonists in the treatment of hyperprolactinaemia and inhibition of lactation. Drug Saf 1996; 14:228–38.

38. Krupp P, Monka C. Bromocriptine in pregnancy: safety aspects. Klin Wochenschr 1987;65:823–7.

39. Bronstein MD. Prolactinomas and pregnancy. Pituitary 2005;8:31–8.

40. Stalldecker G, Mallea-Gil MS, Guitelman M, et al. Effects of cabergoline on pregnancy and embryo-fetal development: retrospective study on 103 pregnancies and a review of the literature. Pituitary 2010;13(4):345–50.

41. Ono M, Miki N, Amano K, et al. Individualized high-dose cabergoline therapy for hyperprolactinemic infertility in women with micro- and macroprolactinomas. J Clin Endocrinol Metab 2010;95:2672–9.

42. Lebbe M, Hubinont C, Bernard P, et al. Outcome of 100 pregnancies initiated under treatment with cabergoline in hyperprolactinemic women. Clin Endocrinol 2010;73:236–42.

43. Barker FG II, Klibanski A, Swearingen B. Transsphenoidal surgery for pituitary tumors in the United States, 1996-2000: mortality, morbidity and the effects of hospital and surgeon volume. J Clin Endocrinol Metab 2003;88:4709–19.

44. Dinc H, Esen F, Demirci A, et al. Pituitary dimensions and volume measurements in pregnancy and post partum. MR assessment. Acta Radiol 1998;39:64–9.

45. Molitch ME. Pregnancy and the hyperprolactinemic woman. N Engl J Med 1985; 312:1364–70.

46. Konopka P, Raymond JP, Merceron RE, et al. Continuous administration of bromocriptine in the prevention of neurological complications in pregnant women with prolactinomas. Am J Obstet Gynecol 1983;146:935–8.

47. Weil C. The safety of bromocriptine in long-term use: a review of the literature. Curr Med Res Opin 1986;10:25–51.

48. Brodsky JB, Cohen EN, Brown BW Jr. Surgery during pregnancy and fetal outcome. Am J Obstet Gynecol 1980;138:1165–7.

49. Holmgren U, Bergstrand G, Hagenfeldt K, et al. Women with prolactinoma–effect of pregnancy and lactation on serum prolactin and on tumor growth. Acta Endocrinol (Copenh) 1986;111:452–9.

50. Jeffcoate WJ, Pound N, Sturrock ND, et al. Long-term follow-up of patients with hyperprolactinaemia. Clin Endocrinol (Oxf) 1996;45:299–303.

51. Schlechte J, Dolan K, Sherman B, et al. The natural history of untreated hyperprolactinemia: a prospective analysis. J Clin Endocrinol Metab 1989;68:412–8.

52. Fathy UM, Foster PA, Torode HW, et al. The effect of combined estrogen/progesterone treatment in women with hyperprolactinemic amenorrhea. Gynecol Endocrinol 1992;6:183–8.

53. Corenblum B, Donovan L. The safety of physiological estrogen plus progestin replacement therapy with oral contraceptive therapy in women with pathological hyperprolactinemia. Fertil Steril 1993;59:671–3.

54. Dekkers OM, Lagro J, Burman P, et al. Recurrence of hyperprolactinemia after withdrawal of dopamine agonists: systemic review and meta-analysis. J Clin Endocrinol Metab 2010;95:43–51.

Hypertension in Pregnancy

Caren G. Solomon, MD, MPH*, Ellen W. Seely, MD

KEYWORDS

- Hypertension • Preeclampsia • Pregnancy
- Gestational hypertension

Hypertensive disorders in pregnancy are commonly classified into 4 categories (**Box 1**).[1] New-onset hypertension in pregnancy includes preeclampsia and gestational hypertension. Both conditions require documentation of at least 2 elevated blood pressures ($\geq$140 mm Hg systolic or $\geq$90 mm Hg diastolic) after the 20th week of gestation in a woman without prior hypertension. In contrast to gestational hypertension, the diagnosis of preeclampsia requires new-onset proteinuria as defined by a 24 hour urine protein of 300 mg or more. A dipstick protein concentration of 1+ or greater[1] or 2+ or greater[2] has alternatively been used to define preeclampsia, although dipstick measurement may be unreliable.[3] An alternative measure of proteinuria endorsed by the National Institute for Health and Clinical Excellence[4] is a spot urine/creatinine ratio greater than 30 mg per millimole. There is ongoing debate as to whether preeclampsia and gestational hypertension are distinct entities or exist on a spectrum.

Hypertension in pregnancy may also reflect preexisting chronic hypertension, defined as a blood pressure greater than or equal to 140/90 mm Hg antedating pregnancy or noted before the 20th week of gestation. Chronic hypertension is complicated in approximately 25% of cases by superimposed preeclampsia.[5]

Because blood pressure characteristically falls in the late first and early second trimester, and then increases to prepregnancy levels later in pregnancy,[6] chronic hypertension may be mistakenly diagnosed as gestational hypertension in women for whom there is no documented prepregnancy or early pregnancy blood pressure measurement available. In these cases, accurate diagnosis may not be made until postpartum; if hypertension does not resolve by 12 weeks postpartum, chronic hypertension is the likely diagnosis.

Women with gestational hypertension or those with essential hypertension not complicated by preeclampsia generally have good pregnancy outcomes. However, preeclampsia is associated with significant risks to the mother and fetus, which are greater when the disease appears earlier in pregnancy.

Department of Medicine, Brigham and Women's Hospital, 75 Francis Street, Boston, MA 02115, USA
* Corresponding author.
E-mail address: cgsolomon@bics.bwh.harvard.edu

Endocrinol Metab Clin N Am 40 (2011) 847–863
doi:10.1016/j.ecl.2011.08.009
0889-8529/11/$ – see front matter © 2011 Elsevier Inc. All rights reserved.

Box 1
Classification of hypertension in pregnancy

Preeclampsia

- Systolic blood pressure >140 mm Hg or diastolic blood pressure >90 mm Hg occurring at or after 20 weeks' gestation in a previously normotensive woman

- Proteinuria >300 mg in a 24-hour urine collection

Gestational hypertension

- Systolic blood pressure >140 mm Hg or diastolic blood pressure >90 mm Hg at or after 20 weeks' gestation in a previously normotensive woman, but without proteinuria

Chronic hypertension

- Systolic blood pressure >140 mm Hg or diastolic blood pressure >90 mm Hg that is documented before the 20th week of gestation

Preeclampsia superimposed on chronic hypertension

- New-onset or greatly increased proteinuria

- Sudden exacerbation of hypertension or other signs of multisystem involvement such as thrombocytopenia or elevated transaminase levels in a woman with prior hypertension

Data from Lindheimer MD, Taler SJ, Cunningham FG. American Society of Hypertension. ASH position paper: hypertension in pregnancy. J Clin Hypertens (Greenwich) 2009;11(4):214–25; with permission.

CLINICAL MANIFESTATIONS OF PREECLAMPSIA

In addition to elevated blood pressure and proteinuria (as required for the diagnosis), preeclampsia is commonly associated with multiorgan dysfunction, including renal, hepatic, hematologic, and neurologic manifestations. The fetoplacental unit is also affected.

There is a decrease in creatinine clearance with preeclampsia, with creatinine levels increasing for pregnancy but generally still within the normal range, unless acute tubular necrosis and frank renal failure occur. The characteristic renal lesion in preeclampsia is glomerular endotheliosis. Urinary excretion of uric acid[7] is reduced, leading to uric acid levels that, like creatinine levels, are high for pregnancy though typically still within the normal nonpregnant range. Hypocalciuria also may occur.[8]

Decreased intravascular volume and resultant hemoconcentration are hallmarks of preeclampsia. Thrombocytopenia may occur alone or in combination with disseminated intravascular coagulation. When preeclampsia is complicated by hemolysis, elevated liver enzymes, and low platelet count, it is termed HELLP. Transaminases are sometimes elevated in the absence of frank HELLP syndrome. Cardiac complications are unusual in preeclampsia, but heart failure resulting in pulmonary edema has been described in rare cases.[9]

Eclampsia is diagnosed when seizures complicate preeclampsia. The occurrence of seizure may be preceded by other neurologic symptoms, such as headache, visual changes, or changes in mental status. Eclampsia may occur in the absence of severe hypertension.

Fetus and Placenta

As delivery is the only definitive treatment for preeclampsia, this condition is among the leading causes of prematurity. Preeclampsia is associated with decreased fetoplacental perfusion, which frequently results in intrauterine growth restriction (IUGR) and small for gestational age infants. A greater risk for IUGR is seen with early-onset preeclampsia.[10]

PATHOPHYSIOLOGY OF PREECLAMPSIA

Although the cause or causes of preeclampsia remain unclear, several factors have been implicated in disease pathogenesis, including abnormalities in angiogenesis, immune function, insulin resistance, and inflammation. It is possible that different mechanisms play a role in different phases of disease or in some but not other individuals.

Placental abnormalities have been recognized early in the development of preeclampsia. In normal early pregnancy, trophoblasts invade the spiral arteries, a process that involves decidual immune cells (specifically natural killer cells) and leads to remodeling of these arteries as low-resistance vessels to assure adequate fetal blood flow. Trophoblastic invasion is defective in women who subsequently manifest preeclampsia, leading to relative placental hypoxia and oxidative stress, which is hypothesized to contribute to disease manifestations. Proposed explanations for the poor trophoblastic invasion include dysregulation of angiogenic factors or immunologic factors, or both, leading to inflammation and endothelial dysfunction.[11]

Established preeclampsia is associated with increased circulating levels of soluble fms-like tyrosine kinase-1 (sFlt-1), an antiangiogenic molecule derived from placental trophoblasts, as well as increased placental expression of this protein.[12] sFlt-1 binds to vascular endothelial growth factor (VEGF) and placental growth factor (PlGF) and thereby prevents their binding to their endogenous receptors, with antiangiogenic effects. Elevations in sFlt1 and reductions in PlGF have been reported to precede clinical manifestations of preeclampsia[13]; it remains unclear whether these changes are primary in pathogenesis or secondary to other abnormalities, such as the relative hypoxia caused by poor trophoblastic invasion.[14] In animal models, administration of sFlt-1 causes hypertension, proteinuria, and glomerular endotheliosis consistent with the preeclampsia phenotype.[12]

Increased levels of antibodies to the angiotensin II type 1 receptor have been reported in women with established preeclampsia,[15] and have been shown to correlate with the severity of disease and with sFlt-1 levels.[16] In animal models, these antibodies have been shown to induce clinical features of preeclampsia.[17]

Increased insulin resistance may also play a role in the pathogenesis of preeclampsia.[18] Compared with women with uncomplicated pregnancies, women with established preeclampsia have been reported to have higher levels of glucose, insulin, and triglycerides.[19] Other reports have shown these[20,21] and other markers of insulin resistance (eg, increased levels of free fatty acids[22] and tumor necrosis factor α,[23] and lower levels of high-density lipoprotein [HDL][24] and sex hormone binding globulin[25]) in pregnant women who subsequently develop preeclampsia, in comparison with women with normotensive pregnancy.

Studies have identified associations between preeclampsia and polymorphisms in genes regulating the renin-angiotensin system, cytokines, endothelial function, and thrombophilia, although these findings have been inconsistent across studies.[26,27] Placental genes have also been considered as predisposing factors.

Regardless of the initiating factors, endothelial dysfunction, involving both the placental and maternal systemic circulation, is central to the pathogenesis of preeclampsia.[28] Compared with women who remain normotensive in pregnancy, women who subsequently develop preeclampsia have been reported to have increased levels of serum markers of endothelial dysfunction (such as soluble endo-glin[29] and endothelin[30]) and increased microvascular responses to acetylcholine and sodium nitroprusside[31] prior to clinical manifestations of disease. Endothelial dysfunction may explain the range of systemic manifestations of preeclampsia (eg, hypertension, renal dysfunction, microangiopathic hemolytic anemia), and may also underlie the increased pressor responsiveness to angiotensin II characteristic of women with preeclampsia.[32]

RISK FACTORS FOR PREECLAMPSIA

Several factors are associated with an increased risk of preeclampsia,[33] and their presence may warrant closer surveillance during pregnancy.[34] Among these are primi-parity, preexisting hypertension, and obesity.[35] Higher blood pressures in the normo-tensive range, and higher body mass index (BMI) even within the nonobese range are also associated with higher risks as compared with lower levels of these measures.[20,36] African American women appear to be at higher risk, but it is unclear whether this association is independent of BMI and blood pressure. Other conditions linked to a higher risk of preeclampsia include diabetes mellitus, renal disease, anti-phospholipid antibody syndrome,[34] and possibly polycystic ovary syndrome.[37]

Women with multiple gestations[38,39] and those with a personal or family history of preeclampsia are also at increased risk for preeclampsia. The risk for preeclampsia is increased twofold to threefold in women who have a first-degree relative with a history of preeclampsia, in comparison with women without this history.[40,41] A maternal history of preeclampsia increases the risk of preeclampsia not only in a daughter but also in a son's partner.[42] These observations support a genetic compo-nent to disease pathogenesis, involving both maternal and fetal genes. Some investi-gators have reported a relationship between preeclampsia and behaviors associated with reduced exposure to paternal antigens (eg, use of barrier contraception),[43] sup-porting the hypothesis that immunologic factors play a role in disease pathogenesis. However, these findings have been inconsistent.[44,45] A change in paternity has also been associated with an increased risk for preeclampsia,[46] However, this association may be explained by longer intervals between pregnancies, which may independently predispose to preeclampsia.[47]

Cigarette smoking during pregnancy has been associated with a decreased risk of developing preeclampsia,[48] although a recent report did not find this association in high-risk women.[49] In a large Swedish cohort, risk reductions in preeclampsia associ-ated with smoking persisted after adjustment for early pregnancy BMI and parity, appeared dose dependent, and were limited to smoking in later pregnancy; women who were smokers before pregnancy but quit in early pregnancy had no significant reduction in preeclampsia risk.[50] Possible mechanisms by which cigarette smoking might reduce preeclampsia risk include effects on angiogenic factors (eg, reductions in sFlt-1)[49] or nitric oxide production.

Several biomarkers (eg, hyperinsulinemia, hypertriglyceridemia,[21] increased sFlt-1 and reduced PIGF[13,51]) are associated with increased risk of preeclampsia. However, the overlap in levels between women who do and do not subsequently develop hyper-tensive pregnancy limits their clinical utility.

PREVENTION OF PREECLAMPSIA

Several interventions have been tested for the prevention of preeclampsia. Although preliminary data from small studies suggested that aspirin, calcium, and antioxidants may reduce the risk of preeclampsia, larger randomized trials have not supported a benefit.

Aspirin

The observation that women with established preeclampsia have a higher ratio of thromboxane to prostacyclin than women with uncomplicated pregnancies raised the possibility that aspirin might be useful in prevention. Although initial small trials suggested a preventive effect of aspirin, several large placebo-controlled randomized trials including healthy nulliparous women[52] and women considered at high risk for other reasons (eg, history of IUGR, chronic hypertension, or multiple pregnancy) failed to show a benefit of low-dose aspirin (60 mg/d).[53,54]

Calcium

Calcium supplementation also initially appeared to be a promising preventive strategy in small studies.[55] However, a large placebo-controlled randomized trial of healthy nulliparous women[56] did not demonstrate a reduced risk of preeclampsia with calcium supplementation (2 g of elemental calcium daily). A trial specifically targeted to women with low calcium intake likewise showed no significant reduction in the incidence of preeclampsia with calcium supplementation.[57]

Vitamin D

Low circulating levels of vitamin D[58] and low self-reported intake of vitamin D supplements[59] have been associated with subsequent development of preeclampsia in some but not all studies.[60] Randomized trials are ongoing to assess the effect of vitamin D supplementation on the risk for preeclampsia.

Antioxidants

Given the observation that markers of oxidative stress are increased in women with preeclampsia, studies have assessed the possibility that antioxidants will decrease the risk of preeclampsia. Despite promising results from a small trial of vitamin E and C supplementation in high-risk women,[61] larger randomized trials involving low-risk[62] and high-risk[63,64] women have shown no benefit. In one of these studies,[63] the offspring of women who received vitamin C and E had lower birth weight than offspring of the control group. Based on available data, the use of these antioxidants for the prevention of preeclampsia is not justified.

Lifestyle Modifications

Higher prepregnancy BMI is associated with increased risk for preeclampsia. Evidence suggests that weight loss between pregnancies is associated with lower risk of recurrent preeclampsia in the subsequent pregnancy, whereas weight gain in this interval is associated with increased preeclampsia risk.[65] A retrospective cohort study demonstrated a reduced risk for preeclampsia among obese women who delivered after bariatric surgery, as compared with those who delivered prior to such surgery.[66]

The risk of preeclampsia increases with greater gestational weight gain. In a large Swedish population-based cohort, greater weight gain during pregnancy (more than 16 kg) in normal weight and overweight women was associated with a twofold increased risk of preeclampsia, compared with weight gain of 8 to 16 kg. Among obese women, lower gestational weight gain (<8 kg) was associated with a 50% reduction in the risk of preeclampsia, but was also associated with a higher risk of small for gestational age offspring.[67] Indirect support for a potential benefit of reduced gestational weight gain comes from two randomized trials assessing effects of treatment of mild gestational diabetes, in which women in the intervention arms had a lower risk of preeclampsia, possibly explained by the lesser weight gain in these groups.[68,69]

Some observational studies have suggested inverse associations between levels of physical activity before and/or during pregnancy and the risk of preeclampsia.[70,71] However, other studies have not confirmed these findings.[72–74] In one cohort study in which there was no association between physical activity and preeclampsia over-all,[74] subgroup analyses limited to cases of severe preeclampsia (HELLP or eclampsia) showed an increase in risk among women reporting more than 270 minutes per week of physical activity; however, this report was limited by the lack of consistency in this finding (which was not observed with other categories of vigorous activity or for less severe cases of preeclampsia) and other methodologic issues.

Antihypertensive Therapy in Women with Hypertension in Pregnancy

Randomized trials of antihypertensive therapy have shown no significant reduction in the risk for developing preeclampsia in women with mild to moderate hypertension during pregnancy. In a meta-analysis including 46 randomized trials there was no benefit of antihypertensive therapy when compared with placebo, or of any particular antihypertensive agent over another, in reducing the risk of preeclampsia.[75]

MANAGEMENT OF PREECLAMPSIA

Women with preeclampsia should be closely monitored, with the aim of preventing the development of eclampsia and other maternal and fetal complications. The only "cure" for preeclampsia is delivery of the fetus. Decisions regarding the optimal timing of delivery must balance the risks of prematurity with maternal and fetal risks associated with preeclampsia.

Immediate delivery has been recommended for women who are near term, or earlier in gestation in the setting of severe uncontrolled hypertension; coagulation or liver abnormalities; decreasing renal function; symptoms or signs of impending eclampsia (eg, persistent severe headaches, severe epigastric pain, hyperreflexia); abnormal fetal nonstress testing; or evidence on ultrasonography of severe growth restriction or unfavorable biophysical profile.[1] In the absence of these indications, close monitoring is recommended.

In women with mild apparently stable disease, monitoring is recommended on at least a weekly basis, including measurement of blood pressure, assessment for symptoms (such as headache, visual changes, or abdominal pain), and laboratory testing (urine protein measurement, platelet count, and renal and liver function). Recommended fetal testing includes nonstress testing to assess fetal heart rate reactivity and/or fetal ultrasonography to assess fetal size and well-being (by biophysical profile) and amniotic fluid volume. More frequent testing is recommended for more severe disease.[76]

Hospitalization and expectant management (involving close maternal and fetal monitoring, and antihypertensive therapy where indicated) has been recommended by some experts for women who develop preeclampsia at a gestational age less than 34 weeks.[77] A systematic review of observational studies including more than 4600 women demonstrated prolongation of pregnancy by 7 to 14 days without an increase in complications.[78] Randomized trial data, however, are limited. In one randomized trial comparing expectant management to immediate delivery in 95 women, expectant management resulted in a significantly higher gestational age at delivery (32.9 vs 30.8 weeks), and a significantly lower incidence of admission and duration of stay in the neonatal intensive care unit.[77] However, data are needed from large randomized trials to better inform the benefits and risks of this strategy. A multi-center randomized trial of women 36 weeks' gestation or more demonstrating a significantly greater rate of maternal complications with expectant management supports recommendations for immediate delivery in women at or near term.[79]

Antihypertensive Therapy

There is controversy regarding the criteria for initiating antihypertensive therapy in women with hypertensive pregnancy, although there is general agreement that the threshold is higher than in the nonpregnant state. To reduce the risk of maternal cardiovascular complications, treatment is routinely considered to be warranted when the diastolic blood pressure is at or above 110 mm Hg.[2,80,81] Some experts support consideration of antihypertensive therapy at lower thresholds (for example, diastolic blood pressure between 100 and 109 mm Hg).[82] However, the use of a lower threshold remains controversial given the concern that lowering the mother's systemic blood pressure may reduce fetoplacental perfusion, and the lack of data to show that reducing maternal blood pressure improved perinatal outcomes.[82] In women with mild preeclampsia,[83] antihypertensive therapy may increase the risk of IUGR.

There are no antihypertensive medications that are specifically approved by the Food and Drug Administration (FDA) for use in pregnancy. **Table 1** reviews medications that are commonly used in the management of hypertensive pregnancy.

Of the antihypertensive medications used in pregnancy, experience is greatest with methyldopa, and this agent is considered by some experts to be a first-line choice for management.[1] A study of children of hypertensive women treated with methyldopa during pregnancy demonstrated no significant differences in physical and mental development at up to 7.5 years of age, compared with children of untreated women.[84] β-Adrenergic blockers, as well as the combined α- and β-blocker labetalol, are also used for treatment of hypertension in pregnancy. A meta-analysis suggested that β-blockers were superior to methyldopa in reducing the risk for development of severe hypertension, but rates of developing preeclampsia did not differ between these agents.[75] Limited data have suggested an association between maternal use of some β-blockers in pregnancy and an increased risk of IUGR.[85] Given limitations in the effectiveness and tolerability of methyldopa, and extensive clinical experience with labetalol in pregnancy, labetalol is often recommended as a first-line therapy.[4] Calcium-channel blockers are alternatively used. A theoretical concern has been that the concomitant use of a calcium-channel blocker and magnesium sulfate may lead to hypotension or other serious complications; however, a large retrospective cohort study reported no excess in complications with this combination in comparison with magnesium and other or no antihypertensive therapy.[86]

Angiotensin-converting enzyme inhibitors (ACEI) and angiotensin receptor blockers are generally contraindicated in pregnancy. Fetal and neonatal renal failure has been reported in offspring of mothers treated with these agents.[87,88] In a large database study, the use of ACEIs early in pregnancy was associated with a higher risk of congenital defects.[89]

A large multicenter trial is currently under way to assess effects of tight versus less tight blood pressure control in women with gestational hypertension (or underlying chronic hypertension), the results of which are expected in 2013.[90]

Emergency Treatment of Hypertension in Pregnancy

When severe hypertension (sustained systolic blood pressure $\geq$160 mm Hg and/or diastolic blood pressure $\geq$110 mm Hg) does not respond to oral medications,

Table 1
Pharmacologic therapy for hypertensive pregnancy

Agent	Usual Dose Range[a]	Comments	FDA Classification[b]
Methyldopa	250 mg to 1.5 g by mouth twice a day	Often used as first-line therapy; long-term data available suggesting safety to offspring	B
Labetalol	100–600 mg by mouth twice a day For emergency treatment: 20 mg intravenous (IV) bolus, followed by repeat IV boluses at 20–30-min intervals until desired response or maximum cumulative dose of 300 mg ; or IV infusion: 1–2 mg/min initially, adjusted according to response	Often used as first-line therapy; may exacerbate asthma	C
β-Blockers	Dose varies according to agent used	May exacerbate asthma; possible small increase in IUGR risk	C
Calcium-channel blockers	eg, Long-acting nifedipine 30–120 mg every day	Short-acting nifedipine should generally be avoided given the risk of hypotension	C
Hydralazine	50–300 mg daily in 2–4 divided doses For emergency treatment: 5 mg IV, followed by 5–10 mg every 20–40 min		C

Angiotensin-converting enzyme inhibitors and angiotensin receptor blockers are contraindicated in pregnancy, due to the risk of fetal or neonatal renal failure and other complications (Category D).

[a] Therapy should be initiated at lower doses and adjusted according to response.

[b] FDA Classifications: Category A—Adequate and well-controlled studies have failed to demonstrate a risk to the fetus in the first trimester of pregnancy (and there is no evidence of risk in later trimesters). Category B—Animal reproduction studies have failed to demonstrate a risk to the fetus, and there are no adequate and well-controlled studies in pregnant women. Category C—Animal reproduction studies have shown an adverse effect on the fetus and there are no adequate and well-controlled studies in humans, but potential benefits may warrant use of the drug in pregnant women despite potential risks. Category D—There is positive evidence of human fetal risk based on adverse reaction data from investigational or marketing experience or studies in humans, but potential benefits may warrant use of the drug in pregnant women despite potential risks. Category X—Studies in animals or humans have demonstrated fetal abnormalities and/or there is positive evidence of human fetal risk based on adverse reaction data from investigational or marketing experience, and the risks involved in use of the drug in pregnant women clearly outweigh potential benefits.

Data from Lindheimer MD, Taler SJ, Cunningham FG. American Society of Hypertension. ASH position paper: hypertension in pregnancy. J Clin Hypertens (Greenwich) 2009;11(4):214–25.

intravenous therapy should be initiated with either labetalol or hydralazine.[4] Nitroprusside should be avoided because of the risk of fetal or maternal cyanide toxicity.

Seizure Prophylaxis

Magnesium sulfate is recommended for the prevention of seizures in women with preeclampsia.[91] In a randomized trial including more than 10,000 women with preeclampsia, magnesium sulfate resulted in a significant reduction in the risk for eclampsia (rates 0.8% vs 1.9% in the placebo group). Magnesium sulfate has been demonstrated in randomized trials to be more effective than dilantin[92] or nimodipine[93] in preventing seizures.[94]

PREECLAMPSIA AND FUTURE CARDIOVASCULAR RISK

Although the majority of women diagnosed with preeclampsia have resolution of hypertension by 3 months postpartum, a history of this disorder is associated with metabolic and vascular abnormalities and future risks for hypertension, diabetes mellitus, and cardiovascular and renal disease.[95]

Women with a history of preeclampsia have been reported to have greater insulin resistance as measured by the homeostatic model assessment (HOMA) model,[96] and other features associated with insulin resistance, including lower HDL, higher triglycerides, higher interleukin-6, and higher C-reactive protein levels,[97] compared with women with uncomplicated pregnancy. In addition, abnormal endothelial relaxation[98] and enhanced pressor sensitivity to angiotensin II[99] have been demonstrated in women with prior preeclampsia.

Hypertension

A meta-analysis of 25 studies, overall including more than 3 million women and nearly 200,000 cases of preeclampsia,[100] demonstrated a significantly increased risk of hypertension in women with a history of preeclampsia (relative risk 3.7; 95% confidence interval [CI] 2.7–5). Given the observation that there was significant heterogeneity among studies; the investigators reanalyzed the data, limiting inclusion to studies with more than 200 cases, and found a relative risk for hypertension associated with a history of preeclampsia of 2.4 (95% CI 2.1–2.7). A subsequent large cohort study involving a Danish registry reported a threefold to sixfold increased risk for subsequent hypertension among women with a diagnosis of gestational hypertension or preeclampsia (with higher risk associated with more severe or recurrent preeclampsia).[101]

Cardiovascular Disease

Several studies have reported increased rates of cardiovascular events in women with a history of hypertensive disorders of pregnancy, or specifically preeclampsia, compared with women with an uncomplicated pregnancy.[102] Among a Norwegian cohort involving 626,272 women followed for a median of 13 years, a history of preeclampsia was associated with a relative risk of cardiovascular mortality of 1.6 (95% CI 1.0–2.7)[103]; the risk was substantially higher among women who had preeclampsia complicated by preterm delivery.

In the Cardiovascular Health After Maternal Placental Syndromes (CHAMPS) study,[104] a population-based retrospective cohort study in Canada involving more than 1 million women, the hazard ratio for cardiovascular morbidity or mortality at least 90 days after delivery associated with preeclampsia was 2.1 (95% CI 1.8–2.4) adjusted for age, multiple gestation, GDM, hypertension, diabetes, and obesity, and that associated with gestational hypertension was 1.8 (95% CI 1.4–2.2). The meta-analysis referred to earlier[100] also found significantly increased risks in women with a history of preeclampsia for nonfatal or fatal-ischemic heart disease (relative risk 2.2, 95% CI 1.9–2.5), and fatal and nonfatal stroke (relative risk 1.8, 95% CI 1.5–2.3). In the Danish registry study,[101] a history of hypertensive pregnancy was associated with approximately 70% increased risk for ischemic heart disease and a similar increase in stroke risk.

A limitation of many of the studies was that analyses were adjusted only for age, and thus associated cardiovascular risk factors may have explained at least some of the increase in risks. As the women enrolled in these studies were still relatively young at the time of follow-up, the magnitude of risk associated with a history of hypertensive pregnancy may be underestimated.

Several studies have indicated that the relative risks of later disease appear greater if preeclampsia is severe (vs mild), early in onset, or occurs in more than one pregnancy. Among more than 14,000 women participating in the Child Health and Development Study and followed for a median of 37 years, the relative risk for cardiovascular mortality, adjusting for age, BMI, smoking, and a history of hypertension at study enrollment, was 2.14 (95% CI 1.29–3.57), and appeared considerably higher if the onset of preeclampsia was before 34 weeks' gestation. Even with the prolonged follow-up in this report, the median age at follow-up was only 56 years.[105]

Type 2 Diabetes Mellitus

Some data also suggest increased risk for type 2 diabetes among women with a history of hypertensive pregnancy.[101,106] In the Danish registry study,[101] women with either gestational hypertension or preeclampsia had approximately 3 times the risk of developing type 2 diabetes as women with uncomplicated pregnancy. As is a limitation of the studies of other long-term risks, no adjustment was made for BMI.

Renal Disease

A meta-analysis including 7 small cohort studies of women followed for a mean of 7 years after pregnancy reported increased risks for microalbuminuria among women with a history of preeclampsia (fourfold increased in women with mild preeclampsia and eightfold increased in women with severe preeclampsia).[107] A large population-based study in Norway involving a mean 17 years of follow-up showed more than 3 times the risk for later development of end-stage renal disease in women with a history of preeclampsia, particularly in women with preeclampsia in multiple pregnancies or associated with preterm birth or low birth weight.[108] However, these studies were not able to rule out the possibility of renal disease antedating pregnancy in these women.

Several potential explanations have been proposed for the observed associations between preeclampsia and these later disease risks.[95] One possibility is that women with underlying hypertension may be misdiagnosed with gestational hypertension or preeclampsia. As many women of reproductive age do not see a physician regularly before pregnancy, and the first prenatal appointment is frequently not until the early second trimester when blood pressure normally declines, essential hypertension may be missed. The observation that both preeclampsia and cardiovascular disease share common risk factors (eg, obesity, preexisting hypertension, dyslipidemia) suggests that pregnancy may unmask a propensity to vascular disease in susceptible women. Another possibility is that preeclampsia may cause damage to the vasculature that later presents as cardiovascular and/or renal disease. Reports that severe or early-onset preeclampsia and multiple episodes of preeclampsia are associated with greater risks of later cardiovascular or renal disease could be consistent with either hypothesis.

Although studies are needed to assess the effects of interventions to reduce risks for subsequent hypertension and cardiovascular disease in women with a history of preeclampsia, lifestyle interventions to control BMI and reduce insulin resistance, including dietary changes and increased physical activity, are reasonable and should be encouraged.

Later-Life Risks in the Offspring

Several studies indicate that offspring of hypertensive pregnancies may also have increased risk of hypertension.[109,110] Among more than 6000 children enrolled in a longitudinal study and examined at age 9 years, offspring of pregnancies complicated by preeclampsia or gestational hypertension had significantly higher systolic and diastolic blood pressures than offspring of uncomplicated pregnancies (mean differences 2 mm and 1 mm, respectively), even after adjusting for the child's BMI. However, differences between offspring of preeclamptic and normotensive pregnancies were no longer significant after further adjustment for other variables, including gestational age at birth and birth weight[109]; prematurity and low birth weight have previously been demonstrated to be associated with increased risk for hypertension.

SUMMARY

Hypertension is a common complication of pregnancy. Preeclampsia, in particular, is associated with substantial risk to both the mother and the fetus. Although the cause of preeclampsia is still unknown, abnormalities in angiogenesis, immune function, insulin resistance, and inflammation may play roles in disease pathogenesis. Several risk factors (for example, primiparity, preexisting essential hypertension, obesity) and biomarkers (eg, hyperinsulinemia, hyperlipidemia, elevated levels of sFlt-1, and reduced levels of PlGF) have been recognized to predict risk for preeclampsia. However, at present no biomarkers have sufficient discriminatory ability to be useful in clinical practice. No effective preventive strategies have yet been identified. Preeclampsia is only "cured" by delivery, and thus is associated with a high risk of prematurity and its attendant complications.

Commonly used medications for the treatment of hypertension in pregnancy include methyldopa and labetalol. Blood pressure thresholds for initiating antihypertensive therapy are higher than outside of pregnancy. Angiotensin-converting enzyme inhibitors and angiotensin receptor blockers are contraindicated in pregnancy. Women with prior preeclampsia are at increased risk of hypertension, cardiovascular disease, and renal disease. Further investigation should focus on identifying the cause(s) of preeclampsia and effective strategies for its prevention and treatment.

REFERENCES

1. Lindheimer MD, Taler SJ, Cunningham FG. American Society of Hypertension. ASH position paper: hypertension in pregnancy. J Clin Hypertens (Greenwich) 2009;11(4):214–25.
2. The Society of Obstetricians and Gynaecologists of Canada. Diagnosis, evaluation and management of the hypertensive disorders of pregnancy. SOGC clinical practice guideline. J Obstet Gynaecol Can 2008;30:S1–48.
3. Waugh JJ, Clark TJ, Divakaran TG, et al. Accuracy of urinalysis dipstick technique in predicting significant proteinuria in pregnancy. Obstet Gynecol 2004; 103:769–77.

4. Visintin C, Mugglestone MA, Almerie MQ, et al. Management of hypertensive disorders during pregnancy: summary of NICE guidance. BMJ 2010;341:c2207.

5. Gifford RW, August PA, Cunningham G. Report of the National High Blood Pressure Education Program Working group on High Blood Pressure in Pregnancy. Am J Obstet Gynecol 2000;183:S1–22.

6. Wilson M, Morganti AA, Zervoulakis D, et al. Blood pressure, the renin-angiotensin system and sex steroids throughout normal pregnancy. Am J Med 1980;68:97–104.

7. Fadel HE, Northrup G, Misenhimer HR. Hyperuricemia in pre-eclampsia. A reappraisal. Am J Obstet Gynecol 1976;125(5):640–7.

8. Seely EW, Wood RJ, Brown EM, et al. Lower serum ionized calcium and abnormal calciotropic hormone levels in preeclampsia. J Clin Endocrinol Metab 1992;74:1436–40.

9. Bauer ST, Cleary KL. Cardiopulmonary complications of pre-eclampsia. Semin Perinatol 2009;33(3):158–65.

10. Odegård RA, Vatten LJ, Nilsen ST, et al. Preeclampsia and fetal growth. Obstet Gynecol 2000;96(6):950–5.

11. Young BC, Levin RJ, Karumanchi SA. Pathogenesis of preeclampsia. Annu Rev Pathol 2010;5:173–92.

12. Maynard SE, Min JY, Merchan J, et al. Excess placental soluble fms-like tyrosine kinase 1 (sFlt1) may contribute to endothelial dysfunction, hypertension, and proteinuria in preeclampsia. J Clin Invest 2003;111(5):649–58.

13. Levine RJ, Maynard SE, Qian C, et al. Circulating angiogenic factors and risk of preeclampsia. N Engl J Med 2004;350:672–83.

14. Redman CW, Sargent IL. Latest advances in understanding preeclampsia. Science 2005;308(5728):1592–4.

15. Wallukat G, Homuth V, Fischer T, et al. Patients with preeclampsia develop agonistic autoantibodies against the angiotensin AT1 receptor. J Clin Invest 1999;103(7):945–52.

16. Siddiqui AH, Irani RA, Blackwell SC, et al. Angiotensin receptor agonistic autoantibody is highly prevalent in preeclampsia: correlation with disease severity. Hypertension 2010;55(2):386–93.

17. Zhou CC, Ahmad S, Mi T, et al. Autoantibody from women with preeclampsia induces soluble Fms-like tyrosine kinase-1 production via angiotensin type 1 receptor and calcineurin/nuclear factor of activated T-cells signaling. Hypertension 2008;51(4):1010–9.

18. Seely EW, Solomon CG. Insulin resistance and its potential role in pregnancy-induced hypertension. J Clin Endocrinol Metab 2003;88:2393–8.

19. Lorentzen B, Birkeland KI, Endresen MJ, et al. Glucose intolerance in women with preeclampsia. Acta Obstet Gynecol Scand 1998;77:22–7.

20. Solomon CG, Graves SW, Greene MF, et al. Glucose intolerance as a predictor of hypertension in pregnancy. Hypertension 1994;23:717–21.

21. Solomon CG, Carroll JS, Okumura K, et al. Higher cholesterol and insulin levels are associated with increased risk for pregnancy-induced hypertension. Am J Hypertens 1999;12:276–82.

22. Lorentzen B, Endresen MJ, Clausen T, et al. Fasting serum free fatty acids and triglycerides are increased before 20 weeks of gestation in women who later develop preeclampsia. Hypertens Pregnancy 1994;13:103–9.

23. Serin YS, Ozcelik B, Bapbou M, et al. Predictive value of tumor necrosis factor-[alpha] (TNF-[alpha]) in preeclampsia. Eur J Obstet Gynecol Reprod Biol 2002;100:143–5.

24. Kaaje R, Laivuori H, Laasko M, et al. Evidence of a state of increased insulin resistance in preeclampsia. Metabolism 1999;48:892–6.
25. Wolf M, Sandler L, Muniz K, et al. First trimester insulin resistance and subsequent preeclampsia: prospective study. J Clin Endocrinol Metab 2002;87: 1563–8.
26. GOPEC Consortium. Disentangling fetal and maternal susceptibility for preeclampsia: a British multicenter candidate-gene study. Am J Hum Genet 2005;77(1):127–31.
27. Chappell S, Morgan L. Searching for genetic clues to the causes of preeclampsia. Clin Sci (Lond) 2006;110(4):443–58.
28. Roberts JM, Taylor RN, Musci TJ, et al. Preeclampsia: an endothelial cell disorder. Am J Obstet Gynecol 1989;161:1200–4.
29. Levine RJ, Lam C, Qian C, et al, CPEP Study Group. Soluble endoglin and other circulating antiangiogenic factors in preeclampsia. N Engl J Med 2006;355(10): 992–1005.
30. Gilbert JS, Ryan MJ, LaMarca BB, et al. Pathophysiology of hypertension during preeclampsia: linking placental ischemia with endothelial dysfunction. Am J Physiol Heart Circ Physiol 2008;294(2):H541–50.
31. Khan F, Belch JJ, MacLeod M, et al. Changes in endothelial function precede the clinical disease in women in whom preeclampsia develops. Hypertension 2005;46(5):1123–8.
32. Gant NF, Daley GL, Chand S, et al. A study of angiotensin II pressor response throughout primigravid pregnancy. J Clin Invest 1973;52(11):2682–9.
33. Duckitt K, Harrington D. Risk factors for preeclampsia at antenatal booking: systematic review of controlled studies. BMJ 2005;330:565.
34. Milne F, Redman C, Walker J, et al. The pre-eclampsia community guideline (PRECOG): how to screen for and detect onset of preeclampsia in the community. BMJ 2005;330(7491):576–80.
35. Eskenazi B, Fenster L, Sidney S. A multivariate analysis of risk factors for preeclampsia. JAMA 1991;266:237–41.
36. Bodnar LM, Ness RB, Markovic N, et al. The risk of preeclampsia rises with increasing prepregnancy body mass index. Ann Epidemiol 2005;15(7):475–82.
37. DeVries MJ, Dekker GA, Shoemaker J. Higher risk of preeclampsia in the polycystic ovary syndrome: a case control study. Eur J Obstet Gynecol Reprod Biol 1998;76:91–5.
38. Sibai BM, Hauth J, Caritis S, et al. Hypertensive disorders in twin versus singleton gestations. National Institute of Child Health and Human Development Network of Maternal-Fetal Medicine Units. Am J Obstet Gynecol 2000;182(4): 938–42.
39. Mastrobattista JM, Skupski DW, Monga M, et al. The rate of severe preeclampsia is increased in triplet as compared to twin gestations. Am J Perinatol 1997;14:263–5.
40. Chesley LC, Annitto JE, Cosgrove RA. The familial factor in toxemia of pregnancy. Obstet Gynecol 1968;32(3):303–11.
41. Arngrimsson R, Björnsson S, Geirsson RT, et al. Genetic and familial predisposition to eclampsia and pre-eclampsia in a defined population. Br J Obstet Gynaecol 1990;97(9):762–9.
42. Esplin MS, Fausett MB, Fraser A. Paternal and maternal components of the predisposition to preeclampsia. N Engl J Med 2001;344:867–72.
43. Klonoff-Cohen HS, Savitz DA, Cefalo RC, et al. An epidemiologic study of contraception and preeclampsia. JAMA 1989;262:3143–7.

44. Ness RB, Markovic N, Harger G, et al. Barrier methods, length of preconception intercourse, and preeclampsia. Hypertens Pregnancy 2004;23:227–35.

45. Mills JL, Klebanoff MA, Graubard BI, et al. Barrier contraceptive methods and preeclampsia. JAMA 1991;265(1):70–3.

46. Trupin LS, Simon LP, Eskenazi B. Change in paternity: a risk factor for preeclampsia in multiparas. Epidemiology 1996;7:240–4.

47. Skjærven R, Wilcox AJ, Lie RT. The interval between pregnancies and the risk of preeclampsia. N Engl J Med 2002;346:33–8.

48. Cnattingius S, Mills JL, Yuen J, et al. The paradoxical effect of smoking in preeclamptic pregnancies: smoking reduces the incidence but increases the rates of perinatal mortality, abruptio placentae, and intrauterine growth restriction. Am J Obstet Gynecol 1997;177(1):156–61.

49. Jeyabalan A, Powers RW, Clifton RG, et al. Effect of smoking on circulating angiogenic factors in high risk pregnancies. PLoS One 2010;5(10):e13270.

50. Wikstrom AK, Stephansson O, Cnattingius S. Tobacco use during pregnancy and preeclampsia risk: effects of cigarette smoking and snuff. Hypertension 2010;55:1254–9.

51. Levine RJ, Thadani R, Qian C, et al. Urinary placental growth factor and risk of preeclampsia. JAMA 2005;293:77–85.

52. Sibai BM, Caritis SN, Thom E, et al. Prevention of preeclampsia with low-dose aspirin in healthy, nulliparous pregnant women. The National Institute of Child Health and Human Development Network of Maternal-Fetal Medicine Units. N Engl J Med 1993;329(17):1213–8.

53. CLASP (Collaborative Low-dose Aspirin Study in Pregnancy) Collaborative group. CLASP: a randomized trial of low-dose aspirin for the prevention and treatment of pre-eclampsia among 9364 pregnant women. Lancet 1994;343: 619–29.

54. Caritis S, Sibai B, Hauth J, et al. Low dose aspirin to prevent preeclampsia in women at high risk. N Engl J Med 1998;338:701–5.

55. Sibai BM. Calcium supplementation during pregnancy reduces risk of high blood pressure, pre-eclampsia and premature birth compared with placebo? Evid Based Med 2011;16(2):40–1.

56. Levine RJ, Hauth JC, Curet LB, et al. Trial of calcium to prevent preeclampsia. N Engl J Med 1997;337:69–76.

57. Villar J, Abdel-Aleem H, Merialdi M, et al. World Health Organization randomized trial of calcium supplementation among low calcium intake pregnant women. Am J Obstet Gynecol 2006;194(3):639–49.

58. Bodnar LM, Catov JM, Simhan HN, et al. Maternal vitamin D deficiency increases the risk of preeclampsia. J Clin Endocrinol Metab 2007;92(9): 3517–22.

59. Haugen M, Brantsaeter AL, Trogstad L, et al. Vitamin D supplementation and reduced risk of preeclampsia in nulliparous women. Epidemiology 2009;20(5): 720–6.

60. Powe CE, Seely EW, Rana S, et al. First trimester vitamin D, vitamin D binding protein, and subsequent preeclampsia. Hypertension 2010;56(4):758–63 [Epub 2010 Aug 23].

61. Chappell LC, Seed PT, Briley AL, et al. Effect of antioxidants on the occurrence of pre-eclampsia in women at increased risk: a randomised trial. Lancet 1999; 354(9181):810–6.

62. Roberts JM, Myatt L, Spong CY, et al. Vitamins C and E to prevent complications of pregnancy-associated hypertension. N Engl J Med 2010;362(14):1282–91.

63. Poston L, Briley AL, Seed PT, et al. Vitamin C and vitamin E in pregnant women at risk for pre-eclampsia (VIP trial): randomised placebo-controlled trial. Lancet 2006;367(9517):1145–54.
64. Villar J, Purwar M, Merialdi M, et al, WHO Vitamin C and Vitamin E trial group. World Health Organisation multicentre randomised trial of supplementation with vitamins C and E among pregnant women at high risk for pre-eclampsia in populations of low nutritional status from developing countries. BJOG 2009; 116(6):780–8.
65. Mostello D, Jen Chang J, Allen J, et al. Recurrent preeclampsia: the effect of weight change between pregnancies. Obstet Gynecol 2010;116(3): 667–72.
66. Bennett WL, Gilson MM, Jamshidi R, et al. Impact of bariatric surgery on hypertensive disorders in pregnancy: retrospective analysis of insurance claims data. BMJ 2010;340:c1662.
67. Cedergren M. Effects of gestational weight gain and body mass index on obstetric outcomes in Sweden. Int J Gynaecol Obstet 2006;93:269–74.
68. Landon MB, Spong CY, Thom E, et al, Eunice Kennedy Shriver National Institute of Child Health and Human Development Maternal-Fetal Medicine Units Network. A multicenter, randomized trial of treatment for mild gestational diabetes. N Engl J Med 2009;361(14):1339–48.
69. Crowther CA, Hiller JE, Moss JR, et al. Effect of treatment of gestational diabetes mellitus on pregnancy outcomes. N Engl J Med 2005;352(24): 2477–86.
70. Marcoux S, Brisson J, Fabia J. Effect of leisure time physical activity on the risk of preeclampsia and gestational hypertension. J Epidemiol Community Health 1989;43:147–52.
71. Sorensen TK, Williams MA, Lee IM, et al. Recreational physical activity during pregnancy and risk of preeclampsia. Hypertension 2003;41(6):1273–80.
72. Saftlas AF, Logsden-Sackett N, Wang W, et al. Work, leisure-time physical activity, and risk of preeclampsia and gestational hypertension. Am J Epidemiol 2004;160:758–65.
73. Hegaard HK, Ottesen B, Hedegaard M, et al. The association between leisure time physical activity in the year before pregnancy and pre-eclampsia. J Obstet Gynaecol 2010;30(1):21–4.
74. Østerdal ML, Strøm M, Klemmensen AK, et al. Does leisure time physical activity in early pregnancy protect against pre-eclampsia? Prospective cohort in Danish women. BJOG 2009;116(1):98–107.
75. Abalos E, Duley L, Steyn DW, et al. Antihypertensive drug therapy for mild to moderate hypertension during pregnancy. Cochrane Database Syst Rev 2007;1:CD002252.
76. ACOG Committee on Practice Bulletins–Obstetrics. ACOG practice bulletin. Diagnosis and management of preeclampsia and eclampsia. Obstet Gynecol 2002;99(1):159–67.
77. Sibai BM, Mercer BM, Schiff E, et al. Aggressive versus expectant management of severe preeclampsia at 28 to 32 weeks' gestation: a randomized controlled trial. Am J Obstet Gynecol 1994;171:818–22.
78. Magee LA, Yong PJ, Espinosa V, et al. Expectant management of severe preeclampsia remote from term: a structured systematic review. Hypertens Pregnancy 2009;28(3):312–47.
79. Koopmans CM, Bijlenga D, Groen H, et al, HYPITAT study group. Induction of labour versus expectant monitoring for gestational hypertension or mild

pre-eclampsia after 36 weeks' gestation (HYPITAT): a multicentre, open-label randomised controlled trial. Lancet 2009;374(9694):979–88.

80. Brown MA, Hague WM, Higgins J, et al. The detection, investigation and management of hypertension in pregnancy: full consensus statement. Aust N Z J Obstet Gynaecol 2000;40(2):139–55.

81. ACOG Committee on Practice Bulletin. Chronic hypertension in pregnancy. Obstet Gynecol 2001;98(1):177–85.

82. Sibai BM, Barton JR, Akl S, et al. A randomized prospective comparison of nifedipine and bed rest versus bed rest alone in the management of preeclampsia remote from term. Am J Obstet Gynecol 1992;167:879–84.

83. Sibai BM, Gonzalez AR, Mabie WC, et al. A comparison of labetalol plus hospitalization versus hospitalization alone in the management of preeclampsia remote from term. Obstet Gynecol 1987;70:323–7.

84. Cockburn J, Moar VA, Ounsted M, et al. Final report of study on hypertension during pregnancy: the effects of specific treatment on the growth and development of the children. Lancet 1982;1(8273):647–9.

85. Butters L, Kennedy S, Rubin PC. Atenolol in essential hypertension during pregnancy. BMJ 1990;301:587–9.

86. Magee LA, Miremadi S, Li J, et al. Therapy with both magnesium sulfate and nifedipine does not increase the risk of serious magnesium-related maternal side effects in women with preeclampsia. Am J Obstet Gynecol 2005;193(1):153–63.

87. Hanssens M, Keirse MJ, Vankelecom F, et al. Fetal and neonatal effects of treatment with angiotensin-converting enzyme inhibitors in pregnancy. Obstet Gynecol 1991;78:128–35.

88. Alwan S, Polifka JE, Friedman JM. Angiotensin II receptor antagonist treatment during pregnancy. Birth Defects Res A Clin Mol Teratol 2005;73:123–30.

89. Cooper WO, Hernandez-Diaz S, Arbogast PG, et al. Major congenital malformations after first-trimester exposure to ACE inhibitors. N Engl J Med 2006;354(23):2443–51.

90. Magee LA, von Dadelszen P, Chan S, et al. The control of hypertension in pregnancy study pilot trial. BJOG 2007;114(6): 770, e13–20.

91. Altman D, Carroli G, Duley L. Do women with pre-eclampsia and their babies benefit from magnesium sulfate? The Magpie Trial: a randomised placebo-controlled trial. Lancet 2002;359:1877–90.

92. Lucas MJ, Leveno KJ, Cunningham FG. A comparison of magnesium sulfate with phenytoin for the prevention of eclampsia. N Engl J Med 1995;333:201–5.

93. Belford MA, Anthony J, Saade GR, et al. A comparison of magnesium sulfate and nimodipine for the prevention of eclampsia. N Engl J Med 2003;348:304–11.

94. Duley L, Gülmezoglu AM, Henderson-Smart DJ, et al. Magnesium sulphate and other anticonvulsants for women with pre-eclampsia. Cochrane Database Syst Rev 2010;11:CD000025.

95. Seely EW. Hypertension in pregnancy: a potential window into long-term cardiovascular risk in women. J Clin Endocrinol Metab 1999;84(6):1858–61.

96. Fuh MM, Yin CS, Pei D, et al. Resistance to insulin-mediated glucose uptake and hyperinsulinemia in women who had preeclampsia during pregnancy. Am J Hypertens 1995;8:768–71.

97. Girouard J, Giguère Y, Moutquin JM, et al. Previous hypertensive disease of pregnancy is associated with alterations of markers of insulin resistance. Hypertension 2007;49(5):1056–62.

98. Chambers JC, Fusi L, Malik I, et al. Association of maternal endothelial dysfunction with preeclampsia. JAMA 2001;285:1607–12.
99. Saxena AR, Karumanchi SA, Brown NJ, et al. Increased sensitivity to angiotensin II is present postpartum in women with a history of hypertensive pregnancy. Hypertension 2010;55(5):1239–45.
100. Bellamy L, Casas JP, Hingorani AD, et al. Pre-eclampsia and risk of cardiovascular disease and cancer in later life: systematic review and meta-analysis. BMJ 2007;335(7627):974.
101. Lykke JA, Langhoff-Roos J, Sibai BM, et al. Hypertensive pregnancy disorders and subsequent cardiovascular morbidity and type 2 diabetes mellitus in the mother. Hypertension 2009;53(6):944–51.
102. Kestenbaum B, Seliger SL, Easterling TR, et al. Cardiovascular and thromboembolic events following hypertensive pregnancy. Am J Kidney Dis 2003;42(5): 982–9.
103. Irgens HU, Reisaeter L, Irgens LM, et al. Long term mortality of mothers and fathers after pre-eclampsia: population based cohort study. BMJ 2001; 323(7323):1213–7.
104. Ray JG, Vermeulen MJ, Schull MJ, et al. Cardiovascular Health After Maternal Placental Syndromes (CHAMPS): population-based retrospective cohort study. Lancet 2005;366(9499):1797–803.
105. Mongraw-Chaffin ML, Cirillo PM, Cohn BA. Preeclampsia and cardiovascular disease death: prospective evidence from the child health and development studies cohort. Hypertension 2010;56(1):166–71.
106. Carr DB, Newton KM, Utzschneider KM, et al. Preeclampsia and risk of developing subsequent diabetes. Hypertens Pregnancy 2009;28(4):435–47.
107. McDonald SD, Han Z, Walsh MW, et al. Kidney disease after preeclampsia: a systematic review and meta-analysis. Am J Kidney Dis 2010;55(6):1026–39.
108. Vikse BE, Irgens LM, Leivestad T, et al. Preeclampsia and the risk of end-stage renal disease. N Engl J Med 2008;359(8):800–9.
109. Geelhoed JJ, Fraser A, Tilling K, et al. Preeclampsia and gestational hypertension are associated with childhood blood pressure independently of family adiposity measures: the Avon Longitudinal Study of Parents and Children. Circulation 2010;122(12):1192–9.
110. Palmsten K, Buka SL, Michels KB. Maternal pregnancy-related hypertension and risk for hypertension in offspring later in life. Obstet Gynecol 2010;116(4): 858–64.

Achieving a Successful Pregnancy in Women with Polycystic Ovary Syndrome

Takako Araki, MD[a], Rony Elias, MD[b], Zev Rosenwaks, MD[b], Leonid Poretsky, MD[a],*

KEYWORDS

- Polycystic ovary syndrome (PCOS) • Infertility • Pregnancy

DEFINITION AND EPIDEMIOLOGY OF POLYCYSTIC OVARY SYNDROME

Polycystic ovary syndrome (PCOS), first described by Stein and Leventhal[1] in 1935, is characterized by oligoanovulation, clinical or biochemical hyperandrogenism, and/or polycystic ovaries.[2,3] PCOS is one of the most common endocrinopathies in women of reproductive age, with prevalence estimated between 7% and 8%.[4,5] It is the most common cause of female infertility among reproductive-age women. It is also the leading cause (75%) of anovulatory infertility.[6,7] The prevalence of different phenotypes of PCOS among various populations is affected by ethnic origin, race, and environmental factors.[8]

Currently, there are 3 broadly accepted sets of criteria for diagnosis of PCOS.[2,3] After excluding all other causes of hyperandrogenism and menstrual dysfunction, National Institutes of Health (NIH) criteria (1990) require evidence of hyperandrogenism (clinical or biochemical) and evidence of anovulation or oligo-ovulation. Rotterdam criteria (2003) added the presence of polycystic ovarian morphology as an alternative (2 out of 3 criteria still need to be present for diagnosis of PCOS).[2] The Androgen Excess and PCOS Society criteria (2006) consider polycystic ovarian morphology as an alternative evidence of ovarian dysfunction (**Box 1**).[3] None of these definitions fully addresses the clinical picture of PCOS. For example, none of the sets mentioned earlier includes insulin resistance or increased circulating luteinizing hormone (LH) levels, both common features of PCOS.

Disclosure: The authors have nothing to disclose.
[a] Division of Endocrinology and Metabolism, Beth Israel Medical Center and Albert Einstein College of Medicine, 317 East 17th Street, Fierman Hall 7th Floor, New York, NY 10003, USA
[b] The Ronald O. Perelman and Claudia Cohen Center for Reproductive Medicine, Weill Cornell Medical College, 1305 York Avenue, New York, NY 10021, USA
* Corresponding author.
E-mail address: LPoretsk@chpnet.org

Endocrinol Metab Clin N Am 40 (2011) 865–894
doi:10.1016/j.ecl.2011.08.003
0889-8529/11/$ – see front matter © 2011 Published by Elsevier Inc.

endo.theclinics.com

Box 1
Diagnostic criteria for PCOS

NIH (1990)

Anovulation or oligo-ovulation

Clinical and/or biochemical hyperandrogenism

Rotterdam (2003) (2 out of 3)

Anovulation or oligo-ovulation

Clinical and/or biochemical hyperandrogenism

Polycystic ovaries (morphology)

Androgen Excess and PCOS Society (2006)

Ovarian dysfunction

Either anovulation or oligo-ovulation or polycystic ovaries (morphology)

Clinical and/or biochemical hyperandrogenism

PATHOGENESIS AND MANIFESTATIONS OF PCOS

Women with PCOS may present with multiple manifestations, which include cutaneous, reproductive, and metabolic abnormalities. The symptoms are usually peripubertal in onset. The cutaneous manifestations include hirsutism, acne, and male pattern baldness, and are caused by hyperandrogenism. The reproductive manifestations include menstrual dysfunction (secondary amenorrhea, oligomenorrhea), anovulation, infertility, early pregnancy loss, and other complications of pregnancy, which are discussed in detailed later. Metabolic and endocrine manifestations include increased circulating levels of total and/or free testosterone, androstenedione, dehydroepiandrosterone sulfate (DHEAS); decreased sex hormone-binding globulin (SHBG); increased insulin levels; and increased LH/follicle-stimulating hormone (FSH) ratio.

Hyperandrogenism results from abnormalities at all levels of the hypothalamic-pituitary-ovarian axis. The increased frequency and amplitude of LH pulses in PCOS seems to result from an increased frequency of hypothalamic gonadotropin-releasing hormone (GnRH) pulses.[8] The increased LH secretion stimulates theca cells to increase production of androgens. The hyperandrogenic milieu alters the intrafollicular microenvironment, leading to aberrant folliculogenesis.[9]

Obesity, insulin resistance, and hyperinsulinemia are commonly present in PCOS. Approximately 40% to 50% of women with PCOS are overweight,[4] and a history of weight gain frequently precedes the onset of clinical manifestations of this syndrome. Obese subjects with PCOS tend to have more severe reproductive abnormalities and may be resistant to treatment.

In adolescent and young women, the age of onset of obesity and onset of menstrual irregularities are significantly correlated.[10] A large study conducted in the United Kingdom, which included 5800 women, showed that obesity in childhood and in the early 20s increased the risk of menstrual abnormalities.[11] In the Nurses' Health Study, the risk of anovulatory infertility increased in women with higher body mass indices (BMI).[12]

Hyperinsulinemia is present in about 80% of obese women with PCOS and in approximately 30% to 40% of those with normal weight.[13] Overall, 20% to 50% of women with PCOS have insulin resistance and approximately 10 % of women with PCOS develop type 2 diabetes by 40 years of age.[14–16]

Hyperinsulinemia may affect steroidogenesis in the human ovary both directly and indirectly.[17] Insulin receptors are present in the human ovary[18] and in vitro studies have shown that, in the ovaries of women with PCOS, insulin is capable of stimulating androgen production in the theca cells. In vivo, both acute and chronic hyperinsulinemia stimulate testosterone production in some studies, whereas suppressing insulin levels by any means uniformly decreases circulating androgen concentrations.[19] In spite of systemic insulin resistance, insulin sensitivity seems to be preserved in the human ovary.[20] In the ovaries, insulin can activate both insulin receptor and type 1 insulinlike growth factor (IGF)-1 receptor, leading to excessive stimulation of androgen production. Insulin suppresses insulinlike growth factor-binding protein type 1 (IGFBP-1) production, therefore increasing the bioavailable IGF level, which can further enhance androgen synthesis, particularly because hyperinsulinemia can also upregulate ovarian type 1 IGF receptors.[19]

Systemically, insulin inhibits production of serum SHBG in the liver, further increasing the levels of free testosterone.[21] Thus, the role of hyperinsulinemia in accelerating ovarian androgen production is multifactorial (**Fig. 1**).

The level of circulating estrogens in PCOS is commonly increased because of aromatization from the excess of androgens. High insulin levels may contribute to this process by stimulating aromatase; however, the effect of hyperinsulinemia on aromatase is controversial.[22]

The effect of hyperinsulinemia, if any, on the hypothalamic/pituitary axis in women with PCOS is controversial. Burcelin and colleagues[23] showed that LH secretion can be stimulated by insulin. In contrast, other studies in women with PCOS, as well as in animals, failed to consistently show the stimulatory effect of insulin on LH production or secretion.[24] For example, Moret and colleagues[25] assessed LH levels before and during hyperinsulinemic clamp and showed that LH levels increased in the control group but not in subjects with PCOS. Obese patients with higher insulin levels frequently do not have an increase in LH/FSH ratio.[26] LH levels are commonly low in obese women.[27] LH levels did not increase either tonically on in response to GnRH in female rats with experimental hyperinsulinemia compared with control animals.[28]

The cause of PCOS is not well understood, but it is believed to be multifactorial (**Box 2**). An abnormality in the hypothalamic-pituitary axis is considered to be one of

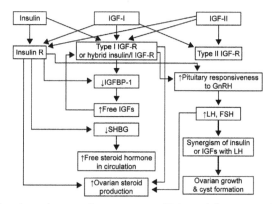

Fig. 1. Insulin-related ovarian regulatory system. (*Adapted from* Poretsky L, Cataldo NA, Rosenwaks Z, et al. The insulin-related ovarian regulatory system in health and disease. Endocr Rev 1999;20:535; with permission.)

> **Box 2**
> **Hypotheses of PCOS pathogenesis**
>
> 1. Central hypothesis[29–31]
> 2. Ovarian hypothesis[33–37]
> 3. Adrenal hypothesis[38–40]
> 4. Dual-defect hypothesis[41]
> 5. Programming hypothesis[41–43]
> 6. Genetic hypothesis[44–46]

many pathogenetic components. It seems that both the frequency and, in particular, the amplitude of LH pulses are increased in PCOS.[29–32] Although the causes of these abnormalities of LH secretion are unclear, they may be primarily caused by increased sensitivity of the pituitary to GnRH.

It has been proposed that intrinsic functional defects of theca cells and granulosa cells may be the primary feature of PCOS. Dysregulation of P-450C17 enzyme is presumed to occur in theca cells, because several studies that used GnRH agonists in PCOS showed hypersecretion of 17-OH progesterone.[33,35,36] The steroidogenic and mitogenic abnormalities have also been found in theca and granulosa cells from patients with PCOS.[47] Aromatase activity was observed to be low in PCOS granulosa cells in vivo, probably reflecting decreased FSH activity in vivo, because aromatase activity seems to be either normal or even exaggerated when granulosa cells from PCOS are examined in vitro.[34,37]

It has been hypothesized that excessive adrenal androgen production during puberty can supply substrate for extragonadal aromatization, resulting in tonic estrogen inhibition of FSH secretion. Premature adrenarche is associated with a higher incidence of functional ovarian hyperandrogenism and insulin resistance.[38–40] Hyperinsulinemia can stimulate adrenal (as well as ovarian) steroidogenesis.[48] It is unknown why pubertal insulin resistance persists in women with PCOS.

There is both in vitro and in vivo evidence that increased circulating levels of LH and hyperinsulinemia may act synergistically to enhance ovarian growth, androgen secretion, and ovarian cyst formation (**Fig. 2**).[19] The dual-defect hypothesis of PCOS postulates the presence of 2 independent primary defects in at least some women with PCOS.[41]

According to the programming hypothesis, the nutritional and endocrine environment in utero can affect development of neuroendocrine systems regulating body

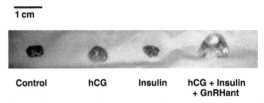

Fig. 2. Synergistic effects of insulin and LH/human chorionic gonadotropin (hCG) on ovarian morphology. (*Adapted from* Poretsky L, Clemons J, Bogovich K. Hyperinsulinemia and human chorionic gonadotropin synergistically promote the growth of ovarian follicular cysts in rats. Metabolism 1992;41:903; with permission.)

weight, food intake, and metabolism. For example, hyperinsulinemia and hyperandrogenism, which can program female reproduction, possibly producing a phenocopy of PCOS.[42,43] A genetic cause has been suspected because PCOS has strong familial clustering[44–46]; however, as discussed later, identifying the specific genetic defects that could lead to the development of PCOS, has been challenging.

INFERTILITY IN PCOS

PCOS is the most common (75%) cause of anovulatory infertility in reproductive-age women.[6,7] Prevalence of infertility among women with PCOS ranges from approximately 40% to 75%.[49–52]

Multiple approaches have been shown effective for the treatment of infertility in women with PCOS. These approaches are based on the pathogenetic mechanisms discussed earlier and include lifestyle modifications, pharmacologic therapy, and surgical interventions.

Lifestyle Modifications

Since the 1990s, when it became apparent that insulin resistance/hyperinsulinemia play a role in the pathogenesis of PCOS, weight loss and exercise have been introduced as potential methods of treatment. It is believed that the primary mechanism by which weight loss can improve reproductive outcomes in PCOS[53–56] involves reducing circulating insulin levels.[57]

Loss of 5% to 10% of initial body weight in 6 months is sufficient to reestablish ovarian function in more than 50% of obese women with PCOS.[58] Even a less significant amount of body weight loss (2%–5%) can result in restoration of regular vaginal bleeding consistent with ovulatory patterns.[55] Short periods (4 weeks) of extremely low-calorie diet (350 kcal/day, 43 g carbohydrate, 33 g protein, 2.9 g fat per 100 g) can decrease fasting insulin and free testosterone levels and increase the levels of SHBG and IGFBP-1.[59,60]

Clark and colleagues[61] conducted an observational study of behavioral modifications (diet/counseling/exercise) in 13 obese women with PCOS. After 6 months, with an average weight loss of 6.3 kg, 12 out of 13 women regained ovulatory cycles, and 11 out of 13 became pregnant. Hollman and colleagues[54] conducted an observational study in 29 obese women with PCOS. With 5.6 kg of mean weight loss in 8 months, the ovulation and pregnancy rates were improved to 80% and 29%, respectively. Fasting insulin, androstenedione, and dihydrotestosterone levels decreased after this intervention, although LH, FSH, dehydroepiandrosterone (DHEA), DHEAS, testosterone, and estrogen levels were unchanged.

Hoeger and colleagues[62] conducted a 48-week trial of diet modification (50% carbohydrate, 25% protein, 25% fat, low-glycemic-index foods) and/or metformin. Ovulation rates were increased equally in all groups, suggesting that reduction of hyperinsulinemia achieved either through lifestyle modification or metformin therapy was equally effective.

There is no clear-cut evidence that exercise, independent of weight loss, improves ovulatory function. However, the potential benefits of exercise can be expected in the overweight PCOS population,[56] because there is evidence that exercise enhances weight loss.[63]

Medical Therapy

Clomiphene citrate

Clomiphene citrate (clomiphene; Clomid), an oral synthetic triphenylethyne, is an inexpensive and safe medication that has been used for ovulation induction since the

1960s.[64] Clomiphene is a partially selective estrogen receptor modulator with antiestrogenic effect in the hypothalamus, where it induces a change in the GnRH pulse frequency. This change results in an increased FSH level, promoting follicular development and estrogen production.[65,66] High ovulation rates of 60% to 85% have been reported with administration of clomiphene[67,68] and a 30% to 40% pregnancy rate can be achieved in the first 3 months of treatment.[69]

Because of a high rate of successful ovulation and cost-effectiveness, the Thessaloniki European Society for Human Reproduction and the American Society of Reproductive Medicine (ESHRE/ASRM) consensus workshop recommended that clomiphene be the first-line therapy for ovulation induction. Clomiphene can be started at 50 mg daily for 5 days beginning on day 2 to 5 of the menstrual cycle, with incremental dose increase to a maximum of 150 mg[70] or 250 mg per day.[71]

There are several limitations to clomiphene use. Clomiphene increases the risk of multiple pregnancies (4%–10%), particularly in obese women with PCOS who are commonly resistant to clomiphene and require a higher dose.[72] Ovarian hyperstimulation syndrome (OHSS) may occur, although the risk of OHSS with clomiphene is less than that with gonadotropin therapy. It is known that obesity and clomiphene resistance correlate, and that hyperinsulinemia may account for the poor responsiveness to clomiphene, possibly because of the alterations in the IGF system.[73,74]

The discrepancy between ovulation rates (60%–85%) and successful pregnancy rates (30%–40%) in patients with PCOS receiving clomiphene therapy may be caused by the antiestrogenic properties of clomiphene, which can cause poor thickening of the cervical mucus and endometrium, rendering the uterine environment hostile for conception.[75]

Gonadotropins/GnRH

Exogenous gonadotropin therapy can be used for ovulation induction in patients who do not conceive after 3 cycles of clomiphene therapy.[76] Gonadotropins have been used in PCOS since the 1960s. Human recombinant FSH, administered subcutaneously, currently is used the most frequently. Gonadotropin ovulation induction is based on the hypothesis that the initiation and maintenance of monofollicular growth may be achieved by a transient increase in FSH to more than the threshold dose for a sufficient duration.

High starting doses of FSH (150 IU daily), which used to be conventional, resulted in high ovulation rates (70%) and a pregnancy rate of about 30%. However, the high-dose protocol increases the risk of multiple pregnancies (25%–30%) and OHSS.[77,78] To avoid these complications, various regimens have been proposed. The step-up low-dose FSH induction protocols (37.5–50 IU daily) have been shown to be safer for monofollicular development.[79] An analysis of 225 women with PCOS treated with low-dose gonadotropin regimens showed high rates of ovulation and pregnancy as well as significantly decreased frequency of multiple pregnancies (6%) and OHSS (8%).[78]

Combination trials involving gonadotropins have been performed. Comparing coadministration of metformin with FSH with FSH monotherapy, one study showed a lower incidence of ovarian hyperstimulation in the combination therapy group,[80] whereas another study showed no significant difference in ovarian response between the 2 groups.[81]

GnRH analogues are used to prevent premature LH surge during ovarian stimulation and are administered before FSH stimulation. Both forms (GnRH agonists and GnRH antagonists) are available. GnRH agonists require a longer period of administration than GnRH antagonists. In initial studies, the concomitant use of GnRH agonists and gonadotropins seemed to increase the risk of OHSS.[82] However, more recent studies showed that there is no significant difference in either reproductive outcomes or overall occurrence of OHSS with the use of either regimen.[83,84]

The drawbacks to gonadotropin therapy include its high cost, the need for frequent monitoring of serum estradiol levels, and the need for frequent ultrasound assessments to minimize the risk of multiple follicles developing.

The Thessaloniki ESHRE/ASRM Consensus Workshop (2007) recommended a low starting dose of FSH (37.5–50.0 IU daily) with a step-up regimen until 6 ovulatory cycles.[70]

Metformin

Because insulin resistance and consequent hyperinsulinemia are considered important factors in the pathogenesis of PCOS, multiple studies attempted to target these metabolic abnormalities to improve ovulation and fertility in women with this syndrome.[85]

In 1994, Velazquez and colleagues[86] published the first trial of metformin in PCOS. This trial included 29 obese women with PCOS who were treated with metformin for 8 weeks and showed improvement in metabolic parameters, as well as a noticeable increase in pregnancy rate. Since then, there have been numerous studies of metformin assessing the metabolic and/or reproductive outcomes on subjects with PCOS. Most of these studies favor metformin use, although there are some that do not.[87]

Metformin is an insulin sensitizer that decreases fasting insulin levels, hepatic gluconeogenesis, and body weight. The mechanisms of the effects of metformin on hyperandrogenism and female reproductive function are not well understood, but are believed to be primarily related to the reduction in hyperinsulinemia. Metformin enhances adenosine monophosphate–activated protein kinase (AMPK) pathway, inhibits IGF-1 signaling[88] and IGFBP-1 production both in the ovary and systemically, and produces increases in SHBG levels.[89] These changes result in improved ovulatory rates.[90]

The first head-to-head randomized controlled trial of metformin and clomiphene was published by Palomba and colleagues[91] in 2005. One hundred nonobese subjects with PCOS without glucose intolerance were randomized into metformin or clomiphene treatment groups. After 6 months, ovulation rates were not significantly different (24.4% vs 31.9%). However, there were striking differences in pregnancy rates (68.9% in the metformin group vs 34% in the clomiphene group). The investigators concluded that metformin was superior to clomiphene as a first-line therapy.

Two years later, a retrospective head-to-head study of 154 patients by Neveu and colleagues[92] showed that metformin was superior to clomiphene in inducing ovulation, but that there was no difference in the pregnancy rate in anovulatory women with PCOS. In contrast, a head-to-head randomized controlled trial by Zain and colleagues[66] in 115 Asian women with PCOS showed that metformin was inferior to clomiphene in ovulation rates but equal to clomiphene in pregnancy rates.

In 2006, Moll and colleagues[93] reported a large multicenter randomized controlled study that compared metformin plus clomiphene versus clomiphene monotherapy in nonobese women with PCOS. Two hundred and twenty-eight women were followed for up to 6 menstrual cycles. The study showed that there were no significant differences in ovulation rates or pregnancy rates between the combination therapy versus clomiphene monotherapy groups, suggesting that addition of metformin provided no benefit.

A meta-analysis by Creanga and colleagues[94] showed that metformin alone improves the odds of ovulation in women with PCOS but it does not improve rates of clinical pregnancy. This meta-analysis suggested that combination therapy increased the likelihood of both ovulation and early pregnancy, compared with clomiphene alone, especially among clomiphene-resistant and obese women with PCOS. However, the combination therapy did not improve the odds of live births.

Another meta-analysis by Moll and colleagues[5] (2007) was limited to the studies using ESHRE/ARSM Rotterdam criteria and compared the live birth rates among patients who received metformin, clomiphene, or their combination, as well as other therapeutic modalities with or without metformin. The investigators analyzed clomiphene-naive and clomiphene-resistant subgroups separately. They concluded that adding metformin did not affect live birth rates in the clomiphene-naive group, whereas there was significant increase in live birth rates in the clomiphene-resistant group.

The largest trial to date (The Pregnancy in Polycystic Ovary Syndrome [PPCOS]) was published in 2007 by Legro and colleagues.[85] This was a prospective randomized controlled trial in 626 anovulatory infertile women with PCOS with live birth rate as the primary outcome. Subjects were randomized to 1 of 3 groups: (1) clomiphene, (2) metformin, (3) clomiphene plus metformin. The live birth rate was 22.5% in the clomiphene group, 7.2% in the metformin group, and 26.8% in the combined group. The difference in live birth rates between the clomiphene group and the metformin group, as well as between the combination group and metformin group, was statistically significant (**Table 1**). There was no significant advantage of the combination therapy compared with clomiphene alone, although, when ovulation was considered to be the outcome, the combination therapy was superior. The investigators concluded that clomiphene, rather than metformin, is the most appropriate first-line treatment in anovulatory women with PCOS.

The combination therapy (clomiphene and metformin) is recommended for a subgroup of patients who have BMI greater than 35 kg/m^2, glucose intolerance, and clomiphene resistance because the only beneficial outcomes in the combination therapy group, compared with clomiphene monotherapy, were decreased BMI and improved insulin resistance, whereas pregnancy rates or live births rates were not affected (see **Table 1**).[85]

To help clinical decision making, a nomogram for clomiphene therapy was created by Imani and colleagues[95] in 2002. This nomogram was designed to predict the

Table 1
Summary of outcomes from PPCOS study

	Clomiphene (C)	Metformin (M)	Combination (comb.)	P value (comb. vs M)	P value (comb. vs C)	P value (C vs M)
N	209	208	209	—	—	—
Ovulation (%)	49	29	60	<.001	.003	<.001
Conception (%)	30	12	38	<.001	.006	<.001
Pregnancy (%)	24	9	31	<.001	.10	<.001
Live birth (%)	23	7	27	<.001	.31	<.001

Data from Legro RS, Barnhart HX, Schlaff WD, et al. Clomiphene, metformin, or both for infertility in the polycystic ovary syndrome. N Engl J Med 2007;356:551.

outcome (chances of ovulation and live birth) with clomiphene induction. The screening characteristics included age, BMI, presence of oligomenorrhea or amenorrhea, and free androgen index. Rausch and colleagues[96] created a more complex live birth prediction chart, using data from a large cohort from PPCOS (**Fig. 3**).[85] This live birth prediction chart was formulated with probabilities of live birth that ranged from 0% to 10% to greater than 60%. The model factored in (1) age, (2) duration of infertility, (3) severity of androgenic manifestations, and (4) BMI. Input of information is based on history and physical examination, and the modalities are not limited to clomiphene, but include the data from metformin monotherapy and combination therapy. Because timing may be a critical factor in treating infertility, the nomograms may help both clinicians and patients to make therapeutic decisions, and, in the case of very low likelihood of successful pregnancy, may help fast-track the treatment.[97]

Metformin is a category B drug for pregnancy. There is no evidence of fetus toxicity in animal studies. In humans, one study reported metformin use throughout the pregnancy in women with type 2 diabetes and gestational diabetes without teratogenic effects or adverse fetal outcomes.[98]

In summary, currently metformin is not recommended as the first-line therapy for infertility in patients with PCOS. The Thessaloniki ESHRE/ARSM Consensus Workshop advised that, thus far, studies do not show an advantage to adding metformin to clomiphene.[70] Remaining areas of uncertainty include the choice of therapy in obese versus nonobese patients with PCOS and in clomiphene-naive versus clomiphene-resistant subgroups.

Thiazolidinediones

Thiazolidinediones (TZDs) are the peroxisome proliferator–activated receptor γ (PPAR-γ) ligands that are being used as insulin sensitizers in individuals with type 2 diabetes. Several studies of troglitazone, the first TZD approved for the treatment of diabetes, have been reported in PCOS. The first pilot study, conducted by Dunaif and colleagues,[99] showed that troglitazone decreased androgen levels in obese

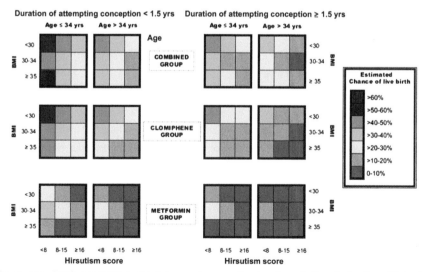

Fig. 3. Live birth prediction chart for various methods of ovulation induction. (*Adapted from* Rausch ME, Legro RS, Barnhart HX, et al. Predictors of pregnancy in women with polycystic ovary syndrome. J Clin Endocrinol Metab 2009;94:3458; with permission.)

women with PCOS. Mitwally and colleagues[100] compared troglitazone plus clomiphene with clomiphene monotherapy and showed significant improvement of ovulation rates in the combination group. A large multicenter trial with more than 400 women with PCOS who received troglitazone in a range of doses (150 mg, 300 mg, and 600 mg daily) for 44 weeks showed a correlation between ovulation rates and the dose of troglitazone.[101] However, troglitazone has been removed from the worldwide market because of its hepatotoxicity. Two other TZDs currently available, rosiglitazone and pioglitazone, have been shown to improve ovulation, hyperandrogenism, and insulin resistance in women with PCOS[102,103]; however, there have been concerns about cardiovascular risks associated with rosiglitazone use,[104] propensity of all TZDs to induce weight gain, and their classification as category C drugs for use in pregnancy.

The mechanism of action of TZDs involves activation of the PPAR-γ ligands, which are present in the human ovary.[105] In vitro, in human ovarian cells, TZDs directly inhibit androgen production. Their action in the ovary involves activation of steroidogenic acute regulatory (StAR) protein[106] and inhibition of 3-β-hydroxysteroid dehydrogenase[107] and aromatase.[108] Systemically, TZDs reduce circulating insulin levels, which further contributes to the reduction of ovarian androgen synthesis (**Box 3**).[17]

Glucagonlike peptide-1 agonists

Glucagonlike peptide-1 (GLP-1) is an incretin, which enhances glucose-dependent insulin secretion, delays gastric emptying, and centrally controls appetite, therefore producing weight loss.[109]

Box 3
Effects of TZDs related to ovarian function

Direct: can be observed in vitro; may be present in vivo

Insulin independent

　↑ Progesterone

　↓ Testosterone

　↓ Estradiol

　↑ IGFBP-1 (in the absence of insulin)

Insulin sensitizing (enhanced insulin effect)

　↓ IGFBP-1 production

　↑ Estradiol production (in vivo, in a setting of high-dose insulin infusion)

Indirect: observed in vivo; caused by systemic insulin-sensitizing action and reduction of hyperinsulinemia

↓ Testosterone

↑ IGFBP-1

↑ SHBG

↓ Free testosterone

Data from Seto-Young D, Paliou M, Schlosser J, et al. Direct thiazolidinedione action in the human ovary: insulin-independent and insulin-sensitizing effects on steroidogenesis and insulin-like growth factor-binding protein-1 production. J Clin Endocrinol Metab 2005; 90:6099.

Several studies have examined GLP-1 levels in women with PCOS. One study showed that there was no difference in circulating GLP-1 levels between women with PCOS and healthy subjects.[110] In another study, Vrbikova and colleagues[111] assessed incretin levels in 34 lean women with PCOS compared with control subjects. In the early phase of the oral glucose tolerance test (OGTT), GLP-1 levels were similar in both women with PCOS and controls; however, in the later phase, the PCOS group showed a significant decrease in GLP-1 levels compared with controls matched for BMI and age. A similar postprandial pattern on the OGTT also exists in patients with type 2 diabetes.[112] GLP-1 has been shown to participate in modulation of GnRH secretion[113] and to reduce the pulsatile component of testosterone secretion in healthy men.[114] GLP-1 knockout mice had reduced gonadal weight and delayed onset of puberty in women.[113]

One pilot study compared the GLP-1 agonist exenatide, metformin, and their combination in obese patients with PCOS.[115] After 24 weeks of intervention, ovulation rates improved by 50%, 29%, and 86%, respectively. The average weight loss was most significant in the combination arm, with 6.0 kg, versus 3.2 kg in the exenatide arm, and 1.6 kg in the metformin arm. Total testosterone levels were reduced in all groups. The preliminary evidence of potential benefits of incretin therapy in PCOS, coupled with the evidence that weight reduction has consistently led to improvement in ovarian function in women with PCOS, suggests that GLP-1 agonists may have a role in therapy for PCOS.

Aromatase inhibitors

Aromatase inhibitors block the biosynthesis of estrogens from androgens. Aromatase inhibitors cause a reversible uncoupling of the hypothalamic/pituitary axis from negative estrogen feedback, leading to FSH and LH secretion and induction of ovulation. Unlike clomiphene, aromatase inhibitors do not block the estrogen receptor, and therefore the potential negative effects on cervical mucus and the endometrium are usually not seen.

Aromatase inhibitors were first introduced for ovulation induction by Mitwally and colleagues[116] in 2001, with promising data. In a prospective study, letrozole, the most commonly used aromatase inhibitor, was administered in the early part of the menstrual cycles to 12 clomiphene-resistant women with PCOS. The results included an ovulation rate of 75% and clinical pregnancy (presence of a gestational sac on ultrasound[117]) rate of 17%. Letrozole treatment also produced a thicker endometrium compared with clomiphene therapy.

Badawy and colleagues[118] compared 115 patients with PCOS given anastrozole 1 mg/d (a third-generation aromatase inhibitor), on cycle days 3 to 7 (for 5 days), to a matched group of 101 patients with PCOS given clomiphene 100 mg/d. The anastrozole group (243 cycles) had a thicker endometrium and fewer mature and growing follicles compared with the clomiphene group (226 cycles). The pregnancy rate per cycle was slightly higher in the anastrozole group but did not reach statistical significance. The investigators concluded that anastrozole should be considered whenever the risks of OHSS and multiple pregnancies are high. Currently, aromatase inhibitors are not recommended for use in treating infertility (except if there is a history of estrogen sensitive tumors), because of the potential embryotoxicity of letrozole.[119]

Glucocorticoids

Glucocorticoids suppress adrenal androgen production and therefore may improve ovulation. Several studies have shown an improvement in reproductive outcomes with glucocorticoid therapy in anovulatory patients, including women with PCOS,[120–122] whereas others have shown no beneficial effects.[123,124] At this time, glucocorticoid therapy is not recommended for treatment of infertility in women with PCOS.

Oral contraceptives/antiandrogens

Oral contraceptives (OCPs) reduce hyperandrogenism via suppression of LH secretion as well as by stimulating SHBG production.[125,126] OCPs can be the first-line therapy for the treatment of hirsutism.[126] Spironolactone, an aldosterone antagonist and competitive inhibitor of the androgen receptor, is also commonly used to treat hirsutism in women with PCOS. A systemic review showed that spironolactone (100 mg daily), compared with placebo, produced a greater reduction in hirsutism (−4.8 in Ferriman-Gallway scores).[127] Cyproterone acetate, a 17-hydroxyprogesterone acetate derivative, blocks androgen receptors and has been used for the treatment of hirsutism and acne; however, it is not currently available in the United States. Finasteride, an inhibitor of 5 α-reductase, produces a 30% to 60% reduction in hirsutism score in most studies.[128] Because none of these agents has been shown to produce consistent improvement in either ovulation or pregnancy rates, and because of concerns regarding their teratogenicity, antiandrogens are not used in treating infertility in PCOS, although contraceptives can be used as part of in vitro fertilization protocols (discussed later).

Surgical management

Surgical management of anovulatory infertility includes traditional ovarian wedge resections, laparoscopic diathermy, and laser drilling.[129] These procedures may restore ovulatory cycles; however, given the invasive nature of these surgical procedures and the development of other medical treatment options, today these surgical management techniques are seldom used for treatment of infertility. In addition, some of the side effects from surgery (pelvic adhesions) may impair fertility.[130] In summary, surgical procedures for treating infertility in PCOS are mostly of historical significance.

In vitro fertilization

In patients with PCOS, in vitro fertilization (IVF) should be considered for the following indications: failure of nonpharmacologic and clomiphene treatment, failure of gonadotropin/intrauterine insemination, or in cases of a high response to FSH (4 or more follicles) despite low gonadotropin dose. As in all patients, when PCOS is combined with tubal disease, male factor infertility, severe endometriosis, and/or patients requiring a preimplantation genetic diagnosis, IVF should be considered. A limited report with a small number of patients (N = 16) suggested that, in women who are older than 30 years and who have increased androgen levels, proceeding directly to IVF may be most cost-effective once clomiphene treatment fails.[131]

A variety of stimulation regimens for patients with PCOS undergoing IVF have been reported, including protocols based on GnRH agonists and GnRH antagonist. Before the use of GnRH antagonists in IVF stimulation, we developed a protocol that involves dual pituitary suppression with oral contraceptives for 28 days with a GnRH agonist overlap during the last 7 days of the OCP (**Fig. 4**).[132] Low-dose stimulation with FSH (150 IU/d) is started on the third day of withdrawal bleeding. Among 73 patients with a total of 99 cycles, only 13 cycles (13.1%) were canceled before embryo transfer. The causes for cancellation included poor response (low estrogen level and few follicles), hyperresponse (>25 follicles with a high estrogen level of >3000 pg/mL), or estrogen reduction of more than 20% after human chorionic gonadotropin (hCG) trigger. Eight patients experienced mild to moderate OHSS. The clinical and ongoing pregnancy rates were 46.5% and 40.4%, respectively.

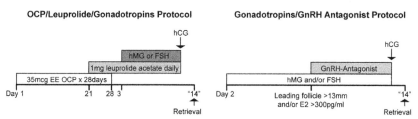

Fig. 4. Representative IVF ovulation induction protocols used at the Center for Reproductive Medicine at Weill Cornell Medical College.

Recently, a randomized controlled trial comparing GnRH agonist–based versus GnRH antagonist–based protocols in 220 women with PCOS showed that the clinical pregnancy rates were similar in the two groups (50.9% vs 47.3%, respectively).[133] However, the incidence of moderate OHSS was higher in the agonist, compared with the antagonist, group (60% vs 40%, respectively, P<.01).

Ovarian stimulation for IVF can be achieved using pure FSH,[134] human menopausal hormones (hMG) alone,[135] or a combination of the two.[136] Addition of clomiphene (100 mg, cycle days 3 to 7, for 5 days) to hMG/GnRH antagonist may produce improved results.[137] A meta-analysis that compared the overall IVF outcome in women with PCOS using different stimulation protocols with controls without PCOS, revealed a higher cancellation rate, an increased number of oocytes per retrieval and a lower fertilization rate in the PCOS group.[138] However, both groups had a similar clinical pregnancy and live birth rates. Regardless of the type of gonadotropins used (pure FSH or hMG, with or without clomiphene), GnRH antagonist–based protocols significantly reduce the incidence of OHSS,[133,139] especially if GnRH agonist is used to trigger ovulation.[140,141] Metformin cotreatment before or during IVF stimulation also reduces the risk of OHSS.[142]

An early report of patients with PCOS undergoing IVF showed that stimulation of ovulation was associated with a sharp increase of E2 levels and an exceedingly high number of developing follicles. The excessively high follicle number and E2 levels are associated with a high incidence of severe OHSS after hCG administration.[143] Several approaches have been suggested to decrease the incidence of OHSS in patients with PCOS. Our approach includes individualization of stimulation protocols (using the lowest effective gonadotropin dose) based on antral follicle count and anti-mullerian hormone levels, using antagonist-based protocols with a GnRH agonist triggering, and coasting. Coasting is a term to describe the technique of withholding gonadotropins when E2 levels exceed 3000 pg/mL during stimulation in an effort to starve small follicles and allow larger follicles to continue to develop. Coasting seems to reduce (but not to eliminate) the incidence of OHSS.

More recently, the advent of GnRH antagonist protocols has allowed us to trigger an endogenous LH surge with GnRH agonist, resulting in a short-lived LH surge compared with the longer surge observed after hCG, which has a longer half-life.[144] If the E2 level is more than 3000 pg/mL on the triggering day, we recommend using GnRH agonists instead of hCG to trigger ovulation. When a GnRH agonist trigger is used, luteal estrogen and progesterone supplementation should be prescribed.[140]

In vitro maturation (IVM) involves the recovery of immature oocytes from women with PCOS on cycle day 10 to 14 after a withdrawal bleed.[145] The immature oocytes are then incubated in maturation medium in the presence of FSH and LH. Following maturation, the oocytes are fertilized by intracytoplasmic sperm injection (ICSI), and the

resulting embryo is transferred into the uterus on day 2 or 3 after ICSI.[145] Before immature oocyte retrieval, FSH priming has been reported to produce varying results.[146,147]
Compared with conventional IVF, the advantages of IVM include lower risk of OHSS,
less complicated stimulation procedures, and reduced cost. At experienced centers,
the clinical pregnancy and implantation rates in women with PCOS following IVM are
30% to 35% and 10% to 15%, respectively.[146] Despite the lack of randomized trials
comparing IVM with conventional IVF in women with PCOS,[148] we suggest that IVM
should be considered if the patient has a history of poor oocyte quality.

Currently, we recommend the use of an antagonist-based protocol with and without
clomiphene. We initiate coasting when the E2 level exceeds 3000 pg/mL, as
mentioned earlier, or in the setting of numerous immature follicles (<16 mm) with
a rapidly increasing E2 level. If the E2 level does not decrease to less than 3000 pg/
mL after 4 days of coasting, we cancel the cycle. If the patient has progressive clinical
signs of OHSS after oocyte retrieval, we consider canceling the transfer and freezing
all the embryos. In the absence of pregnancy, OHSS is generally limited to the luteal
phase in the setting of a conservative stimulation protocol. The avoidance of hyperstimulation syndrome is most effectively accomplished with a conservative approach
to stimulation. Once hCG is administered in the setting of greater than 30 follicles or E2
greater than 6000 pg/mL, OHSS is almost unavoidable, even in the absence of
pregnancy.

RISK OF PCOS FOR THE OFFSPRING DURING PREGNANCY AND BEYOND

During pregnancy, women with PCOS have a significantly increased risk of complications, both maternal and fetal. These complications include early pregnancy loss,
gestational diabetes mellitus (GDM), pregnancy-induced hypertension, preeclampsia,
delivery by cesarean section, premature delivery, and increased perinatal mortality.

Early Pregnancy Loss

Early pregnancy loss, defined as miscarriage of a clinically recognized pregnancy
during the first trimester, occurs in 30% to 50% of women with PCOS compared
with 10% to 15% of women without PCOS.[149–151]

Mechanisms of early pregnancy loss in women with PCOS are not well understood.
Obesity and hyperinsulinemia (insulin resistance) are independent risk factors for early
pregnancy loss.[152] Decreased levels of glycodelin, a glycoprotein produced from
endometrium to protect the embryo from immune response, and reduced IGFBP-1,
as well as increased levels of plasminogen activator inhibitor-1 (PAI-1), seem to
increase the risk of early pregnancy loss.[153,154] Previous studies have suggested
that women who hypersecrete LH are at increased risk for miscarriage[149]; however,
a study by Clifford and colleagues[155] failed to show an improvement in miscarriage
rates after suppression of endogenous LH before conception.

Small studies have suggested a protective effect of metformin on early pregnancy
loss in women with PCOS. For example, in a study by Glueck and colleagues,[156]
the rate of first-trimester pregnancy loss was significantly decreased to 11% in the
metformin group, whereas it was 39% in the control group. In a retrospective study,
Jakubowicz and colleagues[150] reported 8.8% pregnancy loss in the metformin group
compared with 41.9% in the control group. The mechanism of metformin action
responsible for the reduced early pregnancy loss is not understood but may include
reduced glucose and insulin levels as well as PAI-1 activity. The assessment of the
effect of metformin withdrawal on pregnancy is further complicated by the possibility

of metformin withdrawal unmasking preexisting diabetes. Further studies are needed to examine the effect of metformin therapy on early pregnancy loss.

GDM

Insulin resistance develops during pregnancy because of the secretion of human placental lactogen (hPL). Because women with PCOS often have preexisting insulin resistance, they may be at an increased risk of GDM.

Studies of the correlation between GDM and PCOS produced conflicting results. Holte and colleagues[157] found a remarkably high prevalence of PCOS in the GDM population (41%). Other studies have been controversial, with both positive[158,159] and negative correlations between PCOS and GDM reported.[160] Higher incidence of GDM was observed in a lean PCOS population compared with women without PCOS; however, BMI values were not matched in this study (mean BMI 25 kg/m^2 in the PCOS group vs 23 kg/m^2 in the control group).[161] According to the meta-analysis by Boomsma and colleagues,[162] after weight matching, women with PCOS still had a significantly higher chance of developing GDM (odds ratio [OR] 2.94, 95% CI 1.70–5.08), with the increased risk of developing GDM being independent of obesity. However, Toulis and colleagues,[163] in a recent systematic review and meta-analysis, concluded that there was no consistent evidence for a higher risk of GDM in women with PCOS.

These conflicting results may be caused by the heterogeneity of PCOS and the diversity in screening methodology, diagnostic criteria, and predisposing factors for GDM (eg, ethnicity).[164]

In the first study to assess the impact of metformin on the risk of GDM, Glueck and colleagues[165] compared 33 nondiabetic women with PCOS who took metformin throughout the pregnancy versus 28 pregnant women with PCOS who did not receive this intervention. The incidence of GDM decreased significantly in the metformin group compared with the nonmetformin group (3% vs 31% respectively). A recent study in 137 pregnant women with PCOS compared pregnancy complication rates in 3 metformin intervention arms that differed in the duration of metformin therapy (4–8 weeks of gestation, 32 weeks, and throughout the pregnancy).[166] There was no significant difference in occurrence of GDM, but the rate of GDM requiring insulin therapy was significantly lower in the continuous metformin group compared with other groups.

Pregnancy-induced Hypertension and Preeclampsia

Women with PCOS are at high risk of pregnancy-induced hypertension (PIH). PIH occurs in 3% to 5% of pregnancies in previously normotensive women and usually develops during the third trimester.[167] The cause of PIH is likely multifactorial, involving immune, genetic, and placental abnormalities.[168]

The data on the association between PCOS and PIH are still conflicting. Initially, Diamant and colleagues[169] reported an increased incidence of preeclampsia in patients with PCOS, but the groups in this study were not matched for BMI. Gjonnaess[170] suggested that there was increased risk of preeclampsia (13%) in women with PCOS who have moderate to severe obesity. However, Mikola and colleagues[158] showed that PCOS had no predictive value for PIH, regardless of BMI, and a retrospective analysis by Haakova and colleagues[160] showed that there was no statistically significant difference in the rates of occurrence of PIH among PCOS and non-PCOS populations.

More recent studies have shown that PCOS may be an independent risk factor for PIH. Radon and colleagues[159] showed a significant increase in incidence of PIH in women with PCOS (OR 15.0, CI 1.9–121.5) after matching for BMI. Similarly, a recent meta-analysis by Boomsma and colleagues[162] showed a significantly higher chance of developing PIH in pregnant women with PCOS (OR 3.67, 95% CI 1.98–6.81). The rates of preeclampsia in this study were also higher among the women with PCOS (OR 3.47, 95% CI 1.95–6.17). De Vries and colleagues[171] reported a case-controlled study in pregnant women with similar BMI with and without PCOS . In spite of a similar occurrence of PIH, a significantly higher occurrence of preeclampsia was observed in the PCOS group (14%) compared with controls (2.5%).

Several studies noted an association between PIH and hyperinsulinemia. Hamasaki and colleagues[172] conducted a prospective study that showed that hyperinsulinemic pregnant women have higher systolic and diastolic blood pressures, with hyperinsulinemia appearing to constitute an independent risk factor of PIH. The hypothetical mechanisms for this association include endothelial dysfunction caused by hyperinsulinemia, or the stimulatory effect of insulin on blood pressure via stimulation of the sympathetic tone.[173]

Nawaz and colleagues[166] presented data on 137 pregnant women with PCOS divided into 3 different metformin intervention arms to compare pregnancy complications. Rates of PIH were 43.7% in group A (metformin continued until 4–16 weeks of pregnancy), 33% in group B (metformin continued until 32 weeks of pregnancy), and 13.9% in group C (metformin continued throughout the pregnancy), suggesting the benefit of continuous use of metformin during pregnancy for reduction of PIH. There were no adverse fetal or maternal effects of metformin.

Perinatal Care

According to a meta-analysis by Boomsma and colleagues,[162] there is a significantly higher rate of premature delivery (OR 1.75, 95% CI 1.16–2.62), admissions to an neonatal intensive care unit (OR 2.31, 95%CI 1.25–4.26), and perinatal mortality (OR 3.07, 95% CI 1.03–9.21) in PCOS pregnancies. However, there seems to be no significant differences in the rates of cesarean sections,[174] Apgar score,[158] or the occurrence of neonatal malformations.[162]

Birth Weight

It remains controversial whether offspring of women with PCOS are large, normal, or small for gestational age. Several early studies and case reports suggested that offspring of women with PCOS tended to have low gestational weight. Low birth weight has been associated with the development of type 2 diabetes and cardiovascular disease later in life.[175] In contrast, maternal obesity and diabetes are known to pose an increased risk for large fetal size, obesity, and glucose intolerance in the offspring.[176] Several lines of evidence support a hypothesis that there is an association between low birth weight and PCOS.[177] Female sheep treated prenatally with testosterone had reduced birth weight and impaired insulin sensitivity in early postnatal life.[178] Girls with premature pubarche and features of PCOS have a history of being significantly smaller for gestational age.[179,180] A prospective study by Sir-Petermann and colleagues[181] showed that there is increased prevalence of infants who are small for gestational age in women with PCOS compared with normal women.

However, several other studies failed to confirm association between PCOS and alterations in birth weight in singleton pregnancies. According to the meta-analysis by Boomsma and colleagues,[162] when only higher validity studies were considered (for example, those that matched BMI between women with PCOS and controls), no significant difference in birth weight was observed.[162] Legro and colleagues[177] recently published a family-based study of birth weight in PCOS that included approximately 1000 individuals, consisting of both women with PCOS and their family members. Compared with controls, PCOS family members in this study did not have any significant alterations in birth weight.

Risk of PCOS for Female Offspring

Female offspring of women with PCOS may have a higher risk of developing PCOS,[46,182,183] although the precise incidence in the offspring is unknown. The genetic component, supported by strong familial associations,[44–46] and the environmental component, including programming from intrauterine hyperandrogenemia, may affect the risk of developing PCOS.[43]

Prenatally androgenized female monkeys have approximately 40% to 50% fewer menstrual cycles than normal females.[42] In addition, 40% of prenatally androgenized women, compared with ∼14% of controls, have polyfollicular ovaries that resemble the morphology of polycystic ovaries.[42] In one cross-sectional study, daughters of women with PCOS had increased LH and testosterone levels, hyperinsulinemia, and an increase in ovarian size during puberty.[184]

Risk of Metabolic Disorders for the Female Offspring

Offspring of PCOS mothers tend to suffer from metabolic abnormalities in later life.[185,186] Prenatally androgenized female rhesus monkeys develop metabolic problems characteristic of women with PCOS, namely decreased insulin sensitivity and abnormal pancreatic β cell function, as well as increased total body adiposity.[187] The timing of fetal androgen exposure seems to be an important factor in determining phenotypic presentation of the offspring.[42] Eisner and colleagues[188] showed that the offspring of the female monkeys that were treated early (from gestational day 40) had impaired insulin secretion, whereas the offspring of the late-treated (from gestational day 100–115) females showed decrements in insulin sensitivity with increasing adiposity, but preserved normal insulin secretory function.[187] Early androgen–treated female monkeys also had increased visceral fat compared with controls, even after correcting for BMI and total body fat.

Risk for the Male Offspring

Multiple possible phenotypes for male offspring of women with PCOS have been proposed. Manifestations include increased body hair growth, premature male balding, and metabolic abnormalities, such as insulin resistance.[185] There seems to be an increased risk of coronary heart disease in male offspring of mothers with PCOS. The mechanism is not clear, but may involve insulin resistance that develops because of exposure to intrauterine hyperandrogenemia.[43,185] Adult male rhesus monkeys exposed to exogenous testosterone in utero have insulin resistance and impaired insulin secretion.[189]

Norman and colleagues[190] was the first study to report hyperinsulinemia in male first-degree relatives of women with PCOS, although only 5 families were studied. Recabarren and colleagues[185] recently conducted a controlled study of male offspring of women with PCOS (80 boys from women with PCOS vs 56 boys from a control population), to assess the metabolic profiles in different chronologic stages. They found that there was no significant difference in birth weight between the 2 groups; however, there was an increase in body weight in the male offspring of women with PCOS beginning in early infancy (2–3 months). This excessive body weight persisted into adulthood. In addition, insulin resistance developed during adulthood and was independent of body weight.

GENETICS/GENETIC COUNSELING

PCOS has strong familial clustering,[44–46] therefore, as mentioned previously, a genetic cause has been suspected. Several lines of evidence suggest that PCOS is heritable, and various approaches have been used in an attempt to define a specific genetic risk. Despite the extensive studies, the lack of reliable associations between genotype and phenotype raises the possibility that inheritance of PCOS, if any, is probably multifactorial and modified by environmental factors. Thus far, all initial examined candidate genes (**Box 4**), including those involving insulin signaling pathways, regulation of ovarian folliculogenesis, or theca cell androgenesis, have failed to maintain the strong linkage to a PCOS phenotype.[191]

The strongest evidence for an association of a single gene with PCOS is the nucleotide repeat microsatellite marker, D19S884, which lies within intron 55 of the fibrillin-3 gene. This gene is located on chromosome 19, close to the insulin receptor gene and resistin gene, and may relate to insulin resistance and β cell dysfunction.[192,198,209–211] However, because the m-RNA expression of fibrillin-3 in the human ovary is less pronounced than that of other fibrillins (1 or 2), it is still not clear whether or how fibrillin-3 contributes to the pathogenesis of PCOS. Recently, a new single-nucleotide polymorphism linked to PCOS in the pro-opiomelanocortin (POMC) gene

---

Box 4
PCOS candidate genes

Pathway and protein

Insulin secretion and action related

    Insulin receptor (INSR)[191,192]

    Insulin receptor substrate[193]

    Calpain 10 (CAPN10)[194,195]

    PPAR γ[196,197]

Gonadotropin secretion and action

    Follistatin (follistatinlike 3) (FST)[191]

    Activin receptor (ACTR2A)[191]

    Inhibin (INHBA, INHBB)[191]

Obesity and energy metabolism

    Pro-opiomelanocortin (POMC)[198,199]

Androgen biosynthesis

    Androgen receptor (AR)[200]

    Small glutamine-rich tetratricopeptide repeat (TPR)-containing protein α (SGTA)[201]

    Cytochrome P-450c17 (CYP17)[202]

    Cytochrome P-450c11α (CYP11 α)[203,204]

    Sex hormone-binding globulin (SHBG)[205,206]

Others, unclear role

    Feminization-1B (FEM 1A, FEM 1B)[207,208]

    Fibrillin-3 (FBN3)[192,198,209–211]

was also reported[198,199] but, once again, the significance of this finding remains unclear. Similar to other complex diseases, including diabetes, genetic research in PCOS remains challenging and is confounded by the extreme heterogeneity of PCOS.

SUMMARY

PCOS is a complex disease, characterized by variable phenotypes, and whose cause remains unclear. It is characterized by anovulation, hyperandrogenism, and polycystic ovaries. Infertility is commonly present and a variety of methods have been used successfully to achieve pregnancy in women with PCOS. Maintenance of pregnancy is complicated by a higher rate of premature spontaneous abortions and an increased risk of GDM, hypertension, and preeclampsia. However, with careful monitoring and treatment, the outcome of pregnancy in most women with PCOS is excellent.

REFERENCES

1. Stein IF, Leventhal ML. Amenorrhea associated with bilateral polycystic ovaries. Am J Obstet Gynecol 1935;29:181.
2. Rotterdam ESHRE/ASRM-Sponsored PCOS Consensus Workshop Group. Revised 2003 consensus on diagnostic criteria and long-term health risks related to polycystic ovary syndrome. Fertil Steril 2004;81:19.
3. Azziz R, Carmina E, Dewailly D, et al. Positions statement: criteria for defining polycystic ovary syndrome as a predominantly hyperandrogenic syndrome: an Androgen Excess Society guideline. J Clin Endocrinol Metab 2006;91:4237.
4. Azziz R, Woods KS, Reyna R, et al. The prevalence and features of the polycystic ovary syndrome in an unselected population. J Clin Endocrinol Metab 2004;89:2745.
5. Moll E, van der Veen F, van Wely M. The role of metformin in polycystic ovary syndrome: a systematic review. Hum Reprod Update 2007;13:527.
6. Franks S. Polycystic ovary syndrome. N Engl J Med 1995;333:853.
7. Knochenhauer ES, Key TJ, Kahsar-Miller M, et al. Prevalence of the polycystic ovary syndrome in unselected black and white women of the southeastern United States: a prospective study. J Clin Endocrinol Metab 1998;83:3078.
8. Ehrmann DA. Polycystic ovary syndrome. N Engl J Med 2005;352:1223.
9. Patel SS, Carr BR. Oocyte quality in adult polycystic ovary syndrome. Semin Reprod Med 2008;26:196.
10. Pasquali R, Pelusi C, Genghini S, et al. Obesity and reproductive disorders in women. Hum Reprod Update 2003;9:359.
11. Lake JK, Power C, Cole TJ. Women's reproductive health: the role of body mass index in early and adult life. Int J Obes Relat Metab Disord 1997;21:432.
12. Rich-Edwards JW, Goldman MB, Willett WC, et al. Adolescent body mass index and infertility caused by ovulatory disorder. Am J Obstet Gynecol 1994;171:171.
13. Dunaif A, Segal KR, Futterweit W, et al. Profound peripheral insulin resistance, independent of obesity, in polycystic ovary syndrome. Diabetes 1989;38:1165.
14. Dunaif A. Hyperandrogenic anovulation (PCOS): a unique disorder of insulin action associated with an increased risk of non-insulin-dependent diabetes mellitus. Am J Med 1995;98:33S.
15. Legro RS. Polycystic ovary syndrome. Long term sequelae and management. Minerva Ginecol 2002;54:97.
16. Peppard HR, Marfori J, Iuorno MJ, et al. Prevalence of polycystic ovary syndrome among premenopausal women with type 2 diabetes. Diabetes Care 2001;24:1050.

17. Seto-Young D, Paliou M, Schlosser J, et al. Direct thiazolidinedione action in the human ovary: insulin-independent and insulin-sensitizing effects on steroidogenesis and insulin-like growth factor binding protein-1 production. J Clin Endocrinol Metab 2005;90:6099.

18. Poretsky L, Grigorescu F, Seibel M, et al. Distribution and characterization of insulin and insulin-like growth factor I receptors in normal human ovary. J Clin Endocrinol Metab 1985;61:728.

19. Poretsky L, Cataldo NA, Rosenwaks Z, et al. The insulin-related ovarian regulatory system in health and disease. Endocr Rev 1999;20:535.

20. Poretsky L. Polycystic ovary syndrome. In: Principles of diabetes mellitus. 2nd edition. New York: Springer Verlag; 2010. p. 701. Chapter 4.

21. Maciel GA, Soares Junior JM, Alves da Motta EL, et al. Nonobese women with polycystic ovary syndrome respond better than obese women to treatment with metformin. Fertil Steril 2004;81:355.

22. Nestler JE. Regulation of the aromatase activity of human placental cytotrophoblasts by insulin, insulin-like growth factor-I, and -II. J Steroid Biochem Mol Biol 1993;44:449.

23. Burcelin R, Thorens B, Glauser M, et al. Gonadotropin-releasing hormone secretion from hypothalamic neurons: stimulation by insulin and potentiation by leptin. Endocrinology 2003;144:4484.

24. Poretsky L, Clemons J, Bogovich K. Hyperinsulinemia and human chorionic gonadotropin synergistically promote the growth of ovarian follicular cysts in rats. Metabolism 1992;41:903.

25. Moret M, Stettler R, Rodieux F, et al. Insulin modulation of luteinizing hormone secretion in normal female volunteers and lean polycystic ovary syndrome patients. Neuroendocrinology 2009;89:131.

26. Rosenfield RL, Bordini B. Evidence that obesity and androgens have independent and opposing effects on gonadotropin production from puberty to maturity. Brain Res 2010;1364:186–97.

27. Jain A, Polotsky AJ, Rochester D, et al. Pulsatile luteinizing hormone amplitude and progesterone metabolite excretion are reduced in obese women. J Clin Endocrinol Metab 2007;92:2468.

28. Poretsky L, Kalin MF. The gonadotropic function of insulin. Endocr Rev 1987;8:132.

29. Berga SL, Daniels TL. Can polycystic ovary syndrome exist without concomitant hypothalamic dysfunction? Semin Reprod Endocrinol 1997;15:169.

30. Berga SL, Guzick DS, Winters SJ. Increased luteinizing hormone and alpha-subunit secretion in women with hyperandrogenic anovulation. J Clin Endocrinol Metab 1993;77:895.

31. Morales AJ, Laughlin GA, Butzow T, et al. Insulin, somatotropic, and luteinizing hormone axes in lean and obese women with polycystic ovary syndrome: common and distinct features. J Clin Endocrinol Metab 1996;81:2854.

32. Venturoli S, Porcu E, Fabbri R, et al. Episodic pulsatile secretion of FSH, LH, prolactin, oestradiol, oestrone, and LH circadian variations in polycystic ovary syndrome. Clin Endocrinol (Oxf) 1988;28:93.

33. Barnes RB, Rosenfield RL, Burstein S, et al. Pituitary-ovarian responses to nafarelin testing in the polycystic ovary syndrome. N Engl J Med 1989;320:559.

34. Erickson GF, Magoffin DA, Garzo VG, et al. Granulosa cells of polycystic ovaries: are they normal or abnormal? Hum Reprod 1992;7:293.

35. Gilling-Smith C, Story H, Rogers V, et al. Evidence for a primary abnormality of thecal cell steroidogenesis in the polycystic ovary syndrome. Clin Endocrinol (Oxf) 1997;47:93.

36. Ibanez L, Hall JE, Potau N, et al. Ovarian 17-hydroxyprogesterone hyperresponsiveness to gonadotropin-releasing hormone (GnRH) agonist challenge in women with polycystic ovary syndrome is not mediated by luteinizing hormone hypersecretion: evidence from GnRH agonist and human chorionic gonadotropin stimulation testing. J Clin Endocrinol Metab 1996;81:4103.
37. Pierro E, Andreani CL, Lazzarin N, et al. Further evidence of increased aromatase activity in granulosa luteal cells from polycystic ovary. Hum Reprod 1997;12:1890.
38. Ibanez L, Potau N, Virdis R, et al. Postpubertal outcome in girls diagnosed of premature pubarche during childhood: increased frequency of functional ovarian hyperandrogenism. J Clin Endocrinol Metab 1993;76:1599.
39. Ibanez L, Potau N, Zampolli M, et al. Girls diagnosed with premature pubarche show an exaggerated ovarian androgen synthesis from the early stages of puberty: evidence from gonadotropin-releasing hormone agonist testing. Fertil Steril 1997;67:849.
40. Oppenheimer E, Linder B, DiMartino-Nardi J. Decreased insulin sensitivity in prepubertal girls with premature adrenarche and acanthosis nigricans. J Clin Endocrinol Metab 1995;80:614.
41. Poretsky L, Piper B. Insulin resistance, hypersecretion of LH, and a dual-defect hypothesis for the pathogenesis of polycystic ovary syndrome. Obstet Gynecol 1994;84:613.
42. Abbott DH, Barnett DK, Bruns CM, et al. Androgen excess fetal programming of female reproduction: a developmental aetiology for polycystic ovary syndrome? Hum Reprod Update 2005;11:357.
43. Barker DJ. Fetal programming of coronary heart disease. Trends Endocrinol Metab 2002;13:364.
44. Givens JR. Familial polycystic ovarian disease. Endocrinol Metab Clin North Am 1988;17:771.
45. Hague WM, Adams J, Reeders ST, et al. Familial polycystic ovaries: a genetic disease? Clin Endocrinol (Oxf) 1988;29:593.
46. Legro RS, Driscoll D, Strauss JF 3rd, et al. Evidence for a genetic basis for hyperandrogenemia in polycystic ovary syndrome. Proc Natl Acad Sci U S A 1998; 95:14956.
47. Wood JR, Dumesic DA, Abbott DH, et al. Molecular abnormalities in oocytes from women with polycystic ovary syndrome revealed by microarray analysis. J Clin Endocrinol Metab 2007;92:705.
48. Azziz R, Bradley EL Jr, Potter HD, et al. Chronic hyperinsulinemia and the adrenal androgen response to acute corticotropin-(1–24) stimulation in hyperandrogenic women. Am J Obstet Gynecol 1995;172:1251.
49. Goldzieher JW, Green JA. The polycystic ovary. I. Clinical and histologic features. J Clin Endocrinol Metab 1962;22:325.
50. Hull MG. Epidemiology of infertility and polycystic ovarian disease: endocrinological and demographic studies. Gynecol Endocrinol 1987;1:235.
51. Teede H, Deeks A, Moran L. Polycystic ovary syndrome: a complex condition with psychological, reproductive and metabolic manifestations that impacts on health across the lifespan. BMC Med 2010;8:41.
52. Yen. Reproductive endocrinology. 3rd edition. Philadelphia: Saunders; 1991. p. 593.
53. Clark AM, Thornley B, Tomlinson L, et al. Weight loss in obese infertile women results in improvement in reproductive outcome for all forms of fertility treatment. Hum Reprod 1998;13:1502.
54. Hollmann M, Runnebaum B, Gerhard I. Effects of weight loss on the hormonal profile in obese, infertile women. Hum Reprod 1996;11:1884.

55. Huber-Buchholz MM, Carey DG, Norman RJ. Restoration of reproductive potential by lifestyle modification in obese polycystic ovary syndrome: role of insulin sensitivity and luteinizing hormone. J Clin Endocrinol Metab 1999;84:1470.

56. Moran LJ, Brinkworth G, Noakes M, et al. Effects of lifestyle modification in polycystic ovarian syndrome. Reprod Biomed Online 2006;12:569.

57. Kiddy DS, Hamilton-Fairley D, Bush A, et al. Improvement in endocrine and ovarian function during dietary treatment of obese women with polycystic ovary syndrome. Clin Endocrinol (Oxf) 1992;36:105.

58. Homburg R. The management of infertility associated with polycystic ovary syndrome. Reprod Biol Endocrinol 2003;1:109.

59. Hamilton-Fairley D, Kiddy D, Anyaoku V, et al. Response of sex hormone binding globulin and insulin-like growth factor binding protein-1 to an oral glucose tolerance test in obese women with polycystic ovary syndrome before and after calorie restriction. Clin Endocrinol (Oxf) 1993;39:363.

60. Pettigrew R, Hamilton-Fairley D. Obesity and female reproductive function. Br Med Bull 1997;53:341.

61. Clark AM, Ledger W, Galletly C, et al. Weight loss results in significant improvement in pregnancy and ovulation rates in anovulatory obese women. Hum Reprod 1995;10:2705.

62. Hoeger KM, Kochman L, Wixom N, et al. A randomized, 48-week, placebo-controlled trial of intensive lifestyle modification and/or metformin therapy in overweight women with polycystic ovary syndrome: a pilot study. Fertil Steril 2004;82:421.

63. Jacobsen DJ, Donnelly JE, Snyder-Heelan K, et al. Adherence and attrition with intermittent and continuous exercise in overweight women. Int J Sports Med 2003;24:459.

64. Greenblatt RB, Jullien M. [Stimulation of ovulation]. Concours Med 1965;87:1401 [in French].

65. Yildiz BO, Chang W, Azziz R. Polycystic ovary syndrome and ovulation induction. Minerva Ginecol 2003;55:425.

66. Zain MM, Jamaluddin R, Ibrahim A, et al. Comparison of clomiphene citrate, metformin, or the combination of both for first-line ovulation induction, achievement of pregnancy, and live birth in Asian women with polycystic ovary syndrome: a randomized controlled trial. Fertil Steril 2009;91:514.

67. Gorlitsky GA, Kase NG, Speroff L. Ovulation and pregnancy rates with clomiphene citrate. Obstet Gynecol 1978;51:265.

68. Imani B, Eijkemans MJ, te Velde ER, et al. Predictors of patients remaining anovulatory during clomiphene citrate induction of ovulation in normogonadotropic oligoamenorrheic infertility. J Clin Endocrinol Metab 1998;83:2361.

69. Imani B, Eijkemans MJ, te Velde ER, et al. Predictors of chances to conceive in ovulatory patients during clomiphene citrate induction of ovulation in normogonadotropic oligoamenorrheic infertility. J Clin Endocrinol Metab 1999;84:1617.

70. Thessaloniki ESHRE/ASRM-Sponsored PCOS Consensus Workshop Group. Consensus on infertility treatment related to polycystic ovary syndrome. Hum Reprod 2008;23:462.

71. Speroff L. Clinical gynecologic endocrinology and infertility. 7th edition. Philadelphia: Lippincott Williams & Wilkins; 2005. p. 1180.

72. Nestler JE, Stovall D, Akhter N, et al. Strategies for the use of insulin-sensitizing drugs to treat infertility in women with polycystic ovary syndrome. Fertil Steril 2002;77:209.

73. Butzow TL, Kettel LM, Yen SS. Clomiphene citrate reduces serum insulin-like growth factor I and increases sex hormone-binding globulin levels in women with polycystic ovary syndrome. Fertil Steril 1995;63:1200.

74. Nestler JE, Jakubowicz DJ, Evans WS, et al. Effects of metformin on sponta-neous and clomiphene-induced ovulation in the polycystic ovary syndrome. N Engl J Med 1998;338:1876.
75. Gonen Y, Casper RF. Sonographic determination of a possible adverse effect of clomiphene citrate on endometrial growth. Hum Reprod 1990;5:670.
76. Brzechffa PR, Daneshmand S, Buyalos RP. Sequential clomiphene citrate and human menopausal gonadotrophin with intrauterine insemination: the effect of patient age on clinical outcome. Hum Reprod 1998;13:2110.
77. Wang CF, Gemzell C. The use of human gonadotropins for the induction of ovulation in women with polycystic ovarian disease. Fertil Steril 1980;33:479.
78. White DM, Polson DW, Kiddy D, et al. Induction of ovulation with low-dose gonadotropins in polycystic ovary syndrome: an analysis of 109 pregnancies in 225 women. J Clin Endocrinol Metab 1996;81:3821.
79. Christin-Maitre S, Hugues JN. A comparative randomized multicentric study comparing the step-up versus step-down protocol in polycystic ovary syndrome. Hum Reprod 2003;18:1626.
80. De Leo V, la Marca A, Ditto A, et al. Effects of metformin on gonadotropin-induced ovulation in women with polycystic ovary syndrome. Fertil Steril 1999; 72:282.
81. Yarali H, Yildiz BO, Demirol A, et al. Co-administration of metformin during rFSH treatment in patients with clomiphene citrate-resistant polycystic ovarian syndrome: a prospective randomized trial. Hum Reprod 2002;17:289.
82. Fleming R, Haxton MJ, Hamilton MP, et al. Successful treatment of infertile women with oligomenorrhoea using a combination of an LHRH agonist and exogenous gonadotrophins. Br J Obstet Gynaecol 1985;92:369.
83. European and Middle East Orgalutran Study Group. Comparable clinical outcome using the GnRH antagonist ganirelix or a long protocol of the GnRH agonist triptorelin for the prevention of premature LH surges in women under-going ovarian stimulation. Hum Reprod 2001;16:644.
84. Barmat LI, Chantilis SJ, Hurst BS, et al. A randomized prospective trial comparing gonadotropin-releasing hormone (GnRH) antagonist/recombinant follicle-stimulating hormone (rFSH) versus GnRH-agonist/rFSH in women pre-treated with oral contraceptives before in vitro fertilization. Fertil Steril 2005; 83:321.
85. Legro RS, Barnhart HX, Schlaff WD, et al. Clomiphene, metformin, or both for infertility in the polycystic ovary syndrome. N Engl J Med 2007;356:551.
86. Velazquez EM, Mendoza S, Hamer T, et al. Metformin therapy in polycystic ovary syndrome reduces hyperinsulinemia, insulin resistance, hyperandrogenemia, and systolic blood pressure, while facilitating normal menses and pregnancy. Metabolism 1994;43:647.
87. Ng EH, Wat NM, Ho PC. Effects of metformin on ovulation rate, hormonal and metabolic profiles in women with clomiphene-resistant polycystic ovaries: a randomized, double-blinded placebo-controlled trial. Hum Reprod 2001;16: 1625.
88. Ning J, Clemmons DR. AMP-activated protein kinase inhibits IGF-I signaling and protein synthesis in vascular smooth muscle cells via stimulation of insulin receptor substrate 1 S794 and tuberous sclerosis 2 S1345 phosphorylation. Mol Endocrinol 2010;24:1218.
89. Nestler JE, Jakubowicz DJ. Decreases in ovarian cytochrome P450c17 alpha activity and serum free testosterone after reduction of insulin secretion in poly-cystic ovary syndrome. N Engl J Med 1996;335:617.

90. Stadtmauer LA, Toma SK, Riehl RM, et al. Metformin treatment of patients with polycystic ovary syndrome undergoing in vitro fertilization improves outcomes and is associated with modulation of the insulin-like growth factors. Fertil Steril 2001;75:505.

91. Palomba S, Orio F Jr, Falbo A, et al. Prospective parallel randomized, double-blind, double-dummy controlled clinical trial comparing clomiphene citrate and metformin as the first-line treatment for ovulation induction in nonobese anovulatory women with polycystic ovary syndrome. J Clin Endocrinol Metab 2005;90:4068.

92. Neveu N, Granger L, St-Michel P, et al. Comparison of clomiphene citrate, metformin, or the combination of both for first-line ovulation induction and achievement of pregnancy in 154 women with polycystic ovary syndrome. Fertil Steril 2007;87:113.

93. Moll E, Bossuyt PM, Korevaar JC, et al. Effect of clomifene citrate plus metformin and clomifene citrate plus placebo on induction of ovulation in women with newly diagnosed polycystic ovary syndrome: randomised double blind clinical trial. BMJ 2006;332:1485.

94. Creanga AA, Bradley HM, McCormick C, et al. Use of metformin in polycystic ovary syndrome: a metaanalysis. Obstet Gynecol 2008;111:959.

95. Imani B, Eijkemans MJ, te Velde ER, et al. A nomogram to predict the probability of live birth after clomiphene citrate induction of ovulation in normogonadotropic oligoamenorrheic infertility. Fertil Steril 2002;77:91.

96. Rausch ME, Legro RS, Barnhart HX, et al. Predictors of pregnancy in women with polycystic ovary syndrome. J Clin Endocrinol Metab 2009;94:3458.

97. Nader S. Reproductive endocrinology: live birth prediction in polycystic ovary syndrome. Nat Rev Endocrinol 2010;6:64.

98. Coetzee EJ, Jackson WP. Metformin in management of pregnant insulin-independent diabetics. Diabetologia 1979;16:241.

99. Dunaif A, Scott D, Finegood D, et al. The insulin-sensitizing agent troglitazone improves metabolic and reproductive abnormalities in the polycystic ovary syndrome. J Clin Endocrinol Metab 1996;81:3299.

100. Mitwally MF, Kuscu NK, Yalcinkaya TM. High ovulatory rates with use of troglitazone in clomiphene-resistant women with polycystic ovary syndrome. Hum Reprod 1999;14:2700.

101. Azziz R, Ehrmann D, Legro RS, et al. Troglitazone improves ovulation and hirsutism in the polycystic ovary syndrome: a multicenter, double blind, placebo-controlled trial. J Clin Endocrinol Metab 2001;86:1626.

102. Belli SH, Graffigna MN, Oneto A, et al. Effect of rosiglitazone on insulin resistance, growth factors, and reproductive disturbances in women with polycystic ovary syndrome. Fertil Steril 2004;81:624.

103. Glueck CJ, Moreira A, Goldenberg N, et al. Pioglitazone and metformin in obese women with polycystic ovary syndrome not optimally responsive to metformin. Hum Reprod 2003;18:1618.

104. Nissen SE, Wolski K. Rosiglitazone revisited: an updated metaanalysis of risk for myocardial infarction and cardiovascular mortality. Arch Intern Med 2010; 170(14):1191–201.

105. Komar CM, Braissant O, Wahli W, et al. Expression and localization of PPARs in the rat ovary during follicular development and the periovulatory period. Endocrinology 2001;142:4831.

106. Seto-Young D, Avtanski D, Strizhevsky M, et al. Interactions among peroxisome proliferator activated receptor-gamma, insulin signaling pathways, and

steroidogenic acute regulatory protein in human ovarian cells. J Clin Endocrinol Metab 2007;92:2232.

107. Gasic S, Nagamani M, Green A, et al. Troglitazone is a competitive inhibitor of 3beta-hydroxysteroid dehydrogenase enzyme in the ovary. Am J Obstet Gynecol 2001;184:575.

108. Mu YM, Yanase T, Nishi Y, et al. Insulin sensitizer, troglitazone, directly inhibits aromatase activity in human ovarian granulosa cells. Biochem Biophys Res Commun 2000;271:710.

109. DeFronzo RA, Ratner RE, Han J, et al. Effects of exenatide (exendin-4) on glycemic control and weight over 30 weeks in metformin-treated patients with type 2 diabetes. Diabetes Care 2005;28:1092.

110. Gama R, Norris F, Wright J, et al. The entero-insular axis in polycystic ovarian syndrome. Ann Clin Biochem 1996;33(Pt 3):190.

111. Vrbikova J, Hill M, Bendlova B, et al. Incretin levels in polycystic ovary syndrome. Eur J Endocrinol 2008;159:121.

112. Vilsboll T, Krarup T, Deacon CF, et al. Reduced postprandial concentrations of intact biologically active glucagon-like peptide 1 in type 2 diabetic patients. Diabetes 2001;50:609.

113. MacLusky NJ, Cook S, Scrocchi L, et al. Neuroendocrine function and response to stress in mice with complete disruption of glucagon-like peptide-1 receptor signaling. Endocrinology 2000;141:752.

114. Jeibmann A, Zahedi S, Simoni M, et al. Glucagon-like peptide-1 reduces the pulsatile component of testosterone secretion in healthy males. Eur J Clin Invest 2005;35:565.

115. Elkind-Hirsch K, Marrioneaux O, Bhushan M, et al. Comparison of single and combined treatment with exenatide and metformin on menstrual cyclicity in overweight women with polycystic ovary syndrome. J Clin Endocrinol Metab 2008;93:2670.

116. Mitwally MF, Casper RF. Use of an aromatase inhibitor for induction of ovulation in patients with an inadequate response to clomiphene citrate. Fertil Steril 2001; 75:305.

117. Sher G, Keskintepe L, Keskintepe M, et al. Genetic analysis of human embryos by metaphase comparative genomic hybridization (mCGH) improves efficiency of IVF by increasing embryo implantation rate and reducing multiple pregnancies and spontaneous miscarriages. Fertil Steril 2009;92:1886.

118. Badawy A, Abdel Aal I, Abulatta M. Clomiphene citrate or anastrozole for ovulation induction in women with polycystic ovary syndrome? A prospective controlled trial. Fertil Steril 2009;92:860.

119. Health Canada endorsed important safety information on Femara (letrozole) [letter]. 2005. Available at: http://www.hc-sc.gc.ca/dhp-mps/medeff/advisories-avis/public/_2005/femara_pc-cp-eng.php. Accessed August 2, 2011.

120. Daly DC, Walters CA, Soto-Albors CE, et al. A randomized study of dexamethasone in ovulation induction with clomiphene citrate. Fertil Steril 1984;41:844.

121. Evron S, Navot D, Laufer N, et al. Induction of ovulation with combined human gonadotropins and dexamethasone in women with polycystic ovarian disease. Fertil Steril 1983;40:183.

122. Lobo RA, Paul W, March CM, et al. Clomiphene and dexamethasone in women unresponsive to clomiphene alone. Obstet Gynecol 1982;60:497.

123. Bider D, Amoday I, Tur-Kaspa I, et al. The addition of a glucocorticoid to the protocol of programmed oocyte retrieval for in-vitro fertilization–a randomized study. Hum Reprod 1996;11:1606.

124. Rein MS, Jackson KV, Sable DB, et al. Dexamethasone during ovulation induction for in-vitro fertilization: a pilot study. Hum Reprod 1996;11:253.

125. Fitzgerald C, Elstein M, Spona J. Effect of age on the response of the hypothalamo-pituitary-ovarian axis to a combined oral contraceptive. Fertil Steril 1999;71:1079.

126. Martin KA, Chang RJ, Ehrmann DA, et al. Evaluation and treatment of hirsutism in premenopausal women: an endocrine society clinical practice guideline. J Clin Endocrinol Metab 2008;93:1105.

127. Swiglo BA, Cosma M, Flynn DN, et al. Clinical review: antiandrogens for the treatment of hirsutism: a systematic review and metaanalyses of randomized controlled trials. J Clin Endocrinol Metab 2008;93:1153.

128. Townsend KA, Marlowe KF. Relative safety and efficacy of finasteride for treatment of hirsutism. Ann Pharmacother 2004;38:1070.

129. Armar NA, McGarrigle HH, Honour J, et al. Laparoscopic ovarian diathermy in the management of anovulatory infertility in women with polycystic ovaries: endocrine changes and clinical outcome. Fertil Steril 1990;53:45.

130. Gurgan T, Kisnisci H, Yarali H, et al. Evaluation of adhesion formation after laparoscopic treatment of polycystic ovarian disease. Fertil Steril 1991;56:1176.

131. Eijkemans MJ, Polinder S, Mulders AG, et al. Individualized cost-effective conventional ovulation induction treatment in normogonadotrophic anovulatory infertility (WHO group 2). Hum Reprod 2005;20:2830.

132. Damario MA, Barmat L, Liu HC, et al. Dual suppression with oral contraceptives and gonadotrophin releasing-hormone agonists improves in-vitro fertilization outcome in high responder patients. Hum Reprod 1997;12:2359.

133. Lainas TG, Sfontouris IA, Zorzovilis IZ, et al. Flexible GnRH antagonist protocol versus GnRH agonist long protocol in patients with polycystic ovary syndrome treated for IVF: a prospective randomised controlled trial (RCT). Hum Reprod 2010;25:683.

134. Mulders AG, Laven JS, Imani B, et al. IVF outcome in anovulatory infertility (WHO group 2)–including polycystic ovary syndrome–following previous unsuccessful ovulation induction. Reprod Biomed Online 2003;7:50.

135. Sengoku K, Tamate K, Takuma N, et al. The chromosomal normality of unfertilized oocytes from patients with polycystic ovarian syndrome. Hum Reprod 1997;12:474.

136. Kodama H, Fukuda J, Karube H, et al. High incidence of embryo transfer cancellations in patients with polycystic ovarian syndrome. Hum Reprod 1995;10:1962.

137. Lin YH, Seow KM, Hsieh BC, et al. Application of GnRH antagonist in combination with clomiphene citrate and hMG for patients with exaggerated ovarian response in previous IVF/ICSI cycles. J Assist Reprod Genet 2007;24:331.

138. Heijnen EM, Eijkemans MJ, Hughes EG, et al. A metaanalysis of outcomes of conventional IVF in women with polycystic ovary syndrome. Hum Reprod Update 2006;12:13.

139. Kdous M, Chaker A, Bouyahia M, et al. Increased risk of early pregnancy loss and lower live birth rate with GNRH antagonist vs. long GNRH agonist protocol in PCOS women undergoing controlled ovarian hyperstimulation. Tunis Med 2009;87:834 [in French].

140. Engmann L, DiLuigi A, Schmidt D, et al. The use of gonadotropin-releasing hormone (GnRH) agonist to induce oocyte maturation after cotreatment with GnRH antagonist in high-risk patients undergoing in vitro fertilization prevents the risk of ovarian hyperstimulation syndrome: a prospective randomized controlled study. Fertil Steril 2008;89:84.

141. Griesinger G, Diedrich K, Tarlatzis BC, et al. GnRH-antagonists in ovarian stimulation for IVF in patients with poor response to gonadotrophins, polycystic ovary syndrome, and risk of ovarian hyperstimulation: a metaanalysis. Reprod Biomed Online 2006;13:628.
142. Tso LO, Costello MF, Albuquerque LE, et al. Metformin treatment before and during IVF or ICSI in women with polycystic ovary syndrome. Cochrane Database Syst Rev 2009;2:CD006105.
143. Dale PO, Tanbo T, Abyholm T. In-vitro fertilization in infertile women with the polycystic ovarian syndrome. Hum Reprod 1991;6:238.
144. Gonen Y, Balakier H, Powell W, et al. Use of gonadotropin-releasing hormone agonist to trigger follicular maturation for in vitro fertilization. J Clin Endocrinol Metab 1990;71:918.
145. Chian RC, Buckett WM, Tulandi T, et al. Prospective randomized study of human chorionic gonadotrophin priming before immature oocyte retrieval from unstimulated women with polycystic ovarian syndrome. Hum Reprod 2000;15:165.
146. Chian RC. In-vitro maturation of immature oocytes for infertile women with PCOS. Reprod Biomed Online 2004;8:547.
147. Lin YH, Hwang JL, Huang LW, et al. Combination of FSH priming and hCG priming for in-vitro maturation of human oocytes. Hum Reprod 2003;18:1632.
148. Siristatidis CS, Maheshwari A, Bhattacharya S. In vitro maturation in sub fertile women with polycystic ovarian syndrome undergoing assisted reproduction. Cochrane Database Syst Rev 2009;1:CD006606.
149. Homburg R, Armar NA, Eshel A, et al. Influence of serum luteinising hormone concentrations on ovulation, conception, and early pregnancy loss in polycystic ovary syndrome. BMJ 1988;297:1024.
150. Jakubowicz DJ, Iuorno MJ, Jakubowicz S, et al. Effects of metformin on early pregnancy loss in the polycystic ovary syndrome. J Clin Endocrinol Metab 2002;87:524.
151. Sagle M, Bishop K, Ridley N, et al. Recurrent early miscarriage and polycystic ovaries. BMJ 1988;297:1027.
152. Fedorcsak P, Storeng R, Dale PO, et al. Obesity is a risk factor for early pregnancy loss after IVF or ICSI. Acta Obstet Gynecol Scand 2000;79:43.
153. Atiomo WU, Bates SA, Condon JE, et al. The plasminogen activator system in women with polycystic ovary syndrome. Fertil Steril 1998;69:236.
154. Jakubowicz DJ, Seppala M, Jakubowicz S, et al. Insulin reduction with metformin increases luteal phase serum glycodelin and insulin-like growth factor-binding protein 1 concentrations and enhances uterine vascularity and blood flow in the polycystic ovary syndrome. J Clin Endocrinol Metab 2001;86:1126.
155. Clifford K, Rai R, Watson H, et al. Does suppressing luteinising hormone secretion reduce the miscarriage rate? Results of a randomised controlled trial. BMJ 1996;312:1508.
156. Glueck CJ, Phillips H, Cameron D, et al. Continuing metformin throughout pregnancy in women with polycystic ovary syndrome appears to safely reduce first-trimester spontaneous abortion: a pilot study. Fertil Steril 2001;75:46.
157. Holte J, Gennarelli G, Wide L, et al. High prevalence of polycystic ovaries and associated clinical, endocrine, and metabolic features in women with previous gestational diabetes mellitus. J Clin Endocrinol Metab 1998;83:1143.
158. Mikola M, Hiilesmaa V, Halttunen M, et al. Obstetric outcome in women with polycystic ovarian syndrome. Hum Reprod 2001;16:226.
159. Radon PA, McMahon MJ, Meyer WR. Impaired glucose tolerance in pregnant women with polycystic ovary syndrome. Obstet Gynecol 1999;94:194.

160. Haakova L, Cibula D, Rezabek K, et al. Pregnancy outcome in women with PCOS and in controls matched by age and weight. Hum Reprod 2003;18:1438.
161. Urman B, Sarac E, Dogan L, et al. Pregnancy in infertile PCOD patients. Complications and outcome. J Reprod Med 1997;42:501.
162. Boomsma CM, Eijkemans MJ, Hughes EG, et al. A metaanalysis of pregnancy outcomes in women with polycystic ovary syndrome. Hum Reprod Update 2006;12:673.
163. Toulis KA, Goulis DG, Kolibianakis EM, et al. Risk of gestational diabetes mellitus in women with polycystic ovary syndrome: a systematic review and a metaanalysis. Fertil Steril 2009;92:667.
164. Chu SY, Abe K, Hall LR, et al. Gestational diabetes mellitus: all Asians are not alike. Prev Med 2009;49:265.
165. Glueck CJ, Wang P, Kobayashi S, et al. Metformin therapy throughout pregnancy reduces the development of gestational diabetes in women with polycystic ovary syndrome. Fertil Steril 2002;77:520.
166. Nawaz FH, Khalid R, Naru T, et al. Does continuous use of metformin throughout pregnancy improve pregnancy outcomes in women with polycystic ovarian syndrome? J Obstet Gynaecol Res 2008;34:832.
167. Seely EW, Solomon CG. Insulin resistance and its potential role in pregnancy-induced hypertension. J Clin Endocrinol Metab 2003;88:2393.
168. Steegers EA, von Dadelszen P, Duvekot JJ, et al. Pre-eclampsia. Lancet 2010; 376:631.
169. Diamant YZ, Rimon E, Evron S. High incidence of preeclamptic toxemia in patients with polycystic ovarian disease. Eur J Obstet Gynecol Reprod Biol 1982;14:199.
170. Gjonnaess H. The course and outcome of pregnancy after ovarian electrocautery in women with polycystic ovarian syndrome: the influence of body-weight. Br J Obstet Gynaecol 1989;96:714.
171. de Vries MJ, Dekker GA, Schoemaker J. Higher risk of preeclampsia in the polycystic ovary syndrome. A case control study. Eur J Obstet Gynecol Reprod Biol 1998;76:91.
172. Hamasaki T, Yasuhi I, Hirai M, et al. Hyperinsulinemia increases the risk of gestational hypertension. Int J Gynaecol Obstet 1996;55:141.
173. Rowe JW, Young JB, Minaker KL, et al. Effect of insulin and glucose infusions on sympathetic nervous system activity in normal man. Diabetes 1981;30:219.
174. Fridstrom M, Nisell H, Sjoblom P, et al. Are women with polycystic ovary syndrome at an increased risk of pregnancy-induced hypertension and/or preeclampsia? Hypertens Pregnancy 1999;18:73.
175. Hales CN, Barker DJ. The thrifty phenotype hypothesis. Br Med Bull 2001;60:5.
176. Silverman BL, Rizzo TA, Cho NH, et al. Long-term effects of the intrauterine environment. The Northwestern University Diabetes in Pregnancy Center. Diabetes Care 1998;21(Suppl 2):B142.
177. Legro RS, Roller RL, Dodson WC, et al. Associations of birthweight and gestational age with reproductive and metabolic phenotypes in women with polycystic ovarian syndrome and their first-degree relatives. J Clin Endocrinol Metab 2010;95:789.
178. Recabarren SE, Padmanabhan V, Codner E, et al. Postnatal developmental consequences of altered insulin sensitivity in female sheep treated prenatally with testosterone. Am J Physiol Endocrinol Metab 2005;289:E801.
179. Ibanez L, Jaramillo A, Enriquez G, et al. Polycystic ovaries after precocious pubarche: relation to prenatal growth. Hum Reprod 2007;22:395.

180. Ibanez L, Jimenez R, de Zegher F. Early puberty-menarche after precocious pubarche: relation to prenatal growth. Pediatrics 2006;117:117.
181. Sir-Petermann T, Hitchsfeld C, Maliqueo M, et al. Birth weight in offspring of mothers with polycystic ovarian syndrome. Hum Reprod 2005;20:2122.
182. Crosignani PG, Nicolosi AE. Polycystic ovarian disease: heritability and heterogeneity. Hum Reprod Update 2001;7:3.
183. Kahsar-Miller MD, Nixon C, Boots LR, et al. Prevalence of polycystic ovary syndrome (PCOS) in first-degree relatives of patients with PCOS. Fertil Steril 2001;75:53.
184. Sir-Petermann T, Codner E, Perez V, et al. Metabolic and reproductive features before and during puberty in daughters of women with polycystic ovary syndrome. J Clin Endocrinol Metab 2009;94:1923.
185. Recabarren SE, Smith R, Rios R, et al. Metabolic profile in sons of women with polycystic ovary syndrome. J Clin Endocrinol Metab 2008;93:1820.
186. Sir-Petermann T, Maliqueo M, Codner E, et al. Early metabolic derangements in daughters of women with polycystic ovary syndrome. J Clin Endocrinol Metab 2007;92:4637.
187. Eisner JR, Dumesic DA, Kemnitz JW, et al. Timing of prenatal androgen excess determines differential impairment in insulin secretion and action in adult female rhesus monkeys. J Clin Endocrinol Metab 2000;85:1206.
188. Eisner JR, Dumesic DA, Kemnitz JW, et al. Increased adiposity in female rhesus monkeys exposed to androgen excess during early gestation. Obes Res 2003; 11:279.
189. Bruns CM, Baum ST, Colman RJ, et al. Insulin resistance and impaired insulin secretion in prenatally androgenized male rhesus monkeys. J Clin Endocrinol Metab 2004;89:6218.
190. Norman RJ, Masters S, Hague W. Hyperinsulinemia is common in family members of women with polycystic ovary syndrome. Fertil Steril 1996;66:942.
191. Urbanek M, Legro RS, Driscoll DA, et al. Thirty-seven candidate genes for polycystic ovary syndrome: strongest evidence for linkage is with follistatin. Proc Natl Acad Sci U S A 1999;96:8573.
192. Tucci S, Futterweit W, Concepcion ES, et al. Evidence for association of polycystic ovary syndrome in Caucasian women with a marker at the insulin receptor gene locus. J Clin Endocrinol Metab 2001;86:446.
193. Ehrmann DA, Tang X, Yoshiuchi I, et al. Relationship of insulin receptor substrate-1 and -2 genotypes to phenotypic features of polycystic ovary syndrome. J Clin Endocrinol Metab 2002;87:4297.
194. Ehrmann DA, Schwarz PE, Hara M, et al. Relationship of calpain-10 genotype to phenotypic features of polycystic ovary syndrome. J Clin Endocrinol Metab 2002;87:1669.
195. Gonzalez A, Abril E, Roca A, et al. Specific CAPN10 gene haplotypes influence the clinical profile of polycystic ovary patients. J Clin Endocrinol Metab 2003;88: 5529.
196. Hara M, Alcoser SY, Qaadir A, et al. Insulin resistance is attenuated in women with polycystic ovary syndrome with the Pro(12)Ala polymorphism in the PPAR-gamma gene. J Clin Endocrinol Metab 2002;87:772.
197. Yilmaz M, Ergun MA, Karakoc A, et al. Pro12Ala polymorphism of the peroxisome proliferator-activated receptor-gamma gene in women with polycystic ovary syndrome. Gynecol Endocrinol 2006;22:336.
198. Ewens KG, Stewart DR, Ankener W, et al. Family-based analysis of candidate genes for polycystic ovary syndrome. J Clin Endocrinol Metab 2010;95:2306.

199. Eyvazzadeh AD, Pennington KP, Pop-Busui R, et al. The role of the endogenous opioid system in polycystic ovary syndrome. Fertil Steril 2009;92:1.

200. Hickey T, Chandy A, Norman RJ. The androgen receptor CAG repeat polymorphism and X-chromosome inactivation in Australian Caucasian women with infertility related to polycystic ovary syndrome. J Clin Endocrinol Metab 2002; 87:161.

201. Goodarzi MO, Xu N, Cui J, et al. Small glutamine-rich tetratricopeptide repeat-containing protein alpha (SGTA), a candidate gene for polycystic ovary syndrome. Hum Reprod 2008;23:1214.

202. Diamanti-Kandarakis E, Bartzis MI, Zapanti ED, et al. Polymorphism T–>C (-34 bp) of gene CYP17 promoter in Greek patients with polycystic ovary syndrome. Fertil Steril 1999;71:431.

203. Gaasenbeek M, Powell BL, Sovio U, et al. Large-scale analysis of the relationship between CYP11A promoter variation, polycystic ovarian syndrome, and serum testosterone. J Clin Endocrinol Metab 2004;89:2408.

204. Gharani N, Waterworth DM, Batty S, et al. Association of the steroid synthesis gene CYP11a with polycystic ovary syndrome and hyperandrogenism. Hum Mol Genet 1997;6:397.

205. Cousin P, Calemard-Michel L, Lejeune H, et al. Influence of SHBG gene pentanucleotide TAAAA repeat and D327N polymorphism on serum sex hormone-binding globulin concentration in hirsute women. J Clin Endocrinol Metab 2004;89:917.

206. Xita N, Tsatsoulis A, Chatzikyriakidou A, et al. Association of the (TAAAA)n repeat polymorphism in the sex hormone-binding globulin (SHBG) gene with polycystic ovary syndrome and relation to SHBG serum levels. J Clin Endocrinol Metab 2003;88:5976.

207. Goodarzi MO, Maher JF, Cui J, et al. FEM1A and FEM1B: novel candidate genes for polycystic ovary syndrome. Hum Reprod 2008;23:2842.

208. Maher JF, Hines RS, Futterweit W, et al. FEM1A is a candidate gene for polycystic ovary syndrome. Gynecol Endocrinol 2005;21:330.

209. Prodoehl MJ, Hatzirodos N, Irving-Rodgers HF, et al. Genetic and gene expression analyses of the polycystic ovary syndrome candidate gene fibrillin-3 and other fibrillin family members in human ovaries. Mol Hum Reprod 2009;15:829.

210. Urbanek M, Sam S, Legro RS, et al. Identification of a polycystic ovary syndrome susceptibility variant in fibrillin-3 and association with a metabolic phenotype. J Clin Endocrinol Metab 2007;92:4191.

211. Urbanek M, Woodroffe A, Ewens KG, et al. Candidate gene region for polycystic ovary syndrome on chromosome 19p13.2. J Clin Endocrinol Metab 2005;90:6623.

Obesity and Reproductive Dysfunction in Women

Lisa J. Moran, BND (Hons), PhD[a],*,
Jodie Dodd, MBBS, PhD, FRANZCOG, CMFM[b], Victoria Nisenblat, MD[c],
Robert J. Norman, MBChB (Hons), MD, FRANZCOG,
FRCPA, FRCPath, FRCOG, CREI[a]

KEYWORDS

- Obesity • Fertility • Pregnancy • Polycystic ovary syndrome

Obesity represents a significant and increasing health problem and is reported to be the sixth most important risk factor contributing to burden of disease worldwide.[1] There are 3.24 million Australians who are obese (1.72 million or 17% of all women), with a further 25% of women classified as overweight.[2] These figures are similar in the United States, where it is estimated that 66% of adults are overweight or obese.[3] The prevalence of overweight and obesity increased by almost 2.5 times between 1980 and 2000 among women of reproductive age.[4] Obesity presents a significant financial cost to the individual, society, and government. Data from the United States indicates that the treatment of obesity and its related complications rose to $147 billion in 2006, representing 10% of the country's total expenditure on health care.[5] Although the negative effects of obesity on metabolic mortality and morbidity and quality of life are well recognized, obesity additionally interferes with pubertal development, reduces chances for conception, and increases risk of complications in pregnancy for both mother and fetus.

MECHANISMS OF OBESITY AND REPRODUCTIVE DYSFUNCTION

The adverse effects of obesity on reproductive function begin early in life. Childhood and adolescent obesity may modulate timing of puberty and reproductive maturation

Financial disclosures and conflict of interest: the authors have nothing to disclose.
[a] The Robinson Institute, Research Centre for Reproductive Health, School of Paediatrics and Reproductive Health, University of Adelaide, 55 King William Road, North Adelaide, South Australia 5005, Australia
[b] The Robinson Institute, Australian Research Centre for Health of Women and Babies, School of Paediatrics and Reproductive Health, University of Adelaide, 55 King William Road, North Adelaide, South Australia 5005, Australia
[c] The Robinson Institute, School of Paediatrics and Reproductive Health, University of Adelaide, 55 King William Road, North Adelaide, South Australia 5005, Australia
* Corresponding author.
E-mail address: lisa.moran@adelaide.edu.au

Endocrinol Metab Clin N Am 40 (2011) 895–906
doi:10.1016/j.ecl.2011.08.006
0889-8529/11/$ – see front matter © 2011 Elsevier Inc. All rights reserved.

and are linked to earlier puberty in girls.[6] Polycystic ovary syndrome (PCOS) is a common condition affecting 4% to 18% of reproductive-aged women,[7] based on diagnostic features of ultrasonography, hyperandrogenism, or anovulatory irregular periods.[8] Obesity, particularly of abdominal distribution, may be increased in PCOS and worsens clinical reproductive and hormonal features such as menstrual dysfunction and hyperandrogenism.[9] Insulin resistance, with compensatory hyperinsulinemia and hyperandrogenemia, are key contributors to obesity-induced anovulation.[10] This anovulation is believed to be mediated through insulin-enhancing ovarian androgen production as well as a reduction in hepatic sex-hormone binding globulin production. These biochemical features can be present even in the absence of PCOS, with both follicular fluid insulin and markers of bioavailable androgens correlating with body mass index (BMI, calculated as weight in kilograms divided by the square of height in meters) in infertile women.[11] Increased androgens lead to premature follicular atresia, inhibited follicular maturation, and anovulation.[12] Even in the absence of PCOS, the presence of insulin resistance and hyperandrogenism in women may contribute to infertility.

Fertility impairments in obese women cannot be entirely explained by ovulation disorders. A significant decline in fecundity is also reported in ovulating obese women,[13,14] attributed to effects on oocyte development, embryo development, and endometrial receptivity.[15,16] Additional hormonal aberrations in overweight women that may contribute to impairments in reproductive function include adipokines such as such as leptin, tumor necrosis factor alpha (TNF-α), and interleukin-6 (IL-6), which antagonize the effect of insulin, thereby leading to insulin resistance, which sensitizes the body to the effects of insulin (such as adiponectin).[17-19] Alterations in adipokines or other additional factors associated with glucose metabolism or inflammatory markers in pregnancy are less well defined but may provide a plausible explanation for the observed increase in both gestational diabetes mellitus and preeclampsia among obese pregnant women.[20]

OBESITY AND FERTILITY

Obese women are 3 times more likely to present with infertility compared with women of normal BMI,[21] with the infertility rate in obese women increasing by 4% per BMI unit.[13] Young obese women are less likely to conceive within 12 months of unprotected intercourse compared with women within the normal weight range,[22] with a significant correlation between BMI greater than 25 kg/m^2 and a prolonged time to conception.[23] Central obesity has a significant association with infertility with a reported reduction in the probability of conception by 30% per cycle for each 0.1 increase in waist/hip ratio after adjustment for other confounders.[24] The specific reproductive dysfunctions associated with obesity include irregular menstrual cycles, chronic anovulation, and decreased pregnancy and live birth rates in both natural and assisted conception cycles. Infertility in obese women relates primarily to ovulatory dysfunction. The relative risk (RR) of anovulation correlates with the degree of obesity, increasing from 1.3 times (95% confidence interval [CI] 1.2, 1.6) in women with a BMI 24 to 31 kg/m^2 and 2.7 times (95% CI 2.0, 3.7) in infertile women with a BMI greater than 32 kg/m^2 compared with women of normal weight.[21]

Obesity reduces the success of pregnancies associated with assisted reproductive technology (ART).[25] An analysis of 270 ovulation induction cycles with clomiphene citrate or gonadotropins in PCOS indicated that 79% of women with BMI less than 24 kg/m^2 ovulated within 6 months of treatment compared with 15.3% in women with a BMI 30 to 34 kg/m^2 ($P<.001$) and 11.8% in women with a BMI greater than or equal to 35 kg/m^2 (P<.001).[26] This trend is similarly observed following ART treatment in women with PCOS, with 1 unit increase in BMI decreasing the odds for pregnancy by 16% (95% CI 0.73, 0.97).[27] Among 3586 women, 25% of whom had PCOS, the reported chance of achieving pregnancy with ART was significantly reduced with increasing maternal BMI. For women with a BMI between 30 and 34.9 kg/m^2, successful conception was reduced by 27% (95% CI 0.57, 0.96), increasing to 50% (95% CI 0.32, 0.77) for women with a BMI greater than 35 kg/m^2 compared with women of normal BMI.[28] Obese women also require higher clomiphene citrate and gonadotropin doses to achieve ovarian response.[26,29,30] High cycle cancellation rate, reduced responsiveness to stimulation protocols, reduced embryo quality, and impaired implantation with high miscarriage rates all contribute to a reduction in achieving successful pregnancy with ART for women who are overweight or obese.

WEIGHT REDUCTION IN INFERTILE WOMEN

Weight loss in women who are overweight or obese, regardless of whether they have been diagnosed with PCOS, is associated with an increased chance of both spontaneous and treatment-associated conception.[31,32] Even a modest degree of weight loss (5%–10%) can improve insulin resistance, ovulation rate, or conception in women with or without PCOS despite a BMI that remains higher than the healthy range.[31–34]

Weight management should therefore be considered a key aspect of preconception counseling in overweight or obese infertile women. Several international guidelines for obese women of reproductive age advise weight loss before conception[35–37] to both improve the chance of successful conception and reduce the time interval to conception.[38] Furthermore, although favorable reproductive results are achieved with mild weight loss, it has been suggested that severely obese women reduce their BMI at least to 35 kg/m^2 before conception to reduce the risk of pregnancy-associated complications.[39,40] However, there is no consensus as to whether fertility treatment should be withheld based on an individual's weight, or on the optimal BMI for commencement of treatment. Most organizations do not restrict access to fertility treatments on the grounds of excess maternal weight.[41] The American Society for Reproductive Medicine comments that, although some studies recommend that a BMI less than 35 kg/m^2 should be achieved before conception, "the benefits of postponing pregnancy to achieve weight loss must be balanced against the risk of declining fertility with advancing age."[37]

Strategies for Achieving Weight Reduction

Weight reduction is based on a variety of strategies including lifestyle modification, pharmacologic agents, and surgery. Lifestyle modification refers to a multifactorial approach to weight management comprising improvements in diet and exercise in conjunction with behavioral modification. However, the difficulty of sustaining weight loss long-term is well recognized. A systematic review assessed the effect of diet alone or dietary treatment in combination with nonsurgical modalities in adults, most of whom did not have obesity complications (eg, type 2 diabetes). That review identified 17 publications (5 randomized controlled trials [RCT]) with 3030 participants and comparison groups including no diet, no treatment, jaw fixation, or surgical treatment. Only 15% of people undergoing weight loss interventions maintained their reduced weight, reduced their weight further, or had a weight reduction of 9 to 11 kg at a follow-up time of up to 14 years.[42] A recent meta-analysis of RCT assessing weight loss through diet, exercise, or medications compared with minimal advice or varying intensities of diet and exercise or support identified 80 studies with 26,455 adult participants. That study reported maintenance of up to 4.3% weight loss at 48 months following structured diet or exercise regimes, indicating that clinically significant weight loss can be achieved and maintained.[43] Strategies for continued weight loss or prevention of weight regain must be maintained long-term for successful weight maintenance. International and US obesity guidelines recommend that such strategies should target physical activity, dietary change, and behavioral components to support long-term weight loss maintenance.[44,45] The role of pharmacologic agents and surgery for treatment of obesity-associated reproductive impairment is outside the scope of this article and is reviewed extensively elsewhere.[45–49]

Lifestyle Modifications: Diet

Dietary modifications consist of reducing dietary energy intake and/or modifying macronutrient intake. Many studies, both uncontrolled and RCT, have clearly shown the benefits of short-term or long-term (>12 months) energy-restricted diets in overweight and obese women both with or without PCOS in improving reproductive parameters including menstrual abnormalities, ovulation, and pregnancy rates. Longer term benefits include improvements in risk factors for type 2 diabetes mellitus and cardiovascular disease assessed largely by surrogate markers of insulin resistance, glucose intolerance, and dyslipidemia.[46,50,51] Although diets with different macronutrients have been proposed to either enhance weight loss or improve reproductive and metabolic parameters, current guidelines state that reducing energy intake is more important. Dietary interventions should be tailored to individual dietary preferences and calculated to produce an energy deficit of 600 kcal/d.[45,46]

Lifestyle Modifications: Exercise

Physical activity is important in weight loss and maintenance, modifying cardiometabolic risk factors and improving body composition.[52,53] In obese anovulatory women, an exercise training program of 20 to 24 weeks significantly improved hyperandrogenism, menstrual cyclicity, and ovulation and pregnancy rates either as a single intervention or in combination with diet.[31,54,55] Incorporation of physical activity into weight management programs also confers additional benefits to dietary management in isolation and may result in greater reduction of fat mass and maintenance of lean mass compared with diet alone.[55] A recent meta-analysis of RCT of a minimum of 6 months' duration in adult participants also reported that the combination of exercise with diet on weight reduction was more beneficial than diet as sole intervention (15 studies, 1079 subjects, weighed mean difference [WMD] −1.24 kg, 95% CI −0.23, −2.26).[56] Physical activity incorporated in weight-reducing programs also has a favorable impact on eating behaviors, general well-being, and health-related quality of life in obese individuals.[57] Current US physical activity guidelines from the American Colleges of Sports Medicine for weight loss recommend 150 to 225 minutes of moderate-intensity physical activity per week for modest weight loss (approximately 2–3 kg) and greater than 225 to 420 min/wk for clinically significant weight loss (5–7.5 kg).[58]

Lifestyle Modifications: Behavioral Interventions

Depression and low self-esteem may interfere with adherence to short-term weight loss strategies,[59–61] and stress reduction and increase of self-esteem may contribute to the success of weight loss programs. Combining weight management techniques with family and psychological support and incorporation of a group environment into treatment may help improve long-term success and sustainability of weight loss.[62] In support of this concept, a Cochrane review in adults reported that behavioral and cognitive-behavioral strategies are effective weight loss therapies and result in greater weight loss when combined with diet and exercise approaches compared with diet and exercise alone (6 studies, 467 subjects, WMD −4.71 kg, 95% CI −4.97, −4.45).[63] Several studies in PCOS reported the beneficial effects of multifactorial lifestyle interventions on metabolic or reproductive parameters.[31,32,64] This observation has been likewise shown in the general population for reduction in the prevalence of type 2 diabetes mellitus and the metabolic syndrome,[50] indicating the importance of a multidisciplinary approach for weight management.

OBESITY AND PREGNANCY

In addition to effects on fertility, obesity is recognized as a significant health issue for women during pregnancy and childbirth. Recent data suggest that overweight and obesity may affect up to 50% of the pregnant population.[65–67] The risks of adverse health outcomes associated with obesity in pregnancy are well documented, not only for the woman but also for her infant, and increase as BMI increases.[68,69]

Maternal Complications

Women who are overweight or obese are reported to be 1.7 times more likely to suffer a spontaneous miscarriage and 4.7 times more likely to suffer recurrent miscarriage compared with women of a normal BMI.[70] However, recent literature suggests that, following the sonographic detection of a viable pregnancy, early miscarriage is not increased among women with high BMI.[71] Later pregnancy complications include an increased risk of hypertensive conditions and preeclampsia,[68,72–76] gestational diabetes mellitus,[68,72,74,76] infection,[74,76] and thromboembolic events (**Table 1**).[75] There is a reported increased risk of preterm birth,[68] although this primarily seems to be an increase in iatrogenic preterm birth, rather than an increase in spontaneous preterm labor.[69,77] Both antenatal stillbirth and neonatal death are more common among overweight or obese women.[68,77] These increased maternal health complications among overweight or obese women are associated with the use of a greater proportion of health care resources compared with women of normal BMI, representing considerable economic cost to the health care system.[78] Induction of labor is more common

Table 1 Pregnancy and childbirth complications associated with increased maternal BMI	
	Health Outcomes
Pregnancy complications	Gestational diabetes
	Hypertension/preeclampsia
	Iatrogenic preterm birth
	Induction of labor
	Cesarean birth
	Postpartum hemorrhage
	Thromboembolic disease
	Infection
Infant outcomes	Large-for-gestational-age infants
	Neonatal intensive care unit admission
	Congenital anomaly
	Perinatal death
	Treatment of hypoglycemia and jaundice

among overweight or obese women,[79] as is the risk of cesarean section.[68,72,74,76] Approximately 1 in 7 cesarean sections may be directly attributable to maternal obesity,[74] the risk increasing by 7% for each 1 unit increase in maternal BMI.[80] Further compounding this risk is the additive effect of increasing maternal age at the time of conception, with approximately 38% of the increase in primary cesarean section rate attributable to the combination of these 2 factors.[81]

Infant Complications

Compared with women of normal BMI, infants born to overweight or obese women are at considerable risk of adverse health outcomes (see **Table 1**). Infants are more likely to be of high birth weight,[72,80] to require admission to neonatal intensive care units,[68,80] and to require treatment of jaundice or hypoglycemia.[68,79] Infants have also been identified as being at increased risk of congenital anomalies, particularly cardiac malformations and neural tube defects.[68,80] It is unclear whether this association reflects specific nutrient deficiency, including folate,[82] an alteration in the in utero environment (such as is seen among women with preexisting diabetes),[83] ascertainment bias reflecting technical difficulties in the ultrasound examination,[84] or a combination of these factors.

Recommendations for Maternal Weight Gain During Pregnancy

Recommendations by the Institute of Medicine (IOM) relating to maternal weight gain in pregnancy[67,85] remain largely based on observational studies, with a definition of a favorable pregnancy outcome being a gestational age of 39 to 41 weeks, and a birth weight of 3.0 to 4.0 kg.[67,85] The weight gain targets were chosen in an attempt to balance the benefits of increased fetal growth with the risks of complicated labor and delivery, and of postpartum maternal weight retention, while incorporating both the 15th and 85th centiles for weight gain (7.3–18.2 kg) across all women observed.[85] Although the updated IOM recommendations differ little from those previously published,[67] they now provide a gestational weight gain range for women who are either overweight (5.0–9.0 kg) or obese (7.0–11.5 kg).[67] The recommendations acknowledge that there is a relative lack of studies assessing the relationship between gestational weight gain and maternal and childhood health outcomes, with the research agenda published in 1990 indicating this to be a priority.[85] Rigorous evaluation of weight gain targets for women during pregnancy remains a research priority, with particular attention to the relationship between weight gain and maternal and infant health outcomes of clinical importance.

Since 1970, most studies report average weight gains during pregnancy of 10 to 15 kg, with the rate of gain in the last half of pregnancy ranging from 0.45 to 0.52 kg per week.[85] This rate varies more in overweight and obese women.[85] In nonrandomized studies, implementation of recommendations to limit maternal weight gain during pregnancy seem to reduce the risk of birth of a large-for-gestational-age infant.[86–88] Cedergren and colleagues[87,88] published data from Sweden involving in excess of 240,000 pregnant women to assess the effect of gestational weight gain for 5 categories of BMI and 3 of weight gain. Although the risk of large-for-gestational-age infants, preeclampsia, and cesarean birth were reduced among obese women whose weight gain during pregnancy was less than 8 kg, it was at the expense of an increased risk of small-for-gestational-age infants.[87,88] Recommendations have thus been made to restrict weight gain to approximately 5 kg.[88]

Interventions to Improve Health Outcomes in Overweight or Obese Pregnant Women

Despite an extensive body of literature defining the obesity-associated complications of pregnancy and childbirth, there is limited information detailing effective interventions to improve maternal, fetal, and infant health outcomes. Recommendations indicate that, ideally, women should receive prepregnancy counseling to inform about the increased pregnancy risks associated with obesity and encourage lifestyle changes to minimize the development of subsequent complications.[89,90] However, because many women present after conception, an alternate approach is required. Weight loss through dietary interventions has not been widely advocated in pregnancy because the effects of weight loss on maternal and infant health have been poorly investigated to date. Instead, researchers have focused attention on limiting weight gain in pregnancy. A recent systematic review identified 9 RCTs comparing any form of antenatal dietary or lifestyle intervention with no treatment involving 743 women who were overweight or obese during pregnancy.[91] For most pregnancy outcomes, the available sample size was smaller (5 trials, n = 540 women). There were no statistically significant differences identified between women receiving an antenatal intervention or no treatment on the risk of large-for-gestational-age infants (3 studies, 366 women, RR 2.02, 95% CI 0.84, 4.86), or mean gestational weight gain (4 studies, 416 women, WMD −3.10 kg, 95% CI −8.32, 2.13 [random effects model]). Other maternal and infant health outcomes were poorly reported. The effect of providing an antenatal dietary intervention for overweight or obese pregnant women on gestational weight gain and maternal and infant health outcomes remains to be determined.

Box 1
Principles to consider for overweight or obese infertile women

- Addressing reproductive, metabolic, and psychological features associated with increased weight.

- Where possible, discuss weight issues and the importance of weight reduction in both partners before conception at the preconception visits. Overweight or obese women should be counseled about the decrease in spontaneous conception rates and response to fertility treatments conferred by obesity and about the pregnancy-related risks and perinatal consequences aggravated by excessive weight.

- A structured lifestyle modification program to achieve weight loss should be the first-line treatment in overweight or obese women with or without PCOS. To increase success of weight loss and maintenance, a complex approach, based on combination of long-term lifestyle changes with social support, should be adopted at the initial steps of weight reduction programs, incorporating:

  ○ Setting of realistic achievable goals

  ○ Individually based diet with gradual weight loss

  ○ Education for healthy eating habits

  ○ Long-term physical activity program

  ○ Psychological support for stress reduction and increase of self-esteem

  ○ Other lifestyle aspects, such as smoking, illicit drugs, and alcohol consumption, that might have deleterious effect on fertility and pregnancy outcomes, should be avoided to optimize reproductive performance, particularly in women with a priori reduced success rate

SUMMARY

Obesity in women represents a significant problem during preconception, pregnancy, and childbirth, with a well-recognized reduction in chance of conception for both ART and non-ART pregnancies as well as an increased risk of complications during pregnancy and child birth. Although the effect of weight loss on improving reproductive hormone profiles, ovulation, and menstrual irregularity and fertility is shown, the most effective method of achieving and maintaining weight loss is unclear (**Box 1**). Although there is extensive literature identifying and describing obesity-associated risks in pregnancy, there remains more limited information on suitable interventions and strategies that have been rigorously evaluated and are of demonstrable benefit in improving health outcomes for women and their babies.

REFERENCES

1. Ezzati M, Lopez AD, Rodgers A, et al. Selected major risk factors and global and regional burden of disease. Lancet 2002;360:1347–60.
2. Access Economics. The economic costs of obesity. Canberra (Australia): Diabetes Australia; 2006.
3. Centres for Disease Control and Prevention (CDCP). Prevalence of overweight and obesity among adults: United States, 2003-2004. Washington: US Department of Health and Human Services; 2003.
4. Australian Institute of Health and Welfare (AIHW). Health, well-being and body-weight: characteristics of overweight and obesity in Australia. Canberra (Australia): Australian Institute of Health and Welfare; 2001. Bulletin No 13 2001.
5. BMJ News. US soda tax could help tackle obesity, says new director of public health. BMJ 2009;339:b3176.
6. Burt Solorzano CM, McCartney CR. Obesity and the pubertal transition in girls and boys. Reproduction 2010;140:399–410.
7. March WA, Moore VM, Willson KJ, et al. The prevalence of polycystic ovary syndrome in a community sample assessed under contrasting diagnostic criteria. Hum Reprod 2010;25:544–51.
8. Rotterdam ESHRE/ASRM-Sponsored PCOS Consensus Workshop Group. Revised 2003 consensus on diagnostic criteria and long-term health risks related to polycystic ovary syndrome (PCOS). Hum Reprod 2004;19:41–7.
9. Balen AH, Conway GS, Kaltsas G, et al. Polycystic ovary syndrome: the spectrum of the disorder in 1741 patients. Hum Reprod 1995;10:2107–11.
10. Teede H, Hutchison SK, Zoungas S. The management of insulin resistance in polycystic ovary syndrome. Trends Endocrinol Metab 2007;18:273–9.
11. Robker RL, Akison LK, Bennett BD, et al. Obese women exhibit differences in ovarian metabolites, hormones, and gene expression compared with moderate-weight women. J Clin Endocrinol Metab 2009;94:1533–40.
12. Franks S, Stark J, Hardy K. Follicle dynamics and anovulation in polycystic ovary syndrome. Hum Reprod Update 2008;14:367–78.
13. van der Steeg JW, Steures P, Eijkemans MJ, et al. Obesity affects spontaneous pregnancy chances in subfertile, ovulatory women. Hum Reprod 2008;23:324–8.
14. Gesink Law DC, Maclehose RF, Longnecker MP. Obesity and time to pregnancy. Hum Reprod 2007;22:414–20.
15. Brewer CJ, Balen AH. The adverse effects of obesity on conception and implantation. Reproduction 2010;140:347–64.
16. Robker RL. Evidence that obesity alters the quality of oocytes and embryos. Pathophysiology 2008;15:115–21.

17. Han TS, Sattar N, Williams K, et al. Prospective study of C-reactive protein in relation to the development of diabetes and metabolic syndrome in the Mexico City Diabetes Study. Diabetes Care 2002;25:2016–21.
18. Pradhan AD, Manson JE, Rifai N, et al. C-reactive protein, interleukin-6 and risk of developing type 2 diabetes mellitus. JAMA 2001;286:327–34.
19. Greenberg AS, Obin MS. Obesity and the role of adipose tissue in inflammation and metabolism. Am J Clin Nutr 2006;83:461–5.
20. Denison FC, Roberts KA, Barr SM, et al. Obesity, pregnancy, inflammation, and vascular function. Reproduction 2010;140:373–85.
21. Rich-Edwards JW, Goldman MB, Willett WC, et al. Adolescent body mass index and infertility caused by ovulatory disorder. Am J Obstet Gynecol 1994;171:171–7.
22. Lake JK, Power C, Cole TJ. Women's reproductive health: the role of body mass index in early and adult life. Int J Obes Relat Metab Disord 1997;21:432–8.
23. Hassan MA, Killick SR. Negative lifestyle is associated with a significant reduction in fecundity. Fertil Steril 2004;81:384–92.
24. Zaadstra BM, Seidell JC, Van Noord PA, et al. Fat and female fecundity: prospective study of effect of body fat distribution on conception rates. BMJ 1993;306:484–7.
25. Tamer Erel C, Senturk LM. The impact of body mass index on assisted reproduction. Curr Opin Obstet Gynecol 2009;21:228–35.
26. Al-Azemi M, Omu FE, Omu AE. The effect of obesity on the outcome of infertility management in women with polycystic ovary syndrome. Arch Gynecol Obstet 2004;270:205–10.
27. Ferlitsch K, Sator MO, Gruber DM, et al. Body mass index, follicle-stimulating hormone and their predictive value in in vitro fertilization. J Assist Reprod Genet 2004;21:431–6.
28. Wang JX, Davies M, Norman RJ. Body mass and probability of pregnancy during assisted reproduction treatment: retrospective study. BMJ 2000;321:1320–1.
29. Dodson WC, Kunselman AR, Legro RS. Association of obesity with treatment outcomes in ovulatory infertile women undergoing superovulation and intrauterine insemination. Fertil Steril 2006;86:642–6.
30. Fedorcsak P, Dale PO, Storeng R, et al. Impact of overweight and underweight on assisted reproduction treatment. Hum Reprod 2004;19:2523–8.
31. Clark AM, Ledger W, Galletly C, et al. Weight loss results in significant improvement in pregnancy and ovulation rates in anovulatory obese women. Hum Reprod 1995;10:2705–12.
32. Clark AM, Thornley B, Tomlinson L, et al. Weight loss in obese infertile women results in improvement in reproductive outcome for all forms of fertility treatment. Hum Reprod 1998;13:1502–5.
33. Moran LJ, Noakes M, Clifton PM, et al. Dietary composition in restoring reproductive and metabolic physiology in overweight women with polycystic ovary syndrome. J Clin Endocrinol Metab 2003;88:812–9.
34. Hollmann M, Runnebaum B, Gerhard I. Effects of weight loss on the hormonal profile in obese, infertile women. Hum Reprod 1996;11:1884–91.
35. Kennedy R, Kingsland C, Rutherford A, et al. Implementation of the NICE guideline - recommendations from the British Fertility Society for national criteria for NHS funding of assisted conception. Hum Fertil (Camb) 2006;9:181–9.
36. Royal Australian and New Zealand College of Obstetrician and Gynaecologists. RANZCOG statement: ovulation stimulation in infertility. East Melbourne (Australia): Royal Australian and New Zealand College of Obstetrician and Gynaecologists; 2008.
37. The Practice Committee of the American Society for Reproductive Medicine. Obesity and reproduction: an educational bulletin. Fertil Steril 2008;90:S21–9.

38. Fertility: assessment and treatment for people with fertility problems. NICE clinical guideline 11. London: National Institute for Clinical Excellence; 2004. p. 8.
39. Nelson SM, Fleming RF. The preconceptual contraception paradigm: obesity and infertility. Hum Reprod 2007;22:912–5.
40. Balen AH, Dresner M, Scott EM, et al. Should obese women with polycystic ovary syndrome receive treatment for infertility? BMJ 2006;332:434–5.
41. Pandey S, Maheshwari A, Bhattacharya S. Should access to fertility treatment be determined by female body mass index? Hum Reprod 2010;25:815–20.
42. Ayyad C, Andersen T. Long-term efficacy of dietary treatment of obesity: a systematic review of studies published between 1931 and 1999. Obes Rev 2000;1:113–9.
43. Franz MJ, VanWormer JJ, Crain AL, et al. Weight-loss outcomes: a systematic review and meta-analysis of weight-loss clinical trials with a minimum 1-year follow-up. J Am Diet Assoc 2007;107:1755–67.
44. Clinical guidelines on the identification, evaluation, and treatment of overweight and obesity in adults: executive summary. Expert Panel on the Identification, Evaluation, and Treatment of Overweight in Adults. Am J Clin Nutr 1998;68: 899–917.
45. Scottish International Guidelines Network. Management of obesity: a national clinical guideline. Edinburgh (Scotland): Scottish International Guidelines Network; 2010.
46. Moran LJ, Pasquali R, Teede HJ, et al. Treatment of obesity in polycystic ovary syndrome: a position statement of the Androgen Excess and Polycystic Ovary Syndrome Society. Fertil Steril 2009;92:1966–82.
47. Tang T, Lord JM, Norman RJ, et al. Insulin-sensitising drugs (metformin, rosiglitazone, pioglitazone, D-chiro-inositol) for women with polycystic ovary syndrome, oligo amenorrhoea and subfertility. Cochrane Database Syst Rev 2009;4:CD003053.
48. Tso LO, Costello MF, Albuquerque LE, et al. Metformin treatment before and during IVF or ICSI in women with polycystic ovary syndrome. Cochrane Database Syst Rev 2009;2:CD006105.
49. Guelinckx I, Devlieger R, Vansant G. Reproductive outcome after bariatric surgery: a critical review. Hum Reprod Update 2009;15:189–201.
50. Knowler WC, Barrett-Connor E, Fowler SE, et al. Reduction in the incidence of type 2 diabetes with lifestyle intervention or metformin. N Engl J Med 2002;346:393–403.
51. Galletly C, Clark A, Tomlinson L, et al. A group program for obese, infertile women: weight loss and improved psychological health. J Psychosom Obstet Gynaecol 1996;17:125–8.
52. Shaw K, Gennat H, O'Rourke P, et al. Exercise for overweight or obesity. Cochrane Database Syst Rev 2006;4:CD003817.
53. Catenacci VA, Wyatt HR. The role of physical activity in producing and maintaining weight loss. Nat Clin Pract Endocrinol Metab 2007;3:518–29.
54. Palomba S, Giallauria F, Falbo A, et al. Structured exercise training programme versus hypocaloric hyperproteic diet in obese polycystic ovary syndrome patients with anovulatory infertility: a 24-week pilot study. Hum Reprod 2008;23:642–50.
55. Thomson RL, Buckley JD, Noakes M, et al. The effect of a hypocaloric diet with and without exercise training on body composition, cardiometabolic risk profile, and reproductive function in overweight and obese women with polycystic ovary syndrome. J Clin Endocrinol Metab 2008;93:3373–80.
56. Wu T, Gao X, Chen M, et al. Long-term effectiveness of diet-plus-exercise interventions vs. diet-only interventions for weight loss: a meta-analysis. Obes Rev 2009;10:313–23.

57. Lemoine S, Rossell N, Drapeau V, et al. Effect of weight reduction on quality of life and eating behaviors in obese women. Menopause 2007;14:432–40.
58. Donnelly JE, Blair SN, Jakicic JM, et al. American College of Sports Medicine Position Stand. Appropriate physical activity intervention strategies for weight loss and prevention of weight regain for adults. Med Sci Sports Exerc 2009;41: 459–71.
59. Linde JA, Rothman AJ, Baldwin AS, et al. The impact of self-efficacy on behavior change and weight change among overweight participants in a weight loss trial. Health Psychol 2006;25:282–91.
60. Abbot JM, Thomson CA, Ranger-Moore J, et al. Psychosocial and behavioral profile and predictors of self-reported energy underreporting in obese middle-aged women. J Am Diet Assoc 2008;108:114–9.
61. Fabricatore AN, Wadden TA, Moore RH, et al. Predictors of attrition and weight loss success: results from a randomized controlled trial. Behav Res Ther 2009; 47:685–91.
62. Wadden TA, Butryn ML. Behavioral treatment of obesity. Endocrinol Metab Clin North Am 2003;32:981–1003, x.
63. Shaw K, O'Rourke P, Del Mar C, et al. Psychological interventions for overweight or obesity. Cochrane Database Syst Rev 2005;2:CD003818.
64. Hoeger KM, Kochman L, Wixom N, et al. A randomized, 48-week, placebo-controlled trial of intensive lifestyle modification and/or metformin therapy in overweight women with polycystic ovary syndrome: a pilot study. Fertil Steril 2004;82:421–9.
65. Chan A, Scott J, Nguyen AM, et al. Pregnancy outcome in South Australia 2007. Adelaide (Australia): Pregnancy Outcome Unit, South Australian Department of Health; 2009.
66. Chu SY, Kim SY, Bish CL. Prepregnancy obesity prevalence in the United States, 2004-2005. Matern Child Health J 2009;13(5):614–20.
67. National Research Council Institute of Medicine. Weight gain during pregnancy: reexamining the guidelines. In: Rasmussen KM, Yaktine AL, editors. Washington, DC: Institute of Medicine, National Research Council; 2009. p. 241–62.
68. Callaway LK, Prins JB, Chang AM, et al. The prevalence and impact of overweight and obesity in an Australian obstetric population. Med J Aust 2006;184:56–9.
69. Dodd JM, Grivell RM, Ngyuen MA, et al. Maternal and perinatal health outcomes by maternal body mass index category. Aust N Z J Obstet Gynaecol 2011;51: 136–40.
70. Metwally M, Ong KJ, Ledger WL, et al. Does high body mass index increase the risk of miscarriage after spontaneous and assisted conception? A meta-analysis of the evidence. Fertil Steril 2008;90(3):714–26.
71. Turner MJ, Fattah C, O'Connor N, et al. Body mass index and spontaneous miscarriage. Eur J Obstet Gynecol Reprod Biol 2010;151:168–70.
72. Abenhaim HA, Kinch RA, Morin L, et al. Effect of prepregnancy body mass index categories on obstetrical and neonatal outcomes. Arch Gynecol Obstet 2007; 275:39–43.
73. Joglekar CV, Fall CH, Deshpande VU, et al. Newborn size, infant and childhood growth, and body composition and cardiovascular disease risk factors at the age of 6 years: the Pune Maternal Nutrition Study. Int J Obes 2007;31:1534–44.
74. La Coursiere DY, Bloebaum L, Duncan JD, et al. Population-based trends and correlates of maternal overweight and obesity, Utah 1991-2001. Am J Obstet Gynecol 2005;192:832–9.
75. Wolfe H. High prepregnancy body-mass index - a maternal-fetal risk factor. N Engl J Med 1998;338:191–2.

76. Athukorala C, Rumbold AR, Willson KJ, et al. The risk of adverse pregnancy outcomes in women who are overweight or obese. BMC Pregnancy Childbirth 2010;10:56.
77. Smith GC, Shah I, Pell JP, et al. Maternal obesity in early pregnancy and risk of spontaneous and elective preterm deliveries: a retrospective cohort study. Am J Public Health 2007;97:157–62.
78. Chu SY, Bachman DJ, Callaghan WM, et al. Association between obesity during pregnancy and increased use of health care. N Engl J Med 2008;358:1444–53.
79. Doherty DA, Magann EF, Francis J, et al. Pre-pregnancy body mass index and pregnancy outcomes. Int J Gynaecol Obstet 2006;95:242–7.
80. Galtier-Dereure F, Boegner C, Bringer J. Obesity and pregnancy: complications and cost. Am J Clin Nutr 2000;71:1242S–8S.
81. Smith GC, Cordeaux Y, White IR, et al. The effect of delaying childbirth on primary cesarean section rates. PLoS Med 2008;5:e144.
82. Kimmons JE, Blanck HM, Tohill BC, et al. Associations between body mass index and the prevalence of low micronutrient levels among US adults. MedGenMed 2006;8:59.
83. Corrigan N, Brazil DP, McAuliffe F. Fetal cardiac effects of maternal hyperglycemia during pregnancy. Birth Defects Res A Clin Mol Teratol 2009;85:523–30.
84. Aagaard-Tillery KM, Flint Porter T, Malone FD, et al. Influence of maternal BMI on genetic sonography in the FaSTER trial. Prenat Diagn 2010;30:14–22.
85. Institute of Medicine. Subcommittee on Nutritional Status and Weight Gain in Pregnancy. Nutrition during pregnancy. Washington, DC: National Academy Press; 1990.
86. Caufield LE, Stoltzfus RJ, Witter FR. Implications of the Institute of Medicine weight gain recommendations for preventing adverse pregnancy outcomes in black and white women. Am J Public Health 1998;88:1168–74.
87. Cedergren MI. Effects of gestational weight gain and body mass index on obstetric outcomes in Sweden. Int J Gynecol Obstet 2006;93:269–74.
88. Cedergren MI. Optimal gestational weight gain for body mass index categories. Obstet Gynecol 2007;110:759–64.
89. Davies GA, Maxwell C, Gagnon R, et al. Obesity in pregnancy. J Obstet Gynaecol Can 2010;32:165–73.
90. Shaikh H, Robinson S, Teoh TG. Management of maternal obesity prior to and during pregnancy. Semin Fetal Neonatal Med 2010;15:77–82.
91. Dodd JM, Grivell RM, Crowther CA, et al. Antenatal interventions for overweight or obese pregnant women: a systematic review of randomised trials. BJOG 2010; 117(11):1316–26.

Index

Note: Page numbers of article titles are in **boldface** type.

Endocrinol Metab Clin N Am 40 (2011) 907–919
doi:10.1016/S0889-8529(11)00106-X
0889-8529/11/$ – see front matter © 2011 Elsevier Inc. All rights reserved.

endo.theclinics.com

United States Postal Service

Statement of Ownership, Management, and Circulation
(All Periodicals Publications Except Requestor Publications)

1. Publication Title	2. Publication Number	3. Filing Date
Endocrinology and Metabolism Clinics of North America	0 0 0 0 - 2 7 - 5	9/16/11

4. Issue Frequency	5. Number of Issues Published Annually	6. Annual Subscription Price
Mar, Jun, Sep, Dec	4	$290.00

7. Complete Mailing Address of Known Office of Publication (Not printer) (Street, city, county, state, and ZIP+4®)

Elsevier Inc.
360 Park Avenue South
New York, NY 10010-1710

Contact Person: Stephen Bushing

Telephone (Include area code): 215-239-3688

8. Complete Mailing Address of Headquarters or General Business Office of Publisher (Not printer)

Elsevier Inc., 360 Park Avenue South, New York, NY 10010-1710

9. Full Names and Complete Mailing Addresses of Publisher, Editor, and Managing Editor (Do not leave blank)

Publisher (Name and complete mailing address)

Kim Murphy, Elsevier, Inc., 1600 John F. Kennedy Blvd. Suite 1800, Philadelphia, PA 19103-2899

Editor (Name and complete mailing address)

Rachel Glover, Elsevier, Inc., 1600 John F. Kennedy Blvd. Suite 1800, Philadelphia, PA 19103-2899

Managing Editor (Name and complete mailing address)

Sarah Barth, Elsevier, Inc., 1600 John F. Kennedy Blvd. Suite 1800, Philadelphia, PA 19103-2899

10. Owner (Do not leave blank. If the publication is owned by a corporation, give the name and address of the corporation immediately followed by the names and addresses of all stockholders owning or holding 1 percent or more of the total amount of stock. If not owned by a corporation, give the names and addresses of the individual owners. If owned by a partnership or other unincorporated firm, give its name and address as well as those of each individual owner. If the publication is published by a nonprofit organization, give its name and address.)

Full Name	Complete Mailing Address
Wholly owned subsidiary of	4520 East-West Highway
Reed/Elsevier, US holdings	Bethesda, MD 20814

11. Known Bondholders, Mortgagees, and Other Security Holders Owning or Holding 1 Percent or More of Total Amount of Bonds, Mortgages, or Other Securities. If none, check box ☐ None

Full Name	Complete Mailing Address
N/A	

12. Tax Status (For completion by nonprofit organizations authorized to mail at nonprofit rates) (Check one)
The purpose, function, and nonprofit status of this organization and the exempt status for federal income tax purposes:
☐ Has Not Changed During Preceding 12 Months
☐ Has Changed During Preceding 12 Months (Publisher must submit explanation of change with this statement)

PS Form 3526, September 2007 (Page 1 of 3 (Instructions Page 3)) PSN 7530-01-000-9931 PRIVACY NOTICE: See our Privacy policy in www.usps.com

---

13. Publication Title			14. Issue Date for Circulation Data Below
Endocrinology and Metabolism Clinics of North America			September 2011

15. Extent and Nature of Circulation			Average No. Copies Each Issue During Preceding 12 Months	No. Copies of Single Issue Published Nearest to Filing Date
a. Total Number of Copies (Net press run)			1725	1250
b. Paid Circulation (By Mail and Outside the Mail)	(1)	Mailed Outside-County Paid Subscriptions Stated on PS Form 3541. (Include paid distribution above nominal rate, advertiser's proof copies, and exchange copies)	582	557
	(2)	Mailed In-County Paid Subscriptions Stated on PS Form 3541 (Include paid distribution above nominal rate, advertiser's proof copies, and exchange copies)		
	(3)	Paid Distribution Outside the Mails Including Sales Through Dealers and Carriers, Street Vendors, Counter Sales, and Other Paid Distribution Outside USPS®	430	464
	(4)	Paid Distribution by Other Classes Mailed Through the USPS (e.g. First-Class Mail®)		
c. Total Paid Distribution (Sum of 15b (1), (2), (3), and (4))		►	1012	1021
d. Free or Nominal Rate Distribution (By Mail and Outside the Mail)	(1)	Free or Nominal Rate Outside-County Copies Included on PS Form 3541	80	63
	(2)	Free or Nominal Rate In-County Copies Included on PS Form 3541		
	(3)	Free or Nominal Rate Copies Mailed at Other Classes Through the USPS (e.g. First-Class Mail)		
	(4)	Free or Nominal Rate Distribution Outside the Mail (Carriers or other means)		
e. Total Free or Nominal Rate Distribution (Sum of 15d (1), (2), (3) and (4))		►	80	63
f. Total Distribution (Sum of 15c and 15e)		►	1092	1084
g. Copies not Distributed (See instructions to publishers #4 (page 43))		►	633	166
h. Total (Sum of 15f and g)		►	1725	1250
i. Percent Paid (15c divided by 15f times 100)			92.67%	94.19%

16. Publication of Statement of Ownership

☐ If the publication is a general publication, publication of this statement is required. Will be printed in the December 2011 issue of this publication.   ☐ Publication not required

17. Signature and Title of Editor, Publisher, Business Manager, or Owner

[signature]

Stephen R. Bushing – Inventory Distribution Coordinator

Date: September 16, 2011

I certify that all information furnished on this form is true and complete. I understand that anyone who furnishes false or misleading information on this form or who omits material or information requested on the form may be subject to criminal sanctions (including fines and imprisonment) and/or civil sanctions (including civil penalties).

PS Form 3526, September 2007 (Page 2 of 3)

Moving?

Make sure your subscription moves with you!

To notify us of your new address, find your **Clinics Account Number** (located on your mailing label above your name), and contact customer service at:

Email: journalscustomerservice-usa@elsevier.com

800-654-2452 (subscribers in the U.S. & Canada)
314-447-8871 (subscribers outside of the U.S. & Canada)

Fax number: 314-447-8029

Elsevier Health Sciences Division
Subscription Customer Service
3251 Riverport Lane
Maryland Heights, MO 63043

*To ensure uninterrupted delivery of your subscription, please notify us at least 4 weeks in advance of move.

Printed and bound by CPI Group (UK) Ltd, Croydon, CR0 4YY

13/10/2024

01773501-0001